CORONARY ARTERY DISEASE - ASSESSMENT, SURGERY, PREVENTION

Edited by **Kaan Kırali**

Coronary Artery Disease - Assessment, Surgery, Prevention
http://dx.doi.org/10.5772/59455
Edited by Kaan Kırali

Contributors

Ananthasubramaniam, Gurunanthan Palani, Rebecca Baumann, Francesco Formica, Serena Mariani, Giovanni Paolini, Kaan Kirali, Nathan Manghat, Michael Campbell, Stephen Lyen, Mark Hamilton, Jonathan Rodrigues, Juan, Chain-Lin Wu, Takao Hasegawa, Terrence Ruddy, Punitha Arasaratnam, Samy Mcfarlane, Samy I McFarlane, Kendal Endicott, Gregory Trachiotis, Lucia Agoston-Coldea, Oguzhan Yıldız, Melik Seyrek, Kemal Gökhan Ulusoy

Published by InTech

Janeza Trdine 9, 51000 Rijeka, Croatia

Publishing Process Manager Iva Lipovic

Technical Editor InTech DTP team

Cover InTech Design team

First published November, 2015

Printed in Croatia

Additional hard copies can be obtained from orders@intechopen.com

Coronary Artery Disease - Assessment, Surgery, Prevention, Edited by Kaan Kırali

p. cm.

ISBN 978-953-51-2206-7

For EU product safety concerns:
IN TECH d.o.o., Prolaz Marije Krucifikse Kozulić 3, 51000 Rijeka, Croatia,
info@intechopen.com or visit our website at intechopen.com.

Meet the editor

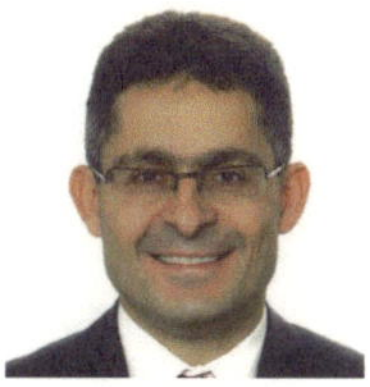

Professor Dr. Kaan Kırali completed his training in Koşuyolu Heart and Research Hospital, Istanbul, Turkey. He became a consultant surgeon in 1997, and has published more than 90 international and 160 national articles. He is the pioneer of awake complete CABG with BIMA. He is also one of the pioneers of aortic root surgery. He has developed a new aortotomy incision, which makes aortic valve interventions simpler. He completed a master's program on preventive medicine in Istanbul University, Istanbul, Turkey. Dr. Kırali is the head of the department of CVS in Sakarya University, Sakarya, Turkey, and the chief of the department of CVS in Koşuyolu Heart and Research Hospital, Istanbul, Turkey. He is also in charge of the heart transplantation mechanical assist device program, and a member of several international societies.

Contents

Preface

Coronary artery atherosclerosis is the most common cardiac pathology, which is the primary cause of acute cardiac mortality. Coronary artery stenosis usually involves the proximal portion of the larger epicardial coronary arteries, but diffuse coronary artery disease is also not rare. Since coronary artery disease is time-consuming, slowly developing occlusions frequently stimulate the formation of collateral vessels that protect against extensive myocardial ischemia. Most of the patients with/without several comorbidities have asymptomatic atherosclerotic lesions in the coronary territory, and hence early assessment of coronary artery pathology is of utmost importance. The noninvasive, but mostly invasive diagnostic tests should be preferred for early diagnosis of the severity of stenotic plaques and viability of the myocardium. These special diagnostic tests can forward cardiac surgeons for early revascularization. Since early surgical intervention is superior to percutaneous interventions, coronary artery bypass grafting is the first choice for the treatment of coronary artery disease. Coronary revascularization can be performed with different approaches according to the patient's risk factors. Off-pump and minimally invasive coronary artery bypass grafting increase the efficiency and hence popularity of surgical therapy over percutaneous treatment modalities. Several aggressive strategies can be used for revascularization in diffuse coronary artery disease. Surgical treatment does not include only myocardial revascularization; surgical therapy for mechanical complications of acute myocardial infarction can be life-saving. Preventive treatment of coronary artery disease should be the basic strategy, and for a healthy system, an aggressive attitude toward the metabolic syndrome and abnormal diet should be taken.

Prof. Dr. Kaan Kırali
Head of Department of Cardiovascular Surgery, Faculty of Medicine, Sakarya University
Chief of Department of Cardiovascular Surgery, Koşuyolu Heart and Research Hospital
Turkey

Section 1

Assessment of Coronary Stenosis

Chapter 1

Regadenoson — Overview of Applications in Cardiology

Gurunanthan Palani, Rebecca Baumann and
Karthik Ananthasubramaniam

Additional information is available at the end of the chapter

http://dx.doi.org/10.5772/61154

Abstract

Coronary artery disease is a leading cause of morbidity and mortality in developed countries. According to a Center for Disease Control report, one out of four deaths is attributed to coronary artery disease. It costs the United States human lives, productivity, and more than 100 billion dollars each year. Due to increased incidence in both men and women and all ethnicities, risk stratification of patients at risk for developing myocardial infarction and death is of paramount importance. Various tests are available for diagnosis and prognosis in coronary heart disease such as exercise treadmill testing, coronary calcium scoring, dobutamine stress echocardiography, exercise, dipyridamole, adenosine or dobutamine stress nuclear myocardial perfusion imaging (MPI), and dobutamine or adenosine stress cardiac magnetic resonance imaging. Since 2008 a new vasodilator, regadenoson (REG), has become available and is now widely used for nuclear perfusion imaging. Pharmacologic stress testing challenges the coronary flow reserve to evaluate the hyperemic capacity of the heart, which can be impaired in significant epicardial stenosis or microvascular dysfunction. In the presence of either of these conditions, ischemia induced by hyperemia manifests as wall motion abnormalities on echocardiography or as perfusion defects in nuclear perfusion imaging.

REG is a selective adenosine A_{2A} receptor agonist, and due to its targeted coronary vasodilator properties and bolus administration of a standard dose in all patients, it has rapidly gained popularity as the preferred MPI stress agent. In this chapter we will review the basis of pharmacologic vasodilator stress imaging starting with a brief discussion of the various adenosine receptors and their function, the structure and mechanism of action of REG, and its development and approval. It will be compared with other myocardial perfusion pharmacologic stress agents like adenosine and dipyridamole in terms of safety, efficacy, and side effect profile. We will also address the utility of REG in special situations like renal disease, chronic obstructive pulmonary disease, heart transplant, left bundle branch block, and paced rhythms. The prognostic value of REG MPI in the general population, its effectiveness with and without exercise, and the emerging applications of REG in other modalities of imaging such as positron emission tomography and stress echocardiography will be discussed.

Keywords: Regadenoson, single photon emission computed tomography, positron emission tomography, stress echocardiography, fractional flow reserve, coronary artery disease

1. Introduction

Cardiovascular disease remains a leading cause of death in the United States. According to a 2009 report by the Center for Disease Control, one out of four deaths is attributable to coronary artery disease (CAD).[1] The increased morbidity and mortality due to CAD poses a huge economic burden. In 2010, CAD alone accounted for over 100 billion dollars in combined direct and indirect (i.e., loss of productivity) costs. This is projected to more than double by 2030.[2] Hence, diagnosing and risk stratifying CAD in its early stages is vital.

Many invasive and noninvasive tests are available to identify patients at high risk of developing CAD. Functional tests include exercise stress testing, exercise or dobutamine stress echocardiography, nuclear myocardial perfusion imaging (MPI) using stress agents such as dipyridamole, adenosine, dobutamine or regadenoson (REG), and vasodilator stress magnetic resonance imaging. Coronary computed tomography angiography (CCTA) and the traditional gold standard, coronary angiography, serve as the two well-established anatomic modalities used for CAD detection. This chapter will focus on REG, the newest of the pharmacologic stress agents, and its applications in myocardial perfusion imaging. It will conclude with a brief overview of some novel applications of REG in cardiology.

2. REG: development, pharmacology, and hemodynamic effects

2.1. Adenosine receptors

Adenosine receptors are located in the myocardium as well as in smooth muscle cells of the coronary arterioles and the bronchial tree. Various subtypes of adenosine receptors exist including A_1 receptors found in the atrioventricular node, A_{2A} receptors present in coronary arteriolar smooth muscle, and A_{2B} and A_3 receptors located in bronchial smooth muscle. The different locations and functions of these receptors have been pivotal in the development of newer pharmacologic stress agents (Figure 1). Adenosine directly and dipyridamole indirectly act on adenosine 2A (A_{2A}) G-protein-coupled receptors found on the cell membrane of coronary arteriolar smooth muscle cells. However, both are nonselective and also activate the other adenosine receptor subtypes causing frequent clinically important side effects (e.g., atrioventricular block due to A_1 activation and bronchoconstriction due to A_{2B} and A_3 receptor activation) as well as other less serious but often unpleasant side effects. In contrast, REG exerts its effect selectively on A_{2A} receptors achieving the coronary dilatation necessary to perform MPI studies while keeping side effects to a minimum.

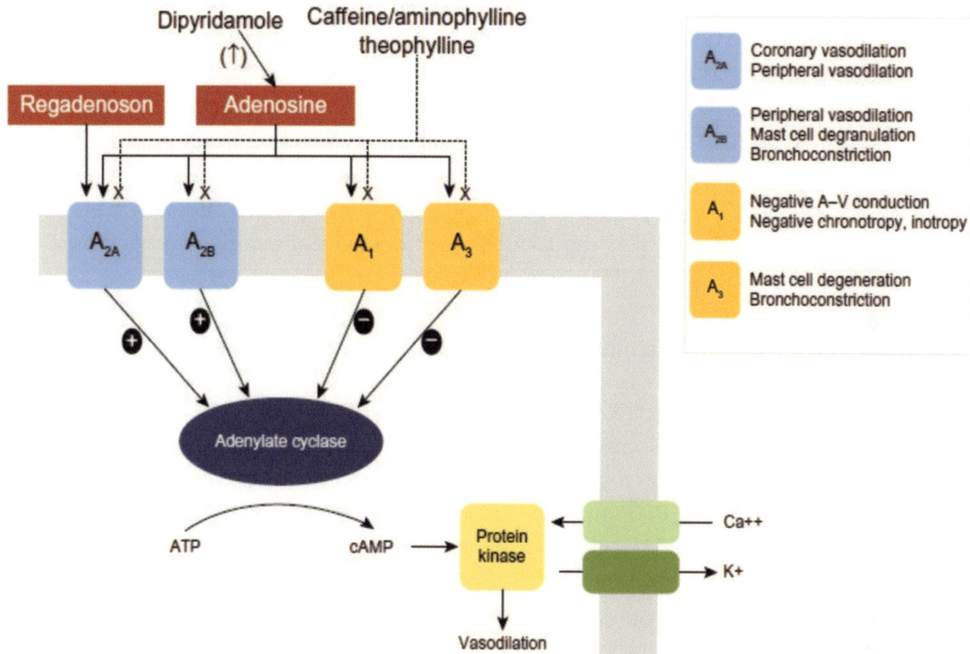

Note: Springer and *J Nucl Cardiol*, 17, 2010, 494-497, The emerging role of the selective A2A agonist in pharmacologic stress testing, Gemignani AS, Abbot BG, Figure 1. With kind permission from Springer Science and Business Media

Figure 1. Types of adenosine receptors, their functions, and activation/inhibition by various pharmacologic agents.

2.2. Development and approval of of REG

Cardiac stress testing is able to identify as well as risk stratify individuals who are at risk for CAD. Vasodilator stress testing challenges the coronary flow reserve in order to evaluate the hyperemic capacity of the heart, which can be impaired in significant epicardial stenosis or microvascular disease and lead to transient ischemia. Ischemic changes manifest either as perfusion or wall motion abnormalities depending on the imaging modality used. The currently available pharmacologic stress agents with primarily vasodilator function are dipyridamole, adenosine, and REG. While dobutamine also vasodilates, it mainly stresses the heart via its positive inotropic and chronotropic effects.

An ideal cardiac stress agent should cause short-lived but maximal coronary vasodilatation. Both of these can be achieved if the stress agent has low affinity for its receptor and the target tissue has many adenosine receptors. The coronary arterial tree has an abundance of A_{2A}

receptors of which only a fraction needs to be activated to elicit the desired coronary vasodilation and produce maximal coronary hyperemia. Given the nonspecific nature of adenosine receptor stimulation by adenosine and dipyridamole leading to undesired side effects, the need existed for the development of an A_{2A}-selective agent largely devoid of significant side effects such as bronchospasm and atrioventricular conduction block. REG (code name CVT 3146) was identified as an agent with A_{2A} selectivity yet with a low affinity for A_{2A} receptors, meaning it dissociates quickly after eliciting maximal coronary vasodilation, thus causing adequate coronary hyperemia for a short period of time. REG underwent preclinical and subsequently randomized clinical studies showing non-inferiority compared to the commonly used vasodilator adenosine. This led to its approval by the Food and Drug Administration in 2008. It is marketed by Astellas Pharma US Inc. under the trade name Lexiscan® in the United States as a cardiac stress agent for MPI studies in patients who are unable to exercise. Following REG administration, coronary hyperemia occurs for approximately 2–5 min, which is adequate for radionuclide uptake and makes it possible to perform stress testing using a single bolus injection.[3]

2.3. Pharmacology and pharmacokinetics of REG

REG is a 2-[*N*-1-(4-*N*-methylcarboxamidopyrazolyl)] adenosine derivative. It is prepared by condensing ethoxycarbonylmalondialdehyde with 2-hydrazinoadenosine in a 1:1 mixture of ethanoic acid and methanol. The resulting ester is then converted directly by aminolysis with methylamine to the amide REG (Figure 2). Alternatively, REG can be prepared from 2-chloro or 2-iodo adenosine derivatives. The amide links at the 4-position of the *N*-pyrazolyl, which has both lipophilic and hydrophilic substituents lending the drug greater affinity for the adenosine 2_A receptor than the other adenosine receptor subtypes.

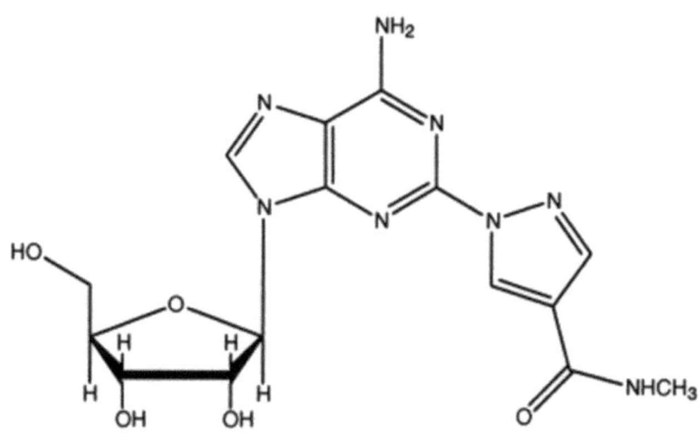

Figure 2. The molecular structure of REG (CVT-3146; (1-[9-[(4S, 2R, 3R, 5R)-3,4-dihydroxy-5-(hydroxymethyl)oxolan-2yl]-6aminopurin-2-yl]pyrazol-4-yl)-*N*-methylcarboxamide).

It is usually given as a single 400-μg (5 mL) intravenous bolus after which it immediately distributes throughout the body. No weight-based dose adjustment is necessary. REG then undergoes three phases of elimination. The first is the phase of maximal coronary hyperemia lasting 2–4 min.[4] The second phase lasts 15–30 min with profound effect on heart rate and blood pressure, and the third phase, which lasts for 33–108 min, is clinically nonsignificant.[5] Much about REG's metabolism remains unknown; however, its excretion is both renal and hepatic. The kidneys remove approximately 60% via tubular secretion, while the liver excretes around 40% of the drug unmetabolized into the bile.

2.4. Hemodynamic effects of REG

As a coronary vasodilator REG is shown to cause tachycardia and changes in blood pressure (both increase and decrease).Trochu et al.[6] showed in animal studies that while adenosine increased left ventricular (LV) systolic pressure, REG did not to any significant degree, and that LV contractility measured by dP/dT increased by 39±7% with REG and 29±7% with adenosine. The ADVANCE MPI studies[7] have shown that the decrease in systolic and diastolic blood pressures (BP) was similar between REG and adenosine (systolic BP drop 14±13 mmHg vs. 13±14 mmHg, P = ns; diastolic BP drop 10±8 mmHg vs. 10±8 mmHg, P = ns). Both drugs increase the heart rate; however, REG more significantly than adenosine (25±11bpm vs. 20±10bpm, $P < 0.001$).

The increase in heart rate with REG is mainly due to direct sympathetic excitation and less so from a baroreceptor reflex induced tachycardia. Dhalla et al.[8] has also suggested that an A_{2A} receptor mediated sinus tachycardia can occur with REG. A blunted heart rate acceleration with both REG and adenosine has also been observed in studies with diabetic patients and is felt to be related to sympathetic denervation.[9]

2.5. Side effect profile of REG

Like other vasodilators, REG is associated with many minor and a few major (albeit to a lesser extent than older vasodilators) side effects of which clinicians need to be aware.[10] Transient side effects included nausea (6%), abdominal pain (5%), headache (26%), and chest tightness (13%). In the randomized studies evaluating REG prior to its FDA approval, atrioventricular (AV) block incidence was <1% with no instances of advanced AV block or asystole in the ADVANCE MPI 3 studies. However, post marketing surveillance has highlighted rare major adverse reactions related to REG such as acute myocardial infarction,[11, 12] atrioventricular block, and asystole.[13] Thus, REG, despite its A_{2A} selectivity, should not be used in patients with greater than the first-degree AV block unless they have a backup pacemaker. Furthermore, cases of syncope[14] and seizures[15] have also been reported following REG administration. Although aminophylline is used for reversal of many REG-induced side effects, it should not be used in the setting of seizures following REG injection as it lowers the seizure threshold. Instead, standard antiseizure therapy with benzodiazepines and agents such as phenytoin should be used.

2.6. Effect of caffeine on REG and clinical implications

Caffeine is an A_{2A} receptor antagonist (Figure 1). Hence, it has the potential to attenuate the hyperemic response, which occurs after vasodilator administration. This is a well-known problem with adenosine and dipyridamole, both of which require abstinence from caffeinated products for at least 24 h prior to stress testing. However, the REG package insert specifies withholding caffeinated products for only 12 h prior to testing. Preclinical animal studies suggested that caffeine attenuated the duration of REG-induced coronary hyperemia in dogs.[16] Subsequent human studies evaluating myocardial blood flow in 41 healthy volunteers using REG with PET imaging showed that moderate caffeine consumption may not interfere with REG-induced coronary hyperemia.[17] Thus, conflicting evidence existed regarding the effect of caffeine on REG stress testing until a multicenter randomized trial on this subject was performed in 2014.

Tejani et al.[18] studied the effects of caffeine on the diagnostic accuracy of REG single proton emissions computed tomography (SPECT) MPI in 207 subjects with documented coronary artery disease on an initial rest-REG SPECT MPI sequence. A third set of SPECT images was acquired in all patients following randomization to two different caffeine doses (200 and 400 mg) or placebo. Previously noted reversible defects were attenuated in patients who consumed both doses of caffeine at least 90 min prior to REG administration, thus diminishing the diagnostic accuracy of the study. There was no difference in adverse effects between the three groups.[18] Current American Society of Nuclear Cardiology (ASNC) guidelines recommend that patients refrain from caffeine consumption for at least 12 h before REG stress testing.

Variable	Regadenoson	Adenosine	Dipyridamole
Brand name	Lexiscan®	Adenocard®/Adenoscan®	Persantine®
Indication	Pharmacologic stress agent in MPI.	Treatment of paroxysmal supraventricular tachycardia, pharmacologic stress agent in MPI	Oral—antithrombotic along with warfarin/aspirin. Intravenous—pharmacologic stress agent in MPI
Mechanism of action	Increases coronary flow reserve (CFR) via selective A_{2A} adenosine receptor agonism	Nonselective adenosine agonist on A_1, A_{2A}, A_{2B}, and A_3 receptors. Increases coronary flow reserve (CFR) via A_{2A}receptor activation.	Increases availability of adenosine by inhibiting adenosine deaminase, which prevents adenosine's breakdown
Potency	10 times more potent than adenosine	Less potent	Less potent
Distribution in body	11.5 L	Unknown	2–3 L
Metabolism	Unknown	In blood and tissue, metabolized by adenosine deaminase into inosine and then adenosine monophosphate and hypoxanthine	Hepatic
Time to peak	1–4 min	30 s	2–2.5 h

http://dx.doi.org/10.5772/61154

Variable	Regadenoson	Adenosine	Dipyridamole
Half-life	Triphasic First phase = 2–4 min Second phase = 15–30 min Third phase = 33–108 min	<10 s	30–45 min
Administration	Bolus	Infusion	Infusion
Dose	400 μg	140 μg/kg/min	0.14 mg/kg/min
Duration of infusion	10-20 s bolus	6 min continuous infusion	4 min continuous infusion
Excretion	57% of drug excreted unchanged in urine via tubular secretion	Cellular uptake	Conjugated by glucuronide and unchanged drug excreted in feces
Safety in pregnancy	Risk cannot be ruled out (Category C)	Risk cannot be ruled out (Category C)	No evidence of human risk in controlled studies (Category B)
Common side effects	Headache 26% , flushing 16%, dyspnea 28%, hypotension 2%	Headache 21%, flushing 35%, dyspnea 19%, hypotension 3%	Headache 12%, flushing 3.4%, dyspnea 2.6%, hypotension 5%
IV tubing	Not needed: only Hep-lock	Needed	Needed
Protocol completion time with radiotracer	Less than 1 min	4–6 min	6–8 min

Table 1. Comparison of the three commonly used vasodilator agents

Compared with the other two agents, REG is more potent, causes more selective coronary vasodilatation, can be injected in a single bolus without weight-based adjustments, and produces SPECT images comparable to adenosine and dipyridamole.

3. REG SPECT MPI in detection of coronary artery disease

3.1. Comparison to adenosine

In a multicenter phase 2 study, REG was tested in 36 patients undergoing SPECT MPI at bolus doses of 400 and 500 μg. Patients with heart transplantation, left bundle branch block, ventricular pacemaker, and low ejection fraction (14 patients) were excluded. This study showed a higher rate of detecting reversible perfusion defects with the lower dose of REG (89% for 400 μg) than with the higher dose (76% for 500 μg).[19] Subsequently, two phase 3 double-blinded, randomized, multicenter trials (ADVANCE-MPI 1 and ADVANCE-MPI 2) demonstrated non-inferiority of REG SPECT MPI to adenosine SPECT MPI. The ADVANCE-MPI 2 trial included 54 sites and 784 patients undergoing clinically indicated adenosine MPI who were blindly randomized 4 weeks later to a second MPI study with REG ($n = 495$) or adenosine ($n = 260$) in a 2:1 ratio. Study images were reported in a blinded fashion by three nuclear cardiology experts unaware of any patient data. The primary aim of the study was to show the strength of agreement between sequential adenosine and REG images, and the non-inferiority of the adenosine-REG sequence to the adenosine-adenosine sequence for consistently detecting reversible perfusion defects. The investigators demonstrated that the overall agreement was not statistically different between sequential adenosine–adenosine images (0.64 ± 0.04) compared to adenosine–REG images (0.63 ± 0.03). Furthermore, there was no significant difference in image quality between the two stress agents, and the patient tolerability questionnaire favored REG in this study. In a subsequent quantitative analysis of the ADVANCE-MPI 2 study, investigators showed that the total perfusion defect size, ischemic perfusion defect size, ejection fraction, and LV volume estimation was similar between REG and adenosine.[20] Thus, cumulative evidence collected from over 2000 patients in these pivotal phase 3 trials demonstrated the non-inferiority of REG to adenosine in SPECT MPI, [7] as well as the effects of age, gender, obesity, and diabetes on the efficacy and safety of REG[21] leading to its approval for clinical use.

3.2. REG in special populations

3.2.1. Renal disease

The predominantly renal excretion of REG (60% of the drug) raises concern for its safety in chronic kidney disease and end stage renal disease patients, including those on dialysis. To date, two major studies and one prognostic study have shown that REG is not associated with any major adverse events in this group.

Ananthasubramaniam et al.[22] conducted a randomized, double-blinded, placebo-controlled multicenter trial to evaluate the safety and tolerability of REG in 432 patients with stage 3 (glomerular filtration rate (GFR) 30–59 mL/min/1.73 m^2) and 72 patients with stage 4 (GFR 15–29 mL/min/1.73 m^2) chronic kidney disease. There were no major adverse events within 24 h of REG injection in the intervention group. Minor adverse effects like headache, dyspnea, chest discomfort, nausea, flushing, and dizziness were more common in the REG group than in the placebo group.

Doukky et al.[23] studied 146 ESRD patients undergoing REG stress testing, which included 131 patients on hemodialysis, 12 patients on peritoneal dialysis, and two not on any dialysis. These were compared with 97 control patients with GFR ≥30 mL/min. The primary end point of the study was patient reported side effects within 24 h following REG administration. There were no statistically significant differences in adverse effects between the groups. Interestingly, end stage renal disease patients tolerated REG stress better than the control group and expressed their willingness to take the test again (117/131 (80%) vs. 63/97 (65%), $P = 0.001$).[23]

3.2.2. Asthma and COPD

Adenosine 2_B and 3 receptors are located in bronchial smooth muscle cells which, when activated, can lead to bronchoconstriction (Figure 1). Although REG is a selective A_{2A} receptor agonist, there is a concern related to its use in patients with asthma and chronic obstructive pulmonary disease (COPD).

More than six studies have been performed to evaluate the safety of REG in this population specifically looking at respiratory symptoms, spirometry parameters, hemodynamic response, and major adverse events. The combined population of these five prospective studies and one retrospective study comprised 686 COPD patients and 695 asthmatics.[24] Respiratory parameters like FEV1, FVC, FEV1/FVC ratio, and patient-reported symptoms were monitored in most of these studies. All showed that REG is safe in COPD and asthmatics. Dyspnea was reported more frequently in COPD and asthmatics, but no significant decline in spirometry measurements occurred among these patients in two double-blinded studies.[25, 26] Of particular note, Kwon et al.[27] demonstrated that patients who underwent low-level exercise in conjunction with REG stress reported fewer respiratory symptoms than those who did not exercise following REG administration.

3.2.3. Pacemaker and left bundle branch block

In patients with left bundle branch block (LBBB), pacemaker, or intrinsic conduction disease, the increased heart rate caused by either exercise, or dobutamine can lead to false-positive septal perfusion defects. This is due to a tachycardia-induced decrease in diastolic perfusion in an already asynchronously activated septum. Multiple studies have compared adenosine and exercise stress tests in these patients. Caner et al.[28–30] showed that dobutamine stress testing is associated with higher false positives in LBBB patients, and similar results were observed in pacemaker patients as well.

The ability of REG to identify perfusion defects in this population was studied by Thomas et al.[31] In their sub-analysis of the ADVANCE MPI 1 and 2 trials, where all 2015 subjects underwent SPECT MPI with adenosine followed by SPECT MPI with either REG or adenosine, 64 patients with LBBB and 93 with pacemakers were identified. Hemodynamic changes, visually assessed summed difference scores (SDS), and quantitative perfusion defects in the LAD territory and septum were compared between REG MPI and adenosine MPI. The study showed that although REG led to a significant increase in heart rate compared with adenosine, it did not cause or exaggerate perfusion defects in the LAD or septal territories either by SDS or quantitative assessment.[31]

3.2.4. Orthotopic heart transplant patients

Orthotopic heart transplant (OHT) patients have a higher incidence of AV block due to denervation supersensitivity. Hence, OHT patients who undergo MPI studies are at increased risk for developing high-grade AV block. Few studies have evaluated the role of MPI in diagnosing cardiac allograft vasculopathy in these patients.

In a retrospective analysis, Al-Mallah et al.[32] identified 102 OHT patients who underwent adenosine MPI and compared them with 204 control patients for heart rate, blood pressure changes, and occurrence of AV block. A threefold increase in the incidence of high-grade AV block (Mobitz type II and third degree) was seen in OHT patients vs. controls. Symptomatic bradyarrhythmias occurred in 2% of OHT patients leading to premature termination of the adenosine infusion.

OHT patients were excluded from the early trials of REG, which led to its approval, and thus the safety of REG in this population was initially unknown. The effects of REG in these patients are particularly relevant, however, given its relative A_{2A} selectivity and the decreased incidence of AV block observed with REG in other populations. Cavalcante et al.[33] identified 40 OHT patients who underwent REG MPI. These results were compared with prior adenosine MPI results in the same patients. There were five episodes of second-degree AV block (Mobitz type II) and three episodes of sinus pause in adenosine MPI compared with only one episode of sinus pause in REG MPI. No major adverse effects such as congestive heart failure or death were reported following REG administration. To reverse REG's side effects, aminophylline was given to four patients (two for severe headache and two for chest pressure). However, REG was largely well tolerated by the OHT patients with no difference in overall adverse effect profile between the two test drugs.

4. REG in positron emission tomography stress myocardial perfusion imaging

Although REG was approved in April 2008 by the U.S. Food and Drug Administration for use in single photon emission computed tomography (SPECT) radionuclide myocardial perfusion imaging (MPI) as a pharmacologic stressor in patients unable to perform exercise stress testing, it has not yet been formally approved for use in positron emission tomography (PET) MPI. Nonetheless, it is increasingly being used in PET MPI in addition to the more established vasodilators, adenosine and dipyridamole. Over the past several years, PET MPI has become more accepted into the mainstream for the diagnosis and management of coronary artery disease (CAD).[34] Furthermore, a recent consensus statement by the American Society of Nuclear Cardiology recommended PET MPI over SPECT MPI as the preferred initial pharmacologic MPI modality if available.[35] The following is a discussion of the current evidence for REG as a pharmacologic stressor in PET MPI.

4.1. Current guidelines

The 2003 ACC/AHA/ASNC Guidelines for Clinical Use of Radionuclide Imaging recommend adenosine or dipyridamole myocardial perfusion PET for diagnosis in patients with an intermediate likelihood of CAD and/or for risk stratification in patients with an intermediate or high likelihood of CAD.[36] The only class I recommendation is in "patients in whom an appropriately indicated myocardial perfusion SPECT study has been found to be equivocal for diagnostic or risk stratification purposes" (Level of Evidence B). Class IIa recommendations for vasodilator PET MPI are identification of "the extent, severity, and location of ischemia as the initial diagnostic test in patients who are unable to exercise" and in "patients who are able to exercise but have LBBB or an electronically-paced rhythm" (both Level of Evidence B). REG is listed as an additional vasodilator in the 2009 American Society of Nuclear Cardiology Guidelines.[37]

4.2. PET vs. SPECT myocardial perfusion imaging: advantages and disadvantages

Cardiac PET imaging always includes concomitant CT acquisition for attenuation correction whereas this is still optional with SPECT. Effective radiation dose is lower with PET despite high positron emission energy due to very short half-life of rubidium-82 (Rb-82), the most commonly used PET radiotracer. Ejection fraction (EF) reserve (stress EF – rest EF) is more accurate with PET than SPECT because PET calculates the EF at peak stress rather than post stress as with SPECT. Coronary blood flow/flow reserve is possible with PET as myocardial uptake of Rb-82 bears a more linear relationship to coronary flow rates whereas the uptake of SPECT tracers plateaus at low flows. This allows for better characterization and localization of CAD. The superior image quality of PET is related to its high spatial resolution, reduced scatter, and the high positron emission energy of Rb-82 (1.52 MeV).

Advantages	Disadvantages
Higher spatial resolution (2–4 mm vs. 6–8 mm) [38-40]	Incompatible with exercise ($t_{1/2}$ of Rb-82 only 75 s)
Better count efficiency (more counts in less time) [38-40]	Insurance coverage not universal
Superior soft tissue attenuation correction [38, 39]	Less availability
Less liver/bowel uptake (less scatter) [40]	Motion artifact affects entire image (360° acquisition)
Shorter scan time (5 vs. 16 min) [40]	Claustrophobia (longer tunnel)
Less radiation (3.7 vs. 10–22 mSv) [40, 41]	
More accurate estimation of EF reserve [42]	
Ability to assess coronary blood flow/coronary flow reserve [34]	
Superior diagnostic sensitivity, specificity, and accuracy [40]	
Superior image quality [40]	
Increased confidence in interpretation [40]	

Table 2. Advantages and disadvantages of Rb-82 PET MPI vs. SPECT MPI

	Sensitivity (PET/SPECT)	Specificity (PET/SPECT)	Accuracy (PET/SPECT)
>70% stenosis	87%/82% (ns)	93%/73% ($P = 0.02$)	89%/79% ($P = 0.03$)
>50% stenosis	86%/81% (ns)	100%/66% ($P = 0.00008$)	87%/71% ($P = 0.003$)

Table 3. Overall sensitivity, specificity, and diagnostic accuracy of PET vs. SPECT MPI for both moderate and severe degrees of coronary stenosis

Comparison of 112 SPECT MPI (using adenosine and Tc-99m) and 112 PET MPI (using dipyridamole and Rb-82) in populations matched for gender, BMI, and presence/extent of

CAD.[40] "Specificity" includes low-likelihood patients who did not undergo angiography in addition to angiographically normal patients. "ns" = not statistically significant.

4.3. Advantages of REG in PET MPI

The increase in coronary blood flow is over 100 times greater with REG than adenosine. Rapid onset of hyperemia (less than 1 min after injection) with peak hyperemia occurring about 2.3 min following injection[3] along with weight-independent standardized dosing make REG well suited for use with short-acting PET radiotracers such as Rb-82 ($t_{1/2}$ = 75 s). Rapid testing is thereby facilitated with the stress portion lasting less than 1 min. When using REG stress together with PET imaging, the entire test duration is only 16–18 min. Figure 3 is a flow diagram of the REG PET MPI protocol used by Hsiao et al.[43]

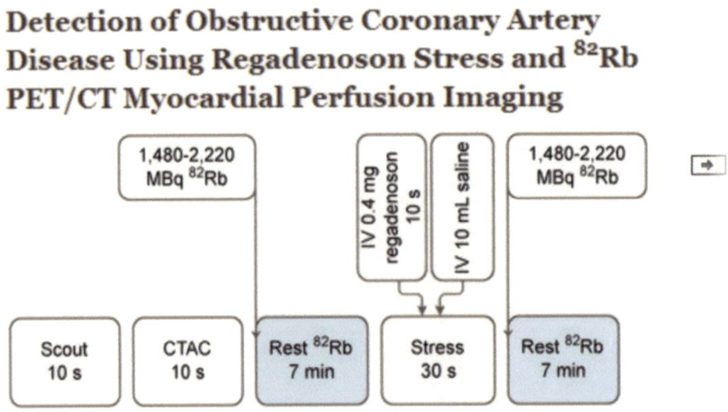

Reproduced with permission. Hsiao E, Ali B, Blankstein R, et al. Detection of obstructive coronary artery disease using regadenoson stress and 82Rb PET/CT myocardial perfusion imaging. J Nucl Med 2013;54:1748–54.

Figure 3. Rest-stress regadenoson [82]Rb PET/CT protocol. After scout CT acquisition (120 kVp, 10 mA), CT transmission scan (CTAC) (140 kVp, 10 mA, pitch of 1.35) was acquired. Patients received 1,480-2,220 MBq of [82]Rb intravenously at rest, and emission images were acquired in 2-dimensional list mode. After rest imaging, patients remained in scanner gantry for stress imaging. Stress was induced with 0.4 mcg of regadenoson given intravenously over 10 s followed by 10-mL flush with normal saline. Immediately after saline flush, second dose of 1,480-2,220 MBq of [82]Rb was administered intravenously approximately 30 s after regadenoson injection and emission images were acquired as previously described. Ordered-subsets expectation maximization (30 iterations and 2 subsets) and 3-dimensional PET filtering (Butterworth filter, cutoff frequency of 10, order of 5) were used for reconstruction of images.[43]

4.4. Coronary flow reserve using PET

The ability to quantitatively assess coronary blood flow (CBF) and coronary flow reserve (CFR) on angiography was discovered by Gould in animal experiments during the mid 1970s.[44] Because PET image acquisition occurs during peak stress, calculation of CFR (peak flow ÷ rest flow) is one of the unique features of PET as opposed to other noninvasive imaging modalities. A "normal range" has proved difficult to define given the disparity between coronary flows in asymptomatic patients. Based on pooled data from nearly 15,000 patients in 252 studies using three different PET isotopes, CFR in patients without CAD is 3.55 ± 1.36. In patients with established coronary disease, this drops to 2.02 ± 0.70.[45] Table 4 displays the range of values for absolute coronary flow and CFR in the presence of CAD risk factors and other forms of cardiac disease. One of the larger studies in the literature, however, identified a CFR of 1.74 as the cutoff for "definite ischemia" below which patients manifest anginal symptoms and/or ischemic ECG changes during vasodilator stress testing matched by a significant perfusion defect on PET imaging.[46]

Population	n	Rest Flow (cc/min/g)	Stress Flow (cc/min/g)	CFR
Normal controls	3,484	0.82 ± 0.06	2.86 ± 1.29	3.55 ± 1.36
Risk factors only	3,592	0.85 ± 0.08	2.25 ± 1.07	2.80 ± 1.39
Established coronary artery disease	1,650	0.83 ± 0.10	1.71 ± 0.71	2.02 ± 0.70
Mixed (risk factors and/or known coronary artery disease)	4,765	0.97 ± 0.10	1.86 ± 0.58	1.93 ± 0.48
Cardiomyopathy	594	0.73 ± 0.07	1.47 ± 0.56	2.02 ± 0.67
Hypertrophic cardiomyopathy	345	0.90 ± 0.10	1.57 ± 0.33	1.84 ± 0.36
Syndrome X	348	1.06 ± 0.11	2.65 ± 1.31	2.54 ± 1.31
After cardiac transplant	184	1.14 ± 0.18	2.44 ± 1.34	2.29 ± 0.86

N = 14,962 from 252 unique publications. N-13 ammonia = 5,541; O-15 water = 3,161; Rb-82 = 6,175.

Reproduced with permission. Gould KL, Johnson NP, Bateman TM, et al. Anatomic versus physiologic assessment of coronary artery disease. Role of coronary flow reserve, fractional flow reserve, and positron emission tomography imaging in revascularization decision-making. J Am CollCardiol2013;62:1639–53.

Table 4. Graded Absolute Flow and Coronary Flow Reserve Across Spectrum of Disease : n=14,962[45]

Not until recently was the clinical utility of PET-derived CFR fully appreciated. A study of 205 patients (using REG in half of these) demonstrated that with a negative predictive value of 97%, normal global CFR virtually assures the absence of high-risk CAD, despite any coexistent abnormal perfusion.[47] However, as a reduced CFR can occur in three different conditions (diffuse non-obstructive atherosclerosis, significant epicardial coronary stenosis, and microvascular disease), it can be somewhat helpful but is not specific for selecting patients likely to have high-risk CAD on angiography. A very recent study of PET-derived CFR further illustrated that low CFR can be seen in patients with systolic cardiomyopathy (EF ≤ 45%) of both ischemic and non-ischemic etiologies.[48] Murthy et al.[49] studied 2783 patients with known or suspected CAD referred for rest/stress PET MPI and then followed over a median of 1.4 years. Those in the lowest CFR tertile (<1.5) had a 16-fold increase in risk of cardiac death versus those in the highest tertile (>2.0). The middle tertile had a 5.7-fold increase in risk compared to the highest tertile. The addition of CFR to clinical and standard MPI factors led to the correct re-categorization of 34.9% of patients in the intermediate-risk group. Patients in this study received one of four different vasodilators (adenosine, dipyridamole, dobutamine, or REG). As resting CBF was similar between all three tertiles, the reduction in CFR was primarily driven by lower CBF with stress suggesting impaired coronary vasodilator function as an etiology. No difference was drawn between the various vasodilators used, however.

Very little has been published on the specific use of REG to assess CFR in Rb-82 PET MPI. Van Tosh et al.[50] used REG alone to show that CFR corresponded with LV dysfunction (LVD) during stress and that regional reductions in CFR were more often present in patients with

LVD than those without, indicating that the phenomenon of coronary steal may be involved in the genesis of LVD.

4.5. REG PET MPI vs. dipyridamole PET MPI

There exist scant data comparing REG and dipyridamole in PET MPI. A recent study retrospectively assessed CBF and CFR using Rb-82 perfusion PET/CT in 104 matched patients with normal stress tests, half with dipyridamole and half with REG. No significant difference in stress CBF and CFR was found between the two vasodilators (Figure 4). Further supporting REG's usefulness as a stress agent was the lack of any correlation between stress CBF or CFR and patient weight or BMI.[51]

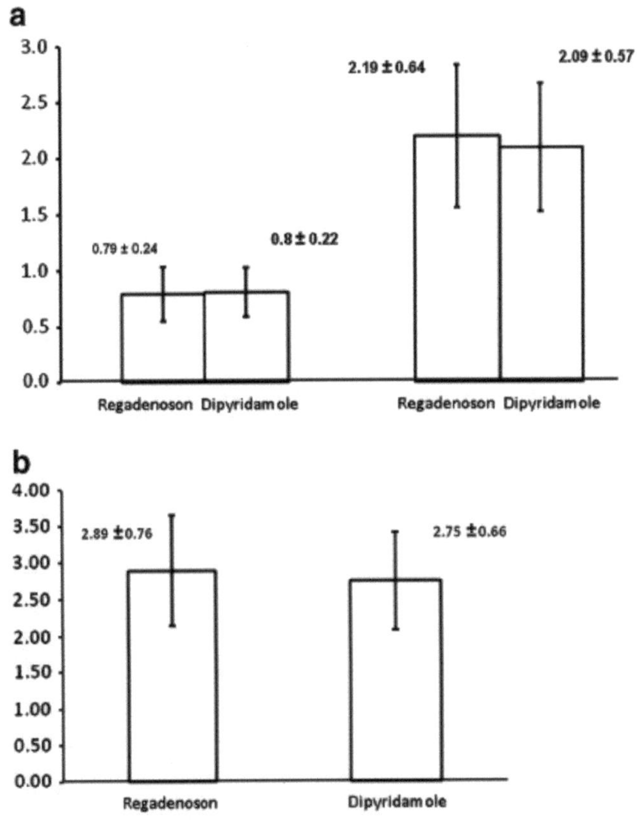

Reproduced with permission. Goudarzi B, Fukushima K, Bravo P, Merrill J, Bengel FM. Comparison of the myocardial blood flow response to regadenoson and dipyridamole: a quantitative analysis in patients referred for clinical 82Rb myocardial perfusion PET. Eur J Nucl Med Mol Imaging2011;38:1908–16.

Figure 4. Myocardial blood flow (MBF) and myocardial flow reserve (MFR) in subjects undergoing pharmacological stress with regadenoson versus dipyridamole. **a** No significant difference in MBF between groups at rest (*left*, p=0.77) or during stress (*right*, p=0.39). **b** No significant difference in MFR (p=0.31).[51]

A very recent study by Johnson and Gould compared CFR in patients undergoing two sequential PET MPIs, either both with dipyridamole (n = 50) or with dipyridamole and REG

(n = 126).[52] In the latter group, various timings between REG administration and activation of the Rb-82 generator were used. It was demonstrated that using the timing recommended in the REG package insert (10–20 s between REG injection and radioisotope injection), the stress CBF and CFR with REG were only 80% of the hyperemia attained with dipyridamole. By increasing this interval to 55 ms, this percentage was increased to 90%. These findings suggest that with the current timing recommendation, REG remains inferior to diypirdamole in detecting stress CBF and CFR.

The shorter duration of peak hyperemia with REG (2.3 min) than dipyridamole has raised some concern as to whether Rb-82 uptake by the myocardium would be sufficient to register perfusion defects or changes in cardiac function with the newer vasodilator. Cullom et al.[53] studied 32 patients, all of whom underwent both REG and dipyridamole PET MPI, and compared summed stress and difference scores, total perfusion deficit, LVEF, LV volumes, and change in stress-rest function. They determined that REG and dipyridamole yielded equivalent measures of cardiac perfusion and function.

To date, there are no published investigations of REG vs. adenosine in PET myocardial perfusion imaging.

4.6. Diagnostic accuracy of REG PET MPI

Studies comparing vasodilator stress SPECT and PET MPI have repeatedly demonstrated slightly higher sensitivity in PET (90%) than SPECT (80–84%) but far greater specificity in PET (89%) than SPECT (53–76%).[34, 38, 39] Table 5 summarizes the results of all published literature on the diagnostic accuracy of PET through 2007. Most of these studies used Rb-82 as a tracer and dipyridamole ± handgrip for stress. One included dipyridamole, adenosine, and dobutamine stress, and one used exercise stress with ammonia-N13 PET imaging.

Reference	No. of patients	Women	Prior CAD	PET radiotracer	Sensitivity	Specificity	PPV	NPV	Accuracy
Sampson et al. (*22*)*	102	0.42	0	^{82}Rb	0.93	0.83	0.80	0.94	0.87
Bateman et al. (*21*)	112	0.46	0.25	^{82}Rb	0.87	0.93	0.95	0.81	0.89
Marwick et al. (*23*)	74	0.19	0.49	^{82}Rb	0.90	1	1	0.36	0.91
Grover-McKay et al. (*24*)	31	0.01	0.13	^{82}Rb	1	0.73	0.80	1	0.87
Stewart et al. (*20*)	81	0.36	0.42	^{82}Rb	0.83	0.86	0.94	0.64	0.84
Go et al. (*19*)	202	NR	0.47	^{82}Rb	0.93	78	0.93	0.80	0.90
Demer et al. (*25*)	193	0.26	0.34	^{82}Rb /^{13}N-ammonia	83	0.95	0.98	0.60	0.85
Tamaki et al. (*26*)	51	NR	0.75	^{13}N-ammonia	0.98	1	1	0.75	0.98
Gould et al. (*27*)	31	NR	NR	^{82}Rb /^{13}N-ammonia	0.95	1	1	0.90	0.97
Weighted summary	877	0.29	0.35		0.90	0.89	0.94	0.73	0.90

*Study using PET/CT (in which CT was used for attenuation correction only).

PPV= positive predictive value; NPV= negative predictive value; NR= not reported. (Reprinted with permission of (28).)

Reproduced with permission. Di Carli MF, Dorbala S, Meserve J, El Fakhri G, Sitek A, Moore SC. Clinical myocardial perfusion PET/CT. J Nucl Med2007;48:783–93.

Table 5. Summary of Published Literature with Regard to Diagnostic Accuracy of PET[34]

Hsiao et al.[43] performed the first and so far only published study to evaluate the diagnostic accuracy of REG in PET MPI. In a relatively small cohort of 134 patients in 98 of whom angiographic data were also available, its accuracy was found to be similar to that of PET MPI using other vasodilators. Sensitivity for obstructive CAD was 92%, and overall specificity was 77% (53% in patients with high likelihood of CAD but no angiographic evidence of obstructive disease and 93% in low likelihood patients who did not go on to angiography [normalcy rate]). The area under the receiver–operator curve was 0.847, comparable to the high accuracy rates of PET in previous studies.

The high sensitivity of PET MPI for detection of obstructive CAD can be further increased by PET's ability to quantify blood flow/flow reserve and to calculate LVEF reserve using peak-stress LVEF.

4.7. Prognostic value of REG PET MPI

It has been shown that the prognostic value of REG is comparable to that of adenosine in patients with normal SPECT myocardial perfusion tests.[54] There are no published data on the prognostic value of REG in PET MPI, nor of REG MPI in patients with abnormal results using either PET or SPECT. Recent studies, however, offer insight as to the prognostic value of LVEF reserve in vasodilator stress PET.

Dorbala et al.[42] established that LVEF reserve (stress LVEF – rest LVEF) is independently predictive of the extent of at-risk myocardium on Rb-82 PET MPI and the extent of CAD on invasive angiography. Based on these results, LVEF reserve >5% essentially rules out severe 3-vessel or left main disease with a negative predictive value of 97%. In 985 patients with gated vasodilator stress Rb-82 PET MPI, nearly half of whom were at intermediate risk for CAD consistent with contemporary practice, the same group of investigators showed that during a mean follow-up period of 1.7 years, the frequency of cardiac events and all-cause death was higher in patients with LVEF reserve <0 than in those with LVEF which either remained the same or augmented with stress.[55] The prognostic value of LVEF reserve was found to be independent of, and incremental to, clinical variables and rest LVEF. These studies, however, included only patients who had received either dipyridamole or adenosine.

Hsiao's was the first group to investigate LVEF reserve using REG PET MPI, albeit in a much smaller cohort of 115 patients. Here, LVEF reserve with REG was inversely related to the severity of reversible perfusion defect (summed difference score) as well as jeopardized myocardium on coronary angiography (Duke Jeopardy Score)[43] (Figures 5 and 6). This suggests that REG may be as useful as dipyridamole or adenosine in determining LVEF reserve; however, further studies are still needed to evaluate its prognostic value.

4.8. Future directions for REG PET MPI

The IDEALPET (Integrated Dual Exercise and Lexiscan PET) study is currently underway and will compare Lexiscan© alone with Lexiscan© plus exercise ("Lexercise") with regards to safety, tolerability, myocardial perfusion image quality, and assessment of relative and absolute myocardial perfusion.[56]

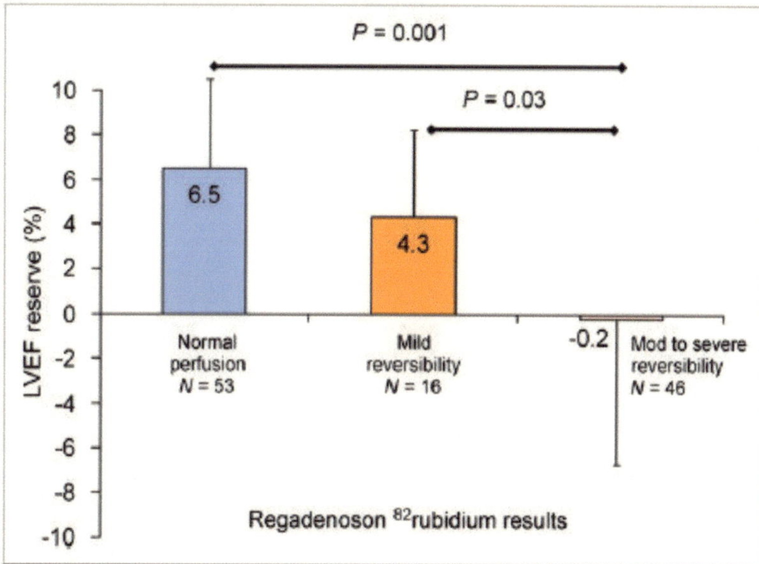

Reproduced with permission. Hsiao E, Ali B, Blankstein R, et al. Detection of obstructive coronary artery disease using regadenoson stress and 82Rb PET/CT myocardial perfusion imaging. J Nucl Med2013;54:1748–54.

Figure 5. Regadenoson LVEF reserve as function of relative MPI results. Mod=moderate.[43]

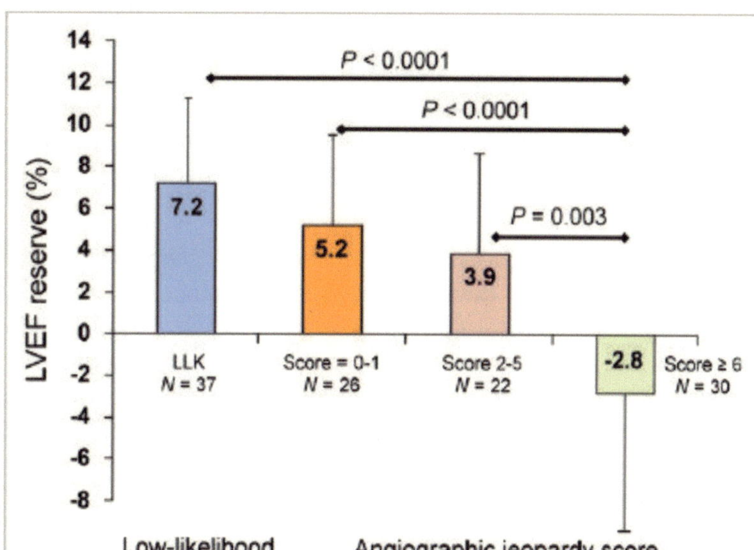

Reproduced with permission. Hsiao E, Ali B, Blankstein R, et al. Detection of obstructive coronary artery disease using regadenoson stress and 82Rb PET/CT myocardial perfusion imaging. J Nucl Med2013;54:1748–54.

Figure 6. Regadenoson LVEF reserve as function of Duke Jeopardy Score. LLK= low likelihood.[43]

As of February 2011 REG was being used in 68% of all pharmacologic stress MPI studies in the United States.[54] Given its already widespread use and favorable profile as a stress agent plus the advantages inherent in Rb-82 PET perfusion imaging (superior image quality, shorter scan time, lower radiation dose to patient, quantitation of myocardial blood flow, measurement of peak LVEF, additional prognostic information), REG PET MPI has the capacity to become the pharmacologic stress test of choice over the next several years.

5. Novel applications of REG

5.1. Adjunct to exercise MPI

Exercise-based testing has been convincingly shown to provide powerful prognostic data and remains the preferred mode of stress testing if patients are capable of exercising.[57, 58] However, about 25% of exercise-based testing may be non-diagnostic due to inability to achieve target heart rates. Two alternatives for these patients have been evaluated in the past: either rescheduling for pharmacologic stress or immediately attempting adjunctive vasodilator stress with agents such as adenosine and dipyridamole.[59, 60] The combination of simultaneous adjunctive low-level exercise with adenosine or dipyridamole helps both to lessen side effects and improve image quality.[61, 62] However, trying to add on adenosine or dipyridamole when exercise testing is submaximal poses major challenges as both are given as an infusion over a few minutes, need to be adjusted for weight or delivered via pump (as in the case of adenosine), and thus are not immediately feasible. In these instances, patients are usually rescheduled for a pharmacologic stress test when exercise testing is submaximal. With the advent of rapid-acting, weight-independent, single-bolus dosing of REG, its use as an adjunct to exercise seemed logistically feasible and potentially convenient. Its administration could result in quick conversion of an otherwise non-diagnostic nuclear exercise stress study due to submaximal heart rate to a diagnostic one. Early data support such a practice.

Thomas et al.[63] evaluated the safety of REG during exercise in a double blind study of 60 patients focusing on image quality, patient acceptance, and detection of perfusion defects. Patients undergoing a clinically indicated adenosine supine MPI were subsequently randomized in a 2:1 fashion to REG with low-level exercise (RegEx) or placebo with low-level exercise (PlcEx). This small study showed no significant differences in blood pressure response between the RegEx and PlcEx groups, although a smaller increase in heart rate was noted in the RegEx than in the PlcEx group. The image quality was better with REGEx compared to the adenosine supine MPI images. Patient tolerability was also reported to be better with RegEx compared to adenosine supine MPI. No significant adverse events, including high-grade AV block, were reported in the RegEx group.

In a subsequent study, Kwon et al.[27] published their retrospective experience with 1263 patients undergoing REG MPI with either adjunctive low-level treadmill exercise (n = 596) or as a standard supine REG stress test (n = 667). Among all participants an asymptomatic drop in systolic blood pressure > 10 mmHg occurred in 51% and > 30 mmHg in 9%. A pressure drop was observed more often in those randomized to REG plus low-level treadmill exercise (56%) than in those undergoing supine REG (47%). In their COPD/asthma patients

(16%), REG with low-level exercise was well tolerated, and they also reported lower incidence of nausea, shortness of breath, transient heart block, palpitations, and dizziness overall in those who underwent low-level exercise.

Our own experience comparing REG MPI (n = 887) to REGWALK MPI (n = 485) (REG with adjunctive low-level exercise) was published as a retrospective series. We showed that REGWALK studies demonstrated higher stress heart rate response, higher heart rate reserve, and higher systolic blood pressure with stress. There was less use of aminophylline for reversal of REG side effects in the REGWALK compared to the REG group. No major adverse events were reported in this series.

No data exist showing improved detection of ischemia/prognosis by combining REG with exercise. A few randomized studies have assessed the safety and efficacy of REG when used as an adjunct to maximal exercise when target heart rate is not achieved. Ross et al.[64] randomized 200 patients undergoing exercise MPI to either adjunctive REG if target heart rate was not achieved at peak exercise or to the discontinuation of exercise with conversion to a standard supine REG stress test. They showed that both approaches were well tolerated without any adverse events. There were no differences in ischemia detection, image quality or referral to cardiac catheterization in either group. Another small randomized study (n = 140) also showed that augmenting submaximal exercise with REG as needed was safe in patients.[65] In an effort to finalize the evaluation of REG's safety as an adjunct to exercise, a large randomized trial has just been completed by Astellas.[66] Results of this study will conclusively address not only the safety of REG with exercise but also the detection of ischemia when compared to REG alone.

5.2. Fractional Flow Reserve (FFR)

The concept of reactive hyperemia is particularly useful in guiding percutaneous coronary intervention (PCI) when intermediate coronary lesions of unclear hemodynamic significance are present on invasive angiography.[67, 68] More recently, seminal studies have firmly established that FFR-guided decision making for coronary lesions of unclear significance is associated with a favorable outcome with PCI being deferred or performed based on FFR values.[69] Most catheterization labs use either intracoronary or intravenous adenosine for assessment of hyperemic response.[70, 71] However recent studies have now shown that REG may be a viable alternative to adenosine with its weight independent bolus and rapid achievement of hyperemia in 33–40 s, thus shortening the entire time needed for FFR assessment.[72, 73] In a study of 25 patients undergoing catheterization, Nair et al.[72] compared the ability of IV adenosine and IV REG to induce coronary hyperemia in assessment of coronary stenosis significance. They found excellent linear correlation for measurement of FFR between the two agents (r = 0.985, P = 0.001). Furthermore, none of the hemodynamically significant lesions (FFR <0.8, 52% of patients) identified by adenosine were reclassified by REG. There were no significant adverse reactions to either drug and REG was overall better tolerated than adenosine.[72] In a more recent study by Prasad et al.,[74] the authors compared 57 patients (60 lesions) undergoing FFR measurements first with adenosine followed by a 10 min washout phase and then with REG. They showed high correlation in hyperemic response between the two drugs (R^2 = 0.93) (Figure 7) and substantially shorter time to peak hyperemia with REG than adenosine as well as a trend to a better side effect profile with REG. One issue of concern raised by these authors has been the potential cost of a single vial of REG (around 250 dollars) compared to a 3-min adenosine infusion (80 dollars). However, such cost differences could be made up by shorter duration of REG administration, no need for infusion pumps and less nursing time for set up. A recent randomized study of 100 patients has also shown that REG is equivalent to central venous infusion of adenosine to induce maximal hyperemia for FFR determination.[75]

In summary, the data accumulated on REG in FFR suggest that it could very well be the preferred agent in the catheterization lab given its ease of use and proven efficacy and comparability to adenosine.

5.3. Stress echocardiography

The detection of CAD using stress echocardiography (SE) is based on the physiologic principle of stress-induced subendocardial ischemia causing wall motion abnormalities in the territory subtended by stenosis. Exercise and dobutamine (DSE) are the main methods of SE in North America,[76] whereas high-dose dipyridamole supplemented with atropine has been the mainstay pharmacologic stressor in Europe.[76, 77]

It is well known that wall motion can be completely normal with DSE despite mild to moderate stenosis and corresponding abnormalities in hyperemic blood flow.[78] Using a newer technique of myocardial contrast echocardiography (MCE), contrast imaging during induced hyperemia allows for the detection of milder degrees of coronary stenosis. Similar to nuclear perfusion imaging, MCE is able to pick up small perfusion abnormalities, which occur prior to ischemic changes in wall motion, in keeping with the "ischemic cascade." Prior studies using adenosine, dobutamine, and exercise with MCE have shown that myocardial contrast perfusion enables detection of moderate stenosis when added to wall motion.[79–81]

Given its ease of use, there has been interest in using REG as a vasodilator to induce hyperemic stress during MCE. In a study of 100 patients undergoing quantitative coronary angiography, Porter et al.[82] performed real-time MCE with Definity 3% infusion at baseline and then at 2-min intervals for up to 6 min after a REG bolus. This study showed that MCE with REG can detect noncritical coronary stenosis (>50% diameter) with sensitivity, specificity, and accuracy of 80%, 74%, and 75%, respectively, which was better than wall motion analysis alone (60%, 70%, and 66%, respectively ($P < 0.001$ for sensitivity)). Furthermore, the authors concluded that the sensitivity was highest when imaging was performed 4–6 min after REG administration.[82] In a recent study performed in 10 dogs with mild to moderate non flow limiting CAD, Le et al.[83] used REG (5 μg/kg, 10-s bolus) along with MCE and assessed myocardial blood volume, flow velocity, and total regional myocardial flow before and after REG administration. REG induced an increase in coronary blood flow for 30 min. This decreased proportionally to stenosis severity, and perfusion defects were visible for up to 10 min after REG bolus. They noted that the optimal time for imaging myocardial perfusion in stress echo with REG was between 3 and 10 min after REG bolus.[83]

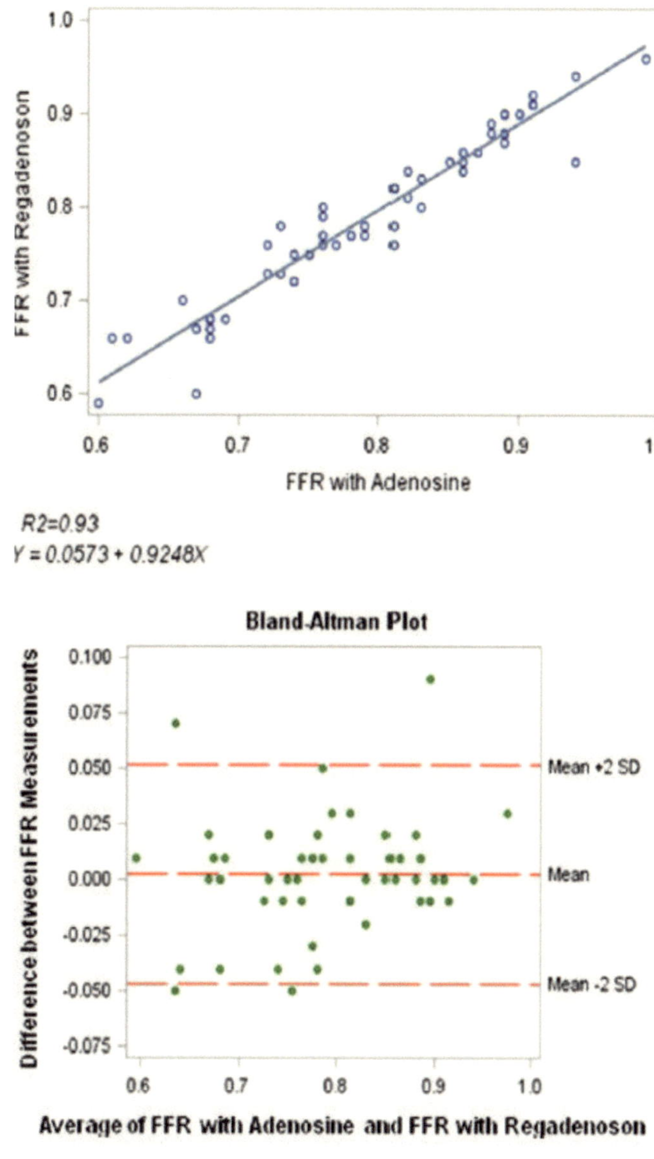

Prasad et al.: CCI; 2014;83;365–74 [74]

Reproduced with permission Prasad A, Zareh M, Doherty R, et al. Use of regadenoson for measurement of fractional flow reserve. Catheter CardiovascInterv2014;83:369–74.

Figure 7. Average of FFR with Adenosine and FFR with Regadenoson[74]

Our group recently reported on 44 patients undergoing diagnostic angiography based on prior abnormal stress testing who also underwent a novel protocol called REGAT (REG + atropine) SE to assess feasibility, safety, and diagnostic accuracy of CAD detection. The testing sequence began with administration of 2 × 1 mg boluses of atropine to induce chronotropy followed by a 400-μg bolus of REG, and then echo imaging at peak stress starting 20 s after the REG bolus. The protocol was found to be safe and well tolerated with no serious adverse effects. The mean duration of REGAT SE was 18 ± 7 min. Significant CAD (≥70% stenosis) by angiography was present in 51.1%. Sensitivity, specificity, and positive and negative predictive values for REGAT SE were 60.9%, 80.4%, 82.4%, and 67.9%, respectively. By coronary territories, the sensitivity, specificity, PPV, and NPV were as follows: left anterior descending artery, 58.8%, 92.9%, 83.3%, and 78.8%; left circumflex artery, 6.7%, 93.3%, 33.3%, and 67.7%; and right coronary artery, 16.7%, 93.9%, 50%, and 75.6%. Over 90% of subjects reported feeling comfortable, with 83% preferring REGAT as a future stress modality. We concluded that although the REGAT protocol was fast, safe, and well-tolerated with good specificity for CAD detection, its low sensitivity and NPV preclude it from routine use. Importantly, contrast was not utilized in our study as we were testing the feasibility of a combination of REG and atropine. Overall evidence indicates that REG in SE may be feasible and safe and, but larger studies are needed in this area as concern still exits that echocardiographic imaging may not detect ischemia induced by vasodilator stress.

5.4. Coronary CT Angiography (CCTA) and stress perfusion

It is now well established that CCTA performs with high diagnostic sensitivity and has excellent negative predictive value for the noninvasive evaluation of CAD[84, 85] However the specificity and positive predictive value have been shown to be less than desired with overestimation of stenosis severity in published studies[86, 87]. When compared to fractional flow reserve or SPECT even apparent high grade stenosis diagnosed on CCTA has not be consistently associated with ischemia[87]. This has raised some concerns that CCTA as a noninvasive modality for CAD may lead to higher false positives and downstream testing. CCTA stenosis detection requires additional physiologic information to correctly identify physiologic significant lesions. Until recently evidence for ischemia evaluation with CCTA has been very limited. The concept of combining stress perfusion with CT (CTP) has been tested and found to be accomplished in many single center studies mainly using adenosine or adenosine triphosphate. This has raised the possibility that a comprehensive anatomic and physiologically CAD assessment could be feasible by CCTA+CTP. [88-90]

Most recently a multicenter study sponsored by Astellas was completed and published evaluating the non-inferiority of REG CTP to REG SPECT. Patients (men > 45 years; women > 50 years) with known or suspected coronary artery disease (n=124) were randomized to 1 of 2 diagnostic sequences: rest/REG SPECT MPI on day 1, then REG/rest CTP on day 2, or REG/rest CTP on day 1 followed by rest/REG SPECT MPI on day 2. CCTA was also performed during the same acquisition as the CTP in both groups. Scanning platforms included 64-, 128-, 256-, and 320-slice systems. The primary analysis examined the agreement rate between CTP and SPECT for detecting or excluding reversible ischemia in 2 myocardial segments as assessed by independent blinded readers. Across the 110 patients included in the final analysis REG CTP was non-inferior to SPECT for detecting or excluding reversible ischemia with an agreement rate of 0.87 (95% confidence interval [CI], 0.77-0.97) and sensitivity and specificity of 0.90 (95% CI, 0.71-1.00) and 0.84 (95% CI, 0.77-0.91), respectively. The agreement rate for

http://dx.doi.org/10.5772/61154

detecting or excluding fixed defects by REG CTP and SPECT was 0.86 (95% CI, 0.74e0.98). With SPECT as the reference standard, the diagnostic accuracies for detecting or excluding ischemia by REG CTP and CTA alone were 0.85 (95% CI, 0.78-0.91) and 0.69 (95% CI, 0.60-0.77), respectively. The authors concluded that REG CTP is non-inferior to SPECT. Thus, CT vasodilator stress perfusion imaging either with REG or adenosine appears to have a promising role in providing physiologic information to clarify anatomic stenosis. Further studies are awaited to establish this modality in clinical practice.

6. Conclusion

We have aimed to provide the reader in this chapter a detailed overview of REG and its current status in cardiac stress testing and other emerging cardiac applications. The role of REG remains to be better defined in cardiac MRI and CT.

Acknowledgements

We thank Stephanie Stebens MLIS AHIP, Sladen Library, Henry Ford Hospital, for her expert assistance in the preparation of this manuscript.

Author details

Gurunanthan Palani[1], Rebecca Baumann[2] and Karthik Ananthasubramaniam[2*]

*Address all correspondence to: kananth1@hfhs.org

1 Department of Internal Medicine, McLaren Regional Medical Center, Michigan State University, Flint, MI, USA

2 Heart and Vascular Institute, Henry Ford Hospital, Detroit MI, USA

Dr. Palani and Dr. Baumann have no disclosures. Dr. Ananthasubramaniam has received research grants from Astellas Pharma US Inc.

References

[1] Kochanek KD, Xu J, Murphy SL, Minino AM, Kung HC. Deaths: final data for 2009. *Natl Vital Stat Rep.* 2011;60(3):1–116.

[2] Heidenreich PA, Trogdon JG, Khavjou OA, et al. Forecasting the future of cardiovascular disease in the United States: a policy statement from the American Heart Association. *Circulation.* 2011;123(8):933–944.

[3] Lieu HD, Shryock JC, von Mering GO, et al. Regadenoson, a selective A2A adenosine receptor agonist, causes dose-dependent increases in coronary blood flow velocity in humans. *J Nucl Cardiol.* 2007;14(4):514–520.

[4] Laighold S, Druz R. Initial clinical experience with a selective A2A receptor agonist, regadenoson, in a patient with end-stage renal disease on hemodialysis. *J Nucl Cardiol.* 2009;16(3):478–480.

[5] Gordi T, Frohna P, Sun HL, Wolff A, Belardinelli L, Lieu H. A population pharmacokinetic/pharmacodynamic analysis of regadenoson, an adenosine A2A-receptor agonist, in healthy male volunteers. *Clin Pharmacokinet.* 2006;45(12):1201–1212.

[6] Trochu JN, Zhao G, Post H, et al. Selective A2A adenosine receptor agonist as a coronary vasodilator in conscious dogs: potential for use in myocardial perfusion imaging. *J Cardiovasc Pharmacol.* 2003;41(1):132–139.

[7] Iskandrian AE, Bateman TM, Belardinelli L, et al. Adenosine versus regadenoson comparative evaluation in myocardial perfusion imaging: results of the ADVANCE phase 3 multicenter international trial. *J Nucl Cardiol.* 2007;14(5):645–658.

[8] Dhalla AK, Wong MY, Wang WQ, Biaggioni I, Belardinelli L. Tachycardia caused by A2A adenosine receptor agonists is mediated by direct sympathoexcitation in awake rats. *J Pharmacol Exp Ther.* 2006;316(2):695–702.

[9] Hage FG, Heo J, Franks B, et al. Differences in heart rate response to adenosine and regadenoson in patients with and without diabetes mellitus. *Am Heart J.* 2009;157(4): 771–776.

[10] Lexiscan (Regadenoson) [package insert]. Northbrook, IL: Astellas Pharma US, Inc.; 2014.

[11] Shah S, Parra D, Rosenstein RS. Acute myocardial infarction during regadenoson myocardial perfusion imaging. *Pharmacotherapy.* 2013;33(6):e90–95.

[12] Hsi DH, Marreddy R, Moshiyakhov M, Luft U. Regadenoson induced acute ST-segment elevation myocardial infarction and multivessel coronary thrombosis. *J Nucl Cardiol.* 2013;20(3):481–484.

[13] Rosenblatt J, Mooney D, Dunn T, Cohen M. Asystole following regadenoson infusion in stable outpatients. *J Nucl Cardiol.* 2014;21(5):862–868.

[14] Agarwal V, DePuey EG. Advanced heart block and unresponsiveness after regadenoson administration during myocardial SPECT study. *Int J Cardiol.* 2014;176(2):e49–51.

[15] Page RL, 2nd, Spurck P, Bainbridge JL, Michalek J, Quaife RA. Seizures associated with regadenoson: a case series. *J Nucl Cardiol.* 2012;19(2):389–391.

[16] Zhao G, Messina E, Xu X, et al. Caffeine attenuates the duration of coronary vasodilation and changes in hemodynamics induced by regadenoson (CVT-3146), a novel adenosine A2A receptor agonist. *J Cardiovasc Pharmacol.* 2007;49(6):369–375.

[17] Gaemperli O, Schepis T, Koepfli P, et al. Interaction of caffeine with regadenoson-induced hyperemic myocardial blood flow as measured by positron emission tomography: a randomized, double-blind, placebo-controlled crossover trial. *J Am Coll Cardiol.* 2008;51(3):328–329.

[18] Tejani FH, Thompson RC, Kristy R, Bukofzer S. Effect of caffeine on SPECT myocardial perfusion imaging during regadenoson pharmacologic stress: a prospective, randomized, multicenter study. *Int J Cardiovasc Imaging.* 2014;30(5):979–989.

[19] Hendel RC, Bateman TM, Cerqueira MD, et al. Initial clinical experience with regadenoson, a novel selective A2A agonist for pharmacologic stress single-photon emission computed tomography myocardial perfusion imaging. *J Am Coll Cardiol.* 2005;46(11):2069–2075.

[20] Mahmarian JJ, Cerqueira MD, Iskandrian AE, et al. Regadenoson induces comparable left ventricular perfusion defects as adenosine: a quantitative analysis from the ADVANCE MPI 2 trial. *JACC Cardiovasc Imaging.* 2009;2(8):959–968.

[21] Cerqueira MD, Nguyen P, Staehr P, Underwood SR, Iskandrian AE. Effects of age, gender, obesity, and diabetes on the efficacy and safety of the selective A2A agonist regadenoson versus adenosine in myocardial perfusion imaging integrated ADVANCE-MPI trial results. *JACC Cardiovasc Imaging.* 2008;1(3):307–316.

[22] Ananthasubramaniam K, Weiss R, McNutt B, Klauke B, Feaheny K, Bukofzer S. A randomized, double-blind, placebo-controlled study of the safety and tolerance of regadenoson in subjects with stage 3 or 4 chronic kidney disease. *J Nucl Cardiol.* 2012;19(2):319–329.

[23] Doukky R, Rangel MO, Wassouf M, Dick R, Alqaid A, Morales Demori R. The safety and tolerability of regadenoson in patients with end-stage renal disease: the first prospective evaluation. *J Nucl Cardiol.* 2013;20(2):205–213.

[24] Golzar Y, Doukky R. Regadenoson use in patients with chronic obstructive pulmonary disease: the state of current knowledge. *Int J Chron Obstruct Pulmon Dis.* 2014;9:129–137.

[25] Prenner BM, Bukofzer S, Behm S, Feaheny K, McNutt BE. A randomized, double-blind, placebo-controlled study assessing the safety and tolerability of regadenoson in subjects with asthma or chronic obstructive pulmonary disease. *J Nucl Cardiol.* 2012;19(4):681–692.

[26] Thomas GS, Tammelin BR, Schiffman GL, et al. Safety of regadenoson, a selective adenosine A2A agonist, in patients with chronic obstructive pulmonary disease: a

randomized, double-blind, placebo-controlled trial (RegCOPD trial). *J Nucl Cardiol.* 2008;15(3):319–328.

[27] Kwon DH, Cerqueira MD, Young R, et al. Lessons from regadenoson and low-level treadmill/regadenoson myocardial perfusion imaging: initial clinical experience in 1263 patients. *J Nucl Cardiol.* 2010;17(5):853–857.

[28] Caner B, Rezaghi C, Uysal U, et al. Dobutamine thallium-201 myocardial SPECT in patients with left bundle branch block and normal coronary arteries. *J Nucl Med.* 1997;38(3):424–427.

[29] O'Keefe JH, Jr., Bateman TM, Barnhart CS. Adenosine thallium-201 is superior to exercise thallium-201 for detecting coronary artery disease in patients with left bundle branch block. *J Am Coll Cardiol.* 1993;21(6):1332–1338.

[30] Lakkis NM, He ZX, Verani MS. Diagnosis of coronary artery disease by exercise thallium-201 tomography in patients with a right ventricular pacemaker. *J Am Coll Cardiol.* 1997;29(6):1221–1225.

[31] Thomas GS, Kinser CR, Kristy R, Xu J, Mahmarian JJ. Is regadenoson an appropriate stressor for MPI in patients with left bundle branch block or pacemakers? *J Nucl Cardiol.* 2013;20(6):1076–1085.

[32] Al-Mallah MH, Arida M, Garcia-Sayan E, et al. Safety of adenosine pharmacologic stress myocardial perfusion imaging in orthotopic cardiac transplant recipients: a single center experience of 102 transplant patients. *Int J Cardiovasc Imaging.* 2011;27(7):1105–1111.

[33] Cavalcante JL, Barboza J, Ananthasubramaniam K. Regadenoson is a safe and well-tolerated pharmacological stress agent for myocardial perfusion imaging in post-heart transplant patients. *J Nucl Cardiol.* 2011;18(4):628–633.

[34] Di Carli MF, Dorbala S, Meserve J, El Fakhri G, Sitek A, Moore SC. Clinical myocardial perfusion PET/CT. *J Nucl Med.* 2007;48(5):783–793.

[35] Cerqueira MD, Allman KC, Ficaro EP, et al. Recommendations for reducing radiation exposure in myocardial perfusion imaging. *J Nucl Cardiol.* 2010;17(4):709–718.

[36] Klocke FJ, Baird MG, Lorell BH, et al. ACC/AHA/ASNC guidelines for the clinical use of cardiac radionuclide imaging—executive summary: a report of the American College of Cardiology/American Heart Association Task Force on Practice Guidelines (ACC/AHA/ASNC Committee to Revise the 1995 Guidelines for the Clinical Use of Cardiac Radionuclide Imaging). *Circulation.* 2003;108(11):1404–1418.

[37] Henzlova MJ, Cerqueira MD, Hansen CL, Taillefer R, Yao S-S. ASNC imaging guidelines for nuclear cardiology procedures, stress protocols and tracers. *J Nucl Cardiol.* 2009;16(2):331.

[38] Stewart RE, Schwaiger M, Molina E, et al. Comparison of rubidium-82 positron emission tomography and thallium-201 SPECT imaging for detection of coronary artery disease. *Am J Cardiol.* 1991;67(16):1303–1310.

[39] Go RT, Marwick TH, MacIntyre WJ, et al. A prospective comparison of rubidium-82 PET and thallium-201 SPECT myocardial perfusion imaging utilizing a single dipyridamole stress in the diagnosis of coronary artery disease. *J Nucl Med.* 1990;31(12): 1899–1905.

[40] Bateman TM, Heller GV, McGhie AI, et al. Diagnostic accuracy of rest/stress ECG-gated Rb-82 myocardial perfusion PET: comparison with ECG-gated Tc-99m sestamibi SPECT. *J Nucl Cardiol.* 2006;13(1):24–33.

[41] Gerber TC, Carr JJ, Arai AE, et al. Ionizing radiation in cardiac imaging: a science advisory from the American Heart Association Committee on Cardiac Imaging of the Council on Clinical Cardiology and Committee on Cardiovascular Imaging and Intervention of the Council on Cardiovascular Radiology and Intervention. *Circulation.* 2009;119(7):1056–1065.

[42] Dorbala S, Vangala D, Sampson U, Limaye A, Kwong R, Di Carli MF. Value of vasodilator left ventricular ejection fraction reserve in evaluating the magnitude of myocardium at risk and the extent of angiographic coronary artery disease: a 82Rb PET/CT study. *J Nucl Med.* 2007;48(3):349–358.

[43] Hsiao E, Ali B, Blankstein R, et al. Detection of obstructive coronary artery disease using regadenoson stress and 82Rb PET/CT myocardial perfusion imaging. *J Nucl Med.* 2013;54(10):1748–1754.

[44] Gould KL. Coronary flow reserve and pharmacologic stress perfusion imaging: beginnings and evolution. *JACC Cardiovasc Imaging.* 2009;2(5):664–669.

[45] Gould KL, Johnson NP, Bateman TM, et al. Anatomic versus physiologic assessment of coronary artery disease. Role of coronary flow reserve, fractional flow reserve, and positron emission tomography imaging in revascularization decision-making. *J Am Coll Cardiol.* 2013;62(18):1639–1653.

[46] Johnson NP, Gould KL. Physiological basis for angina and ST-segment change PET-verified thresholds of quantitative stress myocardial perfusion and coronary flow reserve. *JACC Cardiovasc Imaging.* 2011;4(9):990–998.

[47] Naya M, Murthy VL, Taqueti VR, et al. Preserved coronary flow reserve effectively excludes high-risk coronary artery disease on angiography. *J Nucl Med.* 2014;55(2): 248–255.

[48] Majmudar MD, Murthy VL, Shah RV, et al. Quantification of coronary flow reserve in patients with ischaemic and non-ischaemic cardiomyopathy and its association with clinical outcomes. *Eur Heart J Cardiovasc Imaging.* 2015.

[49] Murthy VL, Naya M, Foster CR, et al. Improved cardiac risk assessment with noninvasive measures of coronary flow reserve. *Circulation.* 2011;124(20):2215–2224.

[50] Van Tosh A, Votaw JR, Reichek N, Palestro CJ, Nichols KJ. The relationship between ischemia-induced left ventricular dysfunction, coronary flow reserve, and coronary steal on regadenoson stress-gated (82)Rb PET myocardial perfusion imaging. *J Nucl Cardiol.* 2013;20(6):1060–1068.

[51] Goudarzi B, Fukushima K, Bravo P, Merrill J, Bengel FM. Comparison of the myocardial blood flow response to regadenoson and dipyridamole: a quantitative analysis in patients referred for clinical 82Rb myocardial perfusion PET. *Eur J Nucl Med Mol Imaging.* 2011;38(10):1908–1916.

[52] Johnson NP, Gould KL. Regadenoson versus dipyridamole hyperemia for cardiac PET imaging. *JACC Cardiovasc Imaging.* 2015.

[53] Cullom SJ, Case JA, Courter SA, McGhie AI, Bateman TM. Regadenoson pharmacologic rubidium-82 PET: a comparison of quantitative perfusion and function to dipyridamole. *J Nucl Cardiol.* 2013;20(1):76–83.

[54] Iqbal FM, Hage FG, Ahmed A, et al. Comparison of the prognostic value of normal regadenoson with normal adenosine myocardial perfusion imaging with propensity score matching. *JACC Cardiovasc Imaging.* 2012;5(10):1014–1021.

[55] Dorbala S, Hachamovitch R, Curillova Z, et al. Incremental prognostic value of gated Rb-82 positron emission tomography myocardial perfusion imaging over clinical variables and rest LVEF. *JACC Cardiovasc Imaging.* 2009;2(7):846–854.

[56] Brigham and Women's Hospital. Integrated Dual Exercise and Lexiscan Positron Emission Tomography: IDEALPET. *ClinicalTrials.gov.* Bethesda, MD: National Library of Medicine; 2010: http://clinicaltrials.gov/show/NCT01109992.

[57] Myers J, Prakash M, Froelicher V, Do D, Partington S, Atwood JE. Exercise capacity and mortality among men referred for exercise testing. *N Engl J Med.* 2002;346(11): 793–801.

[58] Johnson NP, Wu E, Bonow RO, Holly TA. Relation of exercise capacity and body mass index to mortality in patients with intermediate to high risk of coronary artery disease. *Am J Cardiol.* 2008;102(8):1028–1033.

[59] Casale PN, Guiney TE, Strauss HW, Boucher CA. Simultaneous low level treadmill exercise and intravenous dipyridamole stress thallium imaging. *Am J Cardiol.* 1988;62(10 Pt 1):799–802.

[60] Ignaszewski AP, McCormick LX, Heslip PG, McEwan AJ, Humen DP. Safety and clinical utility of combined intravenous dipyridamole/symptom-limited exercise stress test with thallium-201 imaging in patients with known or suspected coronary artery disease. *J Nucl Med.* 1993;34(12):2053–2061.

[61] Holly TA, Satran A, Bromet DS, et al. The impact of adjunctive adenosine infusion during exercise myocardial perfusion imaging: results of the Both Exercise and Adenosine Stress Test (BEAST) trial. *J Nucl Cardiol.* 2003;10(3):291–296.

[62] Elliott MD, Holly TA, Leonard SM, Hendel RC. Impact of an abbreviated adenosine protocol incorporating adjunctive treadmill exercise on adverse effects and image quality in patients undergoing stress myocardial perfusion imaging. *J Nucl Cardiol.* 2000;7(6):584–589.

[63] Thomas GS, Thompson RC, Miyamoto MI, et al. The RegEx trial: a randomized, double-blind, placebo- and active-controlled pilot study combining regadenoson, a selective A(2A) adenosine agonist, with low-level exercise, in patients undergoing myocardial perfusion imaging. *J Nucl Cardiol.* 2009;16(1):63–72.

[64] Ross MI, Wu E, Wilkins JT, et al. Safety and feasibility of adjunctive regadenoson injection at peak exercise during exercise myocardial perfusion imaging: the Both Exercise and Regadenoson Stress Test (BERST) trial. *J Nucl Cardiol.* 2013;20(2):197–204.

[65] Parker MW, Morales DC, Slim HB, et al. A strategy of symptom-limited exercise with regadenoson-as-needed for stress myocardial perfusion imaging: a randomized controlled trial. *J Nucl Cardiol.* 2013;20(2):185–196.

[66] Astellas Pharma Global Development Inc. A Study to Assess Regadenoson Administration following an Inadequate Exercise Stress Test as Compared to Regadenoson Alone for Myocardial Perfusion Imaging (MPI) Using Single Photon Emission Computed Tomography (SPECT). *ClinicalTrials.gov.* Bethesda, MD: National Library of Medicine; 2012: https://clinicaltrials.gov/ct2/show/NCT01618669.

[67] Pijls NH, van Schaardenburgh P, Manoharan G, et al. Percutaneous coronary intervention of functionally nonsignificant stenosis: 5-year follow-up of the DEFER Study. *J Am Coll Cardiol.* 2007;49(21):2105–2111.

[68] Tonino PA, De Bruyne B, Pijls NH, et al. Fractional flow reserve versus angiography for guiding percutaneous coronary intervention. *N Engl J Med.* 2009;360(3):213–224.

[69] De Bruyne B, Pijls NH, Kalesan B, et al. Fractional flow reserve-guided PCI versus medical therapy in stable coronary disease. *N Engl J Med.* 2012;367(11):991–1001.

[70] Jeremias A, Whitbourn RJ, Filardo SD, et al. Adequacy of intracoronary versus intravenous adenosine-induced maximal coronary hyperemia for fractional flow reserve measurements. *Am Heart J.* 2000;140(4):651–657.

[71] Seo MK, Koo BK, Kim JH, et al. Comparison of hyperemic efficacy between central and peripheral venous adenosine infusion for fractional flow reserve measurement. *Circ Cardiovasc Interv.* 2012;5(3):401–405.

[72] Nair PK, Marroquin OC, Mulukutla SR, et al. Clinical utility of regadenoson for assessing fractional flow reserve. *JACC Cardiovasc Interv.* 2011;4(10):1085–1092.

[73] Arumugham P, Figueredo VM, Patel PB, Morris DL. Comparison of intravenous adenosine and intravenous regadenoson for the measurement of pressure-derived coronary fractional flow reserve. *EuroIntervention.* 2013;8(10):1166–1171.

[74] Prasad A, Zareh M, Doherty R, et al. Use of regadenoson for measurement of fractional flow reserve. *Catheter Cardiovasc Interv.* 2014;83(3):369–374.

[75] van Nunen LX, Lenders G, Schampaert S, et al. TCT-619 single bolus regadenoson injection versus central venous infusion of adenosine to induce maximum coronary hyperemia for measurement of FFR. *J Am Coll Cardiol.* 2013;62(18 Suppl 1):B188.

[76] Pellikka PA, Nagueh SF, Elhendy AA, Kuehl CA, Sawada SG. American Society of Echocardiography recommendations for performance, interpretation, and application of stress echocardiography. *J Am Soc Echocardiogr.* 2007;20(9):1021–1041.

[77] Picano E, Molinaro S, Pasanisi E. The diagnostic accuracy of pharmacological stress echocardiography for the assessment of coronary artery disease: a meta-analysis. *Cardiovasc Ultrasound.* 2008;6:30.

[78] Leong-Poi H, Coggins MP, Sklenar J, Jayaweera AR, Wang XQ, Kaul S. Role of collateral blood flow in the apparent disparity between the extent of abnormal wall thickening and perfusion defect size during acute myocardial infarction and demand ischemia. *J Am Coll Cardiol.* 2005;45(4):565–572.

[79] Elhendy A, O'Leary EL, Xie F, McGrain AC, Anderson JR, Porter TR. Comparative accuracy of real-time myocardial contrast perfusion imaging and wall motion analysis during dobutamine stress echocardiography for the diagnosis of coronary artery disease. *J Am Coll Cardiol.* 2004;44(11):2185–2191.

[80] Tsutsui JM, Elhendy A, Anderson JR, Xie F, McGrain AC, Porter TR. Prognostic value of dobutamine stress myocardial contrast perfusion echocardiography. *Circulation.* 2005;112(10):1444–1450.

[81] Miszalski-Jamka T, Kuntz-Hehner S, Schmidt H, et al. Myocardial contrast echocardiography enhances long-term prognostic value of supine bicycle stress two-dimensional echocardiography. *J Am Soc Echocardiogr.* 2009;22(11):1220–1227.

[82] Porter TR, Adolphson M, High RR, et al. Rapid detection of coronary artery stenoses with real-time perfusion echocardiography during regadenoson stress. *Circ Cardiovasc Imaging.* 2011;4(6):628–635.

[83] Le DE, Bragadeesh T, Zhao Y, Wang YG, Zha D, Kaul S. Detection of coronary stenosis with myocardial contrast echocardiography using regadenoson, a selective adenosine A2A receptor agonist. *Eur Heart J Cardiovasc Imaging.* 2012;13(4):298–308.

[84] Meijboom WB, Meijs MF, Chujif JD, et al. Diagnostic accuracy of 64 slice computed tomography coronary angiography ; a prospective multicenter multivendor trial. J Am Coll Cardiol 2008;52;2135-44

[85] Raff GL, Gallagher MJ, O"Neill WW, Goldstein JA. Diagnostic accuracy of noninvasive coronary angiography using 64 slice spiral computed tomography. J Am Coll Cardiol 2005;45;552-57

[86] DiCarli MF, Dorbala S, Currilova Z et al. Relationship between CT coronary angiography and stress perfusion imaging in patients with suspected ischemic heart disease assessed by integrated PET-CT imaging J Nucl Cardjol 2007;14; 799-809

[87] Schujjf JD, Wijns W, Jukema JW, et al. Relationship between noninvasive coronary angiography with multislice computed tomography and myocardial perfusion imaging J Amer Coll Cardiol 2006;48; 2508-2514

[88] George RT, Arbab-Zadeh A, Miller JM ET al. Adenosine stress 64 and 256 row detector computed tomography angiography and perfusion imaging : a pilot study evaluating the transmural extent of perfusion abnormalities to predict atherosclerosis causing myocardial ischemia.Circ Cardiovasc Imaging ;2;174-182

[89] George RT, Arbab-Zadeh A, Miller JM ET al. Computed tomography myocardial perfusion imaging with 320 row computed tomography accurately detects myocardial ischemia in patients with obstructive coronary disease..Circ Cardiovasc Imaging 2012;5;333-340

[90] Kurata A, Mochizuki T, Koyama Y et al. Myocardial perfusion imaging using adenosine triphosphate stress mutltislice spiral computed tomography; alternative to stress myocardial perfusion scintigraphy. Circ J 2005;69;550-557

[91] Cury RC, Kitt TM, Feaheny K et al. A randomized mutlicenter mutlivendor study of myocardial perfusion imaging with regadenoson CT perfusion vs single photon emission CT. J Cardiovasc Comput Tomogr. 2015 Mar-Apr;9(2):103-12

Chapter 2

Noninvasive Imaging for the Assessment of Coronary Artery Disease

Punitha Arasaratnam and Terrence D. Ruddy

Additional information is available at the end of the chapter

http://dx.doi.org/10.5772/61502

Abstract

Noninvasive cardiac imaging is a cornerstone of the diagnostic work-up in patients with suspected coronary artery disease (CAD), cardiomyopathy, heart failure, and congenital heart disease. It is essential for the assessment of CAD from functional and anatomical perspectives, and is considered the gate-keeper to invasive coronary angiography. Cardiac tests include exercise electrocardiography, single photon emission computed tomography myocardial perfusion imaging, positron emission tomography myocardial perfusion imaging, stress echocardiography, coronary computed tomography angiography, and stress cardiac magnetic resonance. The wide range of imaging techniques is advantageous for the detection and management of cardiac diseases, and the implementation of preventive measures that can affect the long-term prognosis of these diseases. However, clinicians face a challenge when deciding which test is most appropriate for a given patient. Basic knowledge of each modality will facilitate the decision-making process in CAD assessment.

Keywords: Noninvasive, imaging, coronary artery disease, assessment, diagnosis

1. Introduction

Noninvasive cardiac imaging is crucial for coronary artery disease (CAD) assessment. The increasing global burden of CAD is a major contributor to the marked growth in the use of noninvasive imaging [1]. In recent years, the development of state-of-the-art hardware and software technologies has broadened the perspective and dimension of noninvasive imaging. This is advantageous to hybrid imaging in CAD assessment, with the introduction of anatomical, physiological, or combined approaches. These techniques allow clinicians to move beyond the dichotomous concept of the presence or absence of CAD by increasing their understanding of the unique pathophysiologic processes in CAD, including subclinical atherosclerosis, plaque vulnerability, myocardial blood flow (MBF), and scar detection.

Invasive coronary angiography (ICA), an anatomical test, is considered the gold standard method for the diagnosis of CAD. Nevertheless, the risk of complications precludes the routine use of ICA and it is only indicated in patients with a high pre-test probability of the disease [2]. Because most patients have low or intermediate pre-test probabilities of disease, noninvasive testing should be considered first, serving as a selection process for ICA. Clinicians can choose from a wide range of noninvasive tests, including exercise electrocardiography (ECG), single photon emission computed tomography (SPECT) myocardial perfusion imaging (MPI), positron emission tomography (PET) MPI, stress echocardiography (SE), coronary computed tomography angiography (CCTA), and stress cardiac magnetic resonance (CMR). Therefore, clinicians are frequently faced with the apparently difficult clinical question: "What is the right test?" However, there are no right tests! The test to be used should be selected for each patient after considering the patient's characteristics, genetic and environmental factors, predisposition, risk factors, and comorbidities. Cardiac testing is generally unnecessary in asymptomatic patients except in high-risk occupations or before starting antiarrhythmic drugs.

A basic understanding of the principles, diagnostic, and prognostic accuracy, and the strengths and limitations of each imaging technique is essential. The clinician must then adopt a structured approach, which will help choose the appropriate test to use after considering the risk and benefit profile of each test. The establishment of a diagnosis of CAD will influence the perceived likelihood of a future cardiac event and warrant secondary prevention to slow or prevent disease progression. The absence of CAD on imaging will reassure the patient, and encourage the clinician to adopt a primary prevention strategy. Hence the ultimate goal is for the chosen test to address the clinical question with a high level of certainty. The theme of this chapter is to provide a comprehensive guide to selecting the appropriate imaging test in patients with suspected CAD.

2. Basic concepts for choosing cardiac imaging tests

2.1. Classification of chest pain

There can be varied presentation of chest pain, including jaw pain, epigastric pain, indigestion, shortness of breath, or reduced effort tolerance. Atypical presentations are commonly seen among diabetics, female, and the elderly. Chest pain can be classified using the criteria below [3]:

Criteria:

1. Substernal chest pain or discomfort

http://dx.doi.org/10.5772/61502

2. Provoked by exertion or emotional stress
3. Relieved by rest ± nitroglycerin

Typical angina: (1) + (2) + (3)

Atypical angina: (1) + (2) or (1) + (3)

Nonanginal chest pain: (1) or none.

2.2. Pre-test and post-test probabilities

Bayes' theorem proposes the use of a combined pre-test probability and test result to determine the post-test probability of disease [4]. This will help the clinician to determine whether a positive test result is a "true positive" or a "false positive" and whether a negative test result is a "true negative" or a "false negative". For example, a positive test result is likely to be a "true positive" result in a 70-year-old patient with typical angina or a "false positive" result in a 40-year-old female with nonanginal chest pain. Meanwhile, a negative test result is likely to be a "true negative" result in a 35-year-old man with atypical chest pain or a "false negative" result in a 60-year-old man with prior myocardial infarction (MI) and typical angina. Pretest probability can be estimated using the Diamond and Forrester classification [5] (Table 1).

Age	Gender	Typical	Atypical	Nonanginal
(years)		Angina	Angina	chest pain
≤ 39	Men	Intermediate	Intermediate	Low
	Women	Intermediate	Very low	Very low
40-49	Men	High	Intermediate	Intermediate
	Women	Intermediate	Low	Very low
50-59	Men	High	Intermediate	Intermediate
	Women	Intermediate	Intermediate	Low
≥ 60	Men	High	Intermediate	Intermediate
	Women	High	Intermediate	Intermediate

Table 1. Diamond and Forrester Pre-Test Probability of Coronary Artery Disease by Age, Sex, and Symptoms. High: >90% pre-test probability. Intermediate: between 10% and 90% pre-test probability. Low: between 5 and 10% pre-test probability. Very low: <5% pre-test probability [5].

2.3. Appropriate use criteria

The appropriate use criteria (AUC) defines appropriate imaging for the different clinical indications. The AUC for test selection among symptomatic patients with suspected CAD [2] (Table 2).

Indication for noninvasive testing in symptomatic patients	Exercise ECG	Stress MPI	Stress Echo	Stress CMR	CCTA
Low pretest probability of CAD ECG interpretable AND able to exercise	A	R	M	R	R
Low pretest probability of CAD ECG uninterpretable OR unable to exercise		A	A	M	M
Intermediate pretest probability of CAD ECG interpretable AND able to exercise	A	A	A	M	M
Intermediate pretest probability of CAD ECG uninterpretable OR unable to exercise		A	A	A	A
High pretest probability of CAD ECG interpretable AND able to exercise	M	A	A	A	M
High pretest probability of CAD ECG uninterpretable OR unable to exercise		A	A	A	M

Table 2. Appropriate Use Criteria for noninvasive testing in symptomatic patients for CAD assessment. A= appropriate, M= maybe appropriate, R= rarely appropriate. Uninterpretable ECG refers to resting abnormalities such as ST-segment depression (≥ 0.10 mV), complete left bundle branch block (LBBB), pre-excitation, digoxin use, or ventricular paced rhythm [2].

3. Non-invasive imaging tests

This section will focus on the unique principles, diagnostic and prognostic accuracy, strengths, limitations, representative cases and clinical pearls for each imaging modality.

3.1. Exercise electrocardiography

3.1.1. Background

Exercise ECG is a well-established and validated functional test used for CAD assessment. It has been used for more than 50 years, despite the increasing use of other imaging modalities. It is the first-line test in patients with suspected CAD who are able to exercise and who have an interpretable resting ECG [2]. Studies have demonstrated a lower diagnostic accuracy of exercise ECG in women because of their lower prevalence of CAD. However the risk of major adverse cardiac events (MACE) in women with good functional capacity and a normal resting ECG was not different between those who underwent exercise ECG compared with exercise SPECT MPI, and exercise ECG was considered a cost-effective strategy [6].

3.1.2. Principles

Exercise ECG evaluates the physiological response of the heart to a controlled level of exercise. The latter can be prescribed using specific exercise protocols such as Bruce and Naughton. Exercise ECG and hemodynamic-specific variables are shown to have diagnostic and prognostic value in the assessment of CAD. These variables include ST deviation, exercise capacity, percentage of the maximum age-predicted target heart rate (HR), heart rate recovery (HRR), blood pressure (BP) response, and the Duke Treadmill Score (DTS) [7].

Abnormal ST deviation is defined as ≥1 mm (0.1 mV) of downsloping or horizontal ST-segment depression (J point + 80 ms); or ≥1 mm of ST segment elevation in leads without pathological Q waves (except aVR). The J-point is defined as the junction of the QRS complex and the ST-segment. The ST deviation should be seen in three or more consecutive beats in the same lead to be considered significant [8, 9]. An upsloping ST-segment depression is considered an "equivocal" response and is not suggestive of myocardial ischemia [10]. High risk features include ST-segment depression ≥ 2mm at < 5 metabolic equivalents (METs) in ≥5 leads and ≥5 minutes into recovery [11]. ST-segment elevation in two or more contiguous leads can help localize the site of significant ischemia, unlike ST-segment depression [12]. In the presence of prior Q waves, ST-segment elevation of > 1.0 mm (J point +60 ms) is considered abnormal. This could represent reversible ischemia in the peri-infarct zone or ventricular dyskinesis or akinesis of a segment of the left ventricle. This finding has been demonstrated among patients with anterior (~30%) and inferior (~15%) infarctions [13, 14].

Exercise capacity (a marker of cardiorespiratory fitness) is an estimate of the maximal oxygen uptake for a given workload, and is measured in METs [15]. The prevalence of significant ischemia was 0.4% and 7.1%, based on the workload achieved (≥10 METs and < 7 METs), respectively, on exercise SPECT MPI [16]. Hence, patients who are able to achieve a high workload (≥10 METs) on exercise ECG, may not require additional functional imaging.

The maximum age-predicted HR is usually described as "220-age". The inability to achieve 85% of the maximum age-predicted HR was associated with decreased survival [17].

HRR is calculated as the peak HR achieved (HR at 1 min) [18]. An abnormal HRR is defined as a decrease in the HR of < 12 bpm in the first minute of recovery, and is predictive of mortality.

A normal blood pressure (BP) response is defined as an increase in systolic BP and an increase or decrease in diastolic BP during exercise. A decrease in systolic BP of >10 mmHg may suggest the presence of acute left ventricular dysfunction owing to ischemia [7]. An abnormal BP response may be a specific marker for left main (LM) or triple vessel disease (TVD) [19].

The DTS is calculated as exercise time (minutes) – (5 x ST depression in mm) – (4 x angina index) (0= no angina; 1= nonlimiting angina; 2= limiting angina) [20]. DTS can be categorized into low risk (≥ +5), intermediate risk (-10 to +4) and high risk (≤ -11).

The absolute and relative contraindications for undergoing and termination of an exercise ECG, respectively, is illustrated in Table 3 and Table 4 [9].

Absolute	Relative
Acute myocardial infarction (<48 hours)	Obstructive left main stenosis
Unstable angina	Moderate aortic stenosis
Decompensated heart failure	Hypertrophic obstructive cardiomyopathy with severe resting gradient
Active endocarditis	
	Significant tachyarrhythmias or bradyarrhythmias
Uncontrolled cardiac arrhythmias	High degree atrioventricular (AV) block
Severe symptomatic aortic stenosis	Recent stroke or transient ischemic attack
Acute pulmonary embolism	Mental impairment with limited ability to cooperate
Acute myocarditis or pericarditis	Uncontrolled BP >200/100 mmHg
Acute aortic dissection	Uncorrected medical conditions, e.g. significant anemia, important electrolyte imbalance, and hyperthyroidism
Physical disability that precludes safe and adequate testing	

Table 3. Absolute and relative contraindications for undergoing exercise ECG [9]

Absolute	Relative
ST segment elevation (> 1.0 mm) in leads without preexisting Q waves (other than aVR, aVL and V1)	Marked ST displacement (horizontal or downsloping of >2 mm measured 60 to 80 ms after the J point
Drop in systolic BP >10 mmHg, despite an increase in workload, in the presence of ischemia	Drop in systolic BP >10 mmHg, despite an increase in workload, in the absence of ischemia
Moderate to severe angina	Worsening chest pain
Central nervous system symptoms (e.g. ataxia, dizziness)	Fatigue, shortness of breath, wheezing, leg cramps or claudication
Signs of poor perfusion	Tachyarrhythmias, including multifocal ectopy, ventricular triplets, supraventricular tachycardia
Sustained ventricular tachycardia (VT), 2nd or 3rd degree AV block	Bradyarrhythmias that potentially become more complex or result in hemodyamic instability
Technical difficulties in monitoring the ECG or BP	BP >250/115 mmHg
Patient's request to stop	Development of bundle branch block which is indistinguishable from VT

Table 4. Absolute and relative indications for termination of exercise ECG [9]

3.1.3. *Diagnostic and prognostic accuracy*

A meta-analysis evaluating the accuracy of exercise ECG reported a sensitivity of 68% and specificity of 77% for the detection of CAD [21]. The discriminatory cut-off point of 1 mm (0.1

mV) of horizontal or downsloping ST-segment depression had a sensitivity of 68% and specificity of 77% [22]. The frequency of significant CAD in patients with low, intermediate, and high DTS was 19.1%, 34.9%, and 89.2%, respectively. In patients with LM or TVD, the frequency of significant CAD was 3.5%, 12.4%, and 46% in patients with low, intermediate, and high DTS, respectively [23]. The 5-year survival rates in patients with a DTS of ≤ -11 and ≥ +7, were 67% and 93%, respectively[24]. In a recent study of 58,020 adults without CAD, the peak METs and the percentage of the maximum predicted HR were highly predictive of survival [25].

In relation to other imaging modalities, significant risk predictors for hard cardiac events in asymptomatic or symptomatic low-risk patients without CAD included abnormal SPECT findings (hazard ratio [HR] = 1.83), ischemia detected by exercise ECG (HR = 1.70), decreasing exercise capacity (HR = 1.11), decreasing DTS (HR = 1.07), and increasing severity of the coronary calcium score (CS) (HR = 1.29). The CS improved the long-term risk prediction for CAD when stratified according to the Framingham Risk Score [26].

3.1.4. Strengths and limitations

The strengths and limitations of an exercise ECG are shown in Table 5.

Strengths	**Limitations**
Cheap	Low sensitivity
Widely available	Low specificity
No radiation exposure	Unable to localise ischemic territory
No injection	
Short procedural time	
Assess exercise capacity	

Table 5. Strengths and limitations of exercise ECG

3.1.5. Case example 1

A 71-year-old man presents with atypical chest pain, able to exercise, and a normal resting ECG. Risk factors include ex-smoker and hypertension. Pretest probability of CAD is intermediate. Based on the AUC, exercise ECG is considered an appropriate test. Resting ECG revealed sinus rhythm at a HR of 61 bpm (Figure 1A). He underwent exercise ECG using Bruce protocol. He exercised for 7 minutes 31 seconds and achieved 10.1 METS. At 6 minutes into the exercise and at a HR of 121 bpm, ECG demonstrated 1 mm horizontal ST-segment depression in leads II, III, aVF, V3 to V6 and reached a maximum of 3 mm at peak stress at HR of 151 bpm in leads II, III, and aVF (Figure 1B). The changes resolved at 1 minutes 50 seconds during recovery. Test was terminated due to fatigue. He developed chest pain at recovery. The calculated DTS = -11.5. Conclusion: Abnormal exercise ECG with a high DTS. He was referred for ICA.

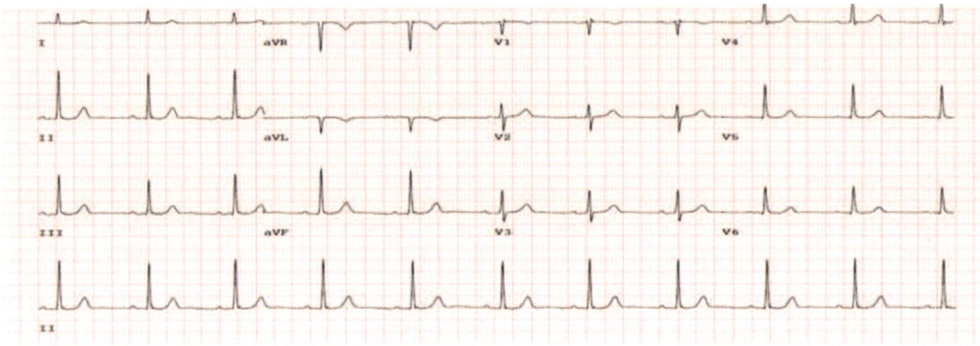

(a)

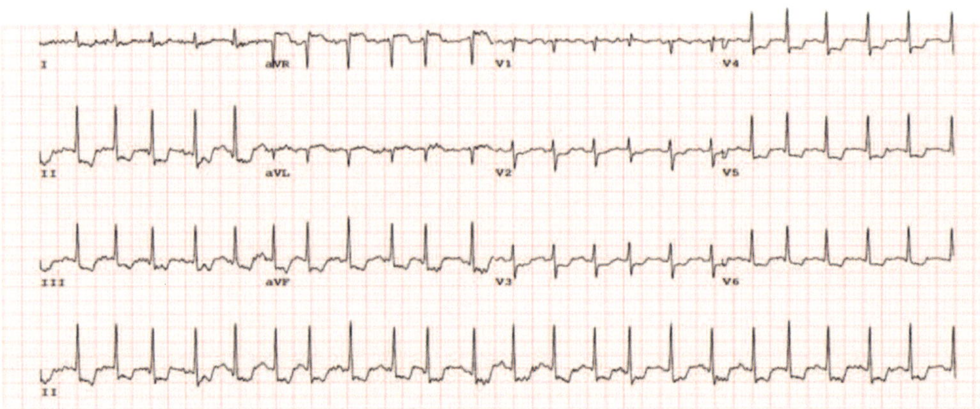

(b)

Figure 1. (a) Normal resting ECG. (b) Maximum of 3 mm horizontal ST segment depression seen in leads II, III and aVF, 2 mm ST segment depression in leads V3 to V6, at peak stress.

3.1.6. Clinical pearls

1. The J-point is defined as the junction of the QRS complex and the ST segment.
2. Achieving 85% of age predicted HR should not be an indication for test termination.
3. Exercise ECG with a high DTS may warrant ICA.
4. Exercise duration and METs achieved are strong predictors of prognosis.
5. The modification in ECG lead placement during exercise ECG compared to standard ECG may result in shift of the frontal axis to the right, increasing the voltage in the inferior leads, disappearance of Q waves in a patient with prior inferior infarct, or produce artifactual Q waves in normal subjects.

http://dx.doi.org/10.5772/61502

3.2. Single photon emission computed tomography

3.2.1. Background

There is robust evidence supporting the use of SPECT MPI in the workup and risk stratification of patients with suspected or known CAD because of its high diagnostic and prognostic value [27]. The development of solid state detector cameras compared with conventional SPECT (Anger) cameras offer improved signal resolution and shorter image acquisition time, which increases laboratory throughput [28, 29]. The switch from the standard, filtered back projection reconstruction method to iterative algorithms, which include depth independent resolution recovery, noise regularization, and scatter and attenuation correction, has improved the signal-to-noise ratio and image quality. This also allows for low-dose imaging using a standard acquisition time with reduced radiation exposure to the patient and operator,without compromising image quality and accuracy in the detection of CAD [30–32]. This is consistent with the American Society of Nuclear Cardiology's goal to reduce the radiation dose to ≤9 mSv in 50% of MPI studies by 2014.

3.2.2. Principles

SPECT MPI uses radionuclide-labeled compounds that emit Y ray photons. SPECT perfusion radiotracers include 201-Thallium (Tl-201, half-life [$t_{½}$] = 73 hours), and 99m-Technetium (^{99m}Tc, $t_{½}$ = 6 hours)-labeled sestamibi or tetrofosmin. Tl-201 is produced from a cyclotron and ^{99m}Tc is produced by a molybdenum-99-^{99m}Tc generator.

SPECT MPI can be performed using exercise or pharmacological stressors. Exercise is preferred for patients who can exercise at an adequate workload, aiming for a minimum of 85% of the maximal age-predicted HR and 5 METs [33]. A submaximal exercise workload decreases the sensitivity of exercise SPECT MPI for the detection of CAD. Exercise usually increases MBF by 2–3 times of resting flow [24, 34].

A pharmacological stressor should be used in patients who are unable to exercise or those with baseline ECG abnormalities (pre-excitation, paced ventricular rhythm, LBBB). Pharmacological stressors include intravenous vasodilators (adenosine, dipyridamole or regadenoson) or dobutamine, a β-adrenoceptor agonist. Vasodilators activate the adenosine A2A receptor and cause coronary arteriolar vasodilatation. Vasodilators increase MBF by 3–5 times in normal coronary vessels, an increase termed as the coronary flow reserve. Meanwhile, dobutamine increases MBF similar to that induced by exercise. In the presence of flow limiting stenosis, the coronary vessel is maximally vasodilated at baseline. Hence, the administration of a vasodilator is unable to augment coronary flow. MPI assesses the regional flow heterogeneity in normal and diseased coronary vessels [35]. Generally, vasodilators do not cause myocardial ischemia because MBF increases, albeit with some variability in all coronary artery beds with a minimal or no increase in the rate-pressure product, a measure of myocardial oxygen demand. In patients with extensive CAD, ischemia can be induced by the coronary steal phenomenon [33]. Vasodilators may also activate other adenosine receptors (A1, A2B, and A3) resulting in bronchospasm (A2B and, A3) or AV conduction delay (A1). Regadenoson is a selective A2A receptor agonist that is better than other vasodilators in patients with moderate chronic obstructive pulmonary disease (COPD) or asthma [36, 37].

For pharmacological stress SPECT MPI, contraindications include asthma or COPD with active wheezing, 2nd or 3rd degree AV block without a pacemaker or sick sinus syndrome, systolic BP <90 mmHg, use of methylxantines (e.g., aminophylline or caffeine) <12 hours, known hypersensitivity to the vasodilator, acute myocardial infarction (MI) and acute coronary syndrome [33].

3.2.3. Diagnostic and prognostic accuracy

The diagnostic accuracy of all noninvasive tests is subject to the post-test referral bias, also known as the verification bias. This increases the sensitivity and reduces the specificity of the test. A normalcy rate is used as a surrogate for specificity. It is defined as the percentage of normal perfusion scans in patients with a low likelihood (<10%) of CAD based on the results of clinical and ECG stress tests [38–40]. A pooled analysis of 4,480 patients with known or suspected CAD showed that exercise SPECT MPI had a mean sensitivity of 87% and a specificity of 73% for the detection of >50% stenosis [41]. The normalcy rate of SPECT MPI is around 84% [38]. Standard MPI studies include a combination of stress and rest protocols. The use of a stress-only protocol with a "normal" stress study can reduce the radiation dose by 40% and detected similar event rates [42–44]. A "normal" stress-only study is defined as homogenous perfusion, summed stress score (SSS) of <3, normal left ventricular (LV) cavity size, function, and wall motion [43].

The prognostic value of a normal pharmacological stress MPI test is independent of the radiopharmaceutical used [45]. A meta-analysis of 19 SPECT MPI studies comprising 39,000 patients demonstrated a low annual event rate of 0.6%, for hard cardiac events such as cardiac death or nonfatal MI in patients with a normal test result [46]. However, the prognostic value is based on the studied population. For example, the annual event rate among individuals with a normal test result was higher among diabetic patients than in non-diabetic subjects (0.5% vs. 1.7%, respectively, $p < 0.005$). Diabetic patients with a LV ejection fraction (LVEF) of $\leq 45\%$ had the worst outcome [47]. High-risk MPI variables include large perfusion defect size and extent, transient ischemic dilatation (TID), post stress stunning, increased right ventricular uptake, and increased lung uptake especially with Tl-201. A normal perfusion on exercise SPECT MPI was associated with a low event rate (<1% per year) in subjects with a low or intermediate DTS, compared in subjects with an intermediate DTS and high-risk SPECT variables or those with a high DTS and a normal perfusion [48].

3.2.4. Strengths and limitations

The strengths and limitations of SPECT using ^{99m}Tc-labeled sestamibi or tetrofosmin are shown in Table 6.

3.2.5. Case example 2

A 60-year-old female with hypertension presented with atypical chest pain. Pre-test probability of CAD is intermediate. Pharmacological (dipyridamole) SPECT MPI was performed due to an uninterpretable resting ECG that showed a LBBB. The test is considered appropriate based on the AUC. SPECT MPI demonstrated normal perfusion (Figure 2).

Strengths	Limitations
Widely available	Low specificity
High sensitivity	Lower spatial resolution
Expensive	Prone to attenuation artifacts
Well validated	Long procedural time (≈4 hrs)
Exercise and pharmacological stress	Longer half life of tracers
Improved specificity with gated SPECT	Increase hepatobiliary uptake
	Radiation exposure

Table 6. Strengths and limitations of ^{99m}Tc-labelled sestamibi or tetrofosmin SPECT MPI

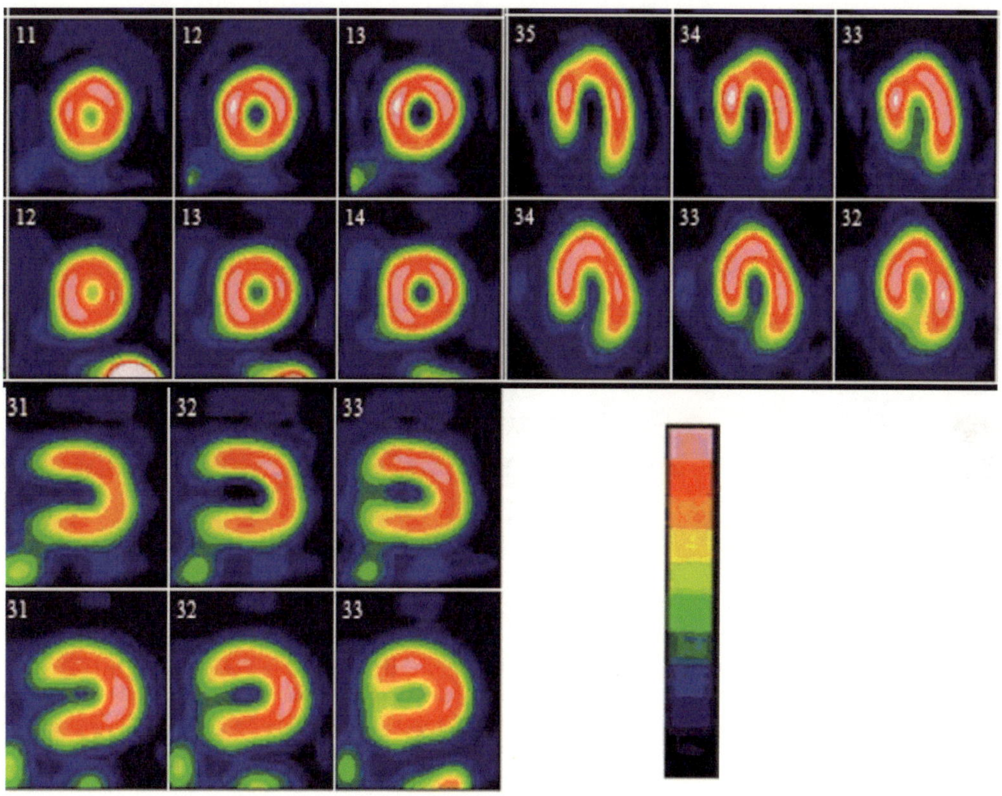

Figure 2. Stress (top row) & Rest (bottom row) images in the short axis (SA), horizontal long axis (HLA) and vertical long axis (VLA) show normal homogenous tracer uptake. Gated images showed normal left ventricular ejection fraction (not shown). This is a normal SPECT MPI study.

3.2.6. *Case example 3*

A 58-year-old man with a history of hyperlipidemia presented with typical angina (Canadian Cardiovascular Society Class 2). Pre-test probability of CAD: High. He underwent exercise SPECT MPI, which is considered an appropriate test based on the AUC. Baseline ECG showed sinus rhythm (Figure 3A) and resting BP of 140/90 mmHg. At 2 minutes in Bruce protocol, he developed significant ST-segment depression (Figure 3B). A significant BP drop from 140/90 mmHg to 80/60 mmHg during exercise was present and the test was terminated. The ECG changes persisted 5:50 minutes into recovery, and BP gradually returned to baseline. He achieved a total of 5 METS. He remained asymptomatic of chest pain. Calculated DTS was -17 (high risk). SPECT MPI findings as described in Figure 3C. He was referred for ICA (Figure 3D).

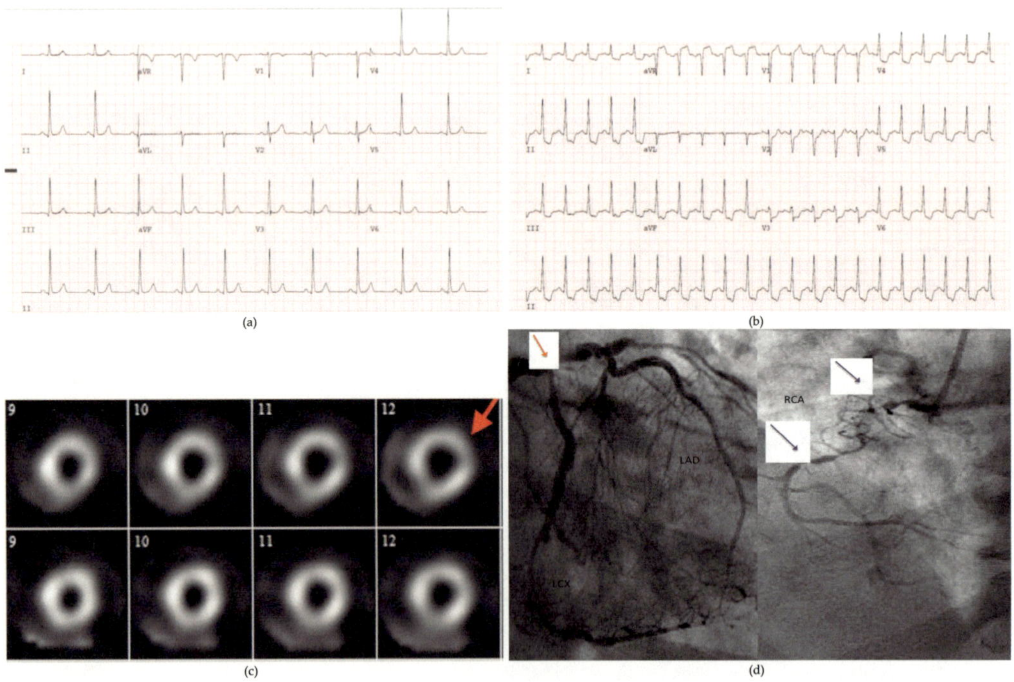

Figure 3. (a) Resting ECG showed normal sinus rhythm (b) ECG showed 3 mm ST segment depression in leads 1, aVF and V3, and a maximum of 4 mm ST segment depression leads II, V4 to V6. (c) Stress (top row), Rest (bottom row) in the SA slices: Mild reduction in tracer uptake in the mid to distal anterolateral walls (arrow) which normalized at rest. This was consistent with mild ischemia in the left circumflex (LCX) artery/ left anterior descending artery territory (LAD). TID is defined as the ratio of ungated LV volumes at stress and rest was present (1.21). TID is due to extensive subendocardial ischemia post stress that resolves on the rest images. ICA showed distal left main 90%, ostial LAD 90%, first diagonal 90%, first obtuse marginal 100%, second obtuse marginal 100%, right coronary artery 100%, and subsequently referred for CABG. This example clearly illustrates, despite a mildly abnormal perfusion (i.e. mild reduction in myocardial tracer uptake), the associated presence of high risk variables such as TID, and a high DTS, identifies a high risk scan. (d) Significant stenosis in the ostial LAD (orange arrow) and occluded proximal RCA with diffuse disease (purple arrows).

http://dx.doi.org/10.5772/61502

4. Clinical pearls

1. Combination of low-level exercise with dipyridamole can improve image quality and reduce symptoms resulting from drug effects.
2. High-risk findings include large defect size and extent, TID, post-stress stunning, increased right ventricular uptake, and increased lung uptake.
3. The prognosis of a normal MPI study is dependent on the study population.
4. A normal SPECT perfusion scan with ischemic ECG changes during vasodilator stress is associated with a significant cardiac event rate (~2% per year) and should be followed up with further cardiac imaging (PET MPI or CCTA).
5. Avoid antianginal medications such as beta-blockers, calcium channel blockers, or nitrates at least 48 hours prior to stress MPI for ischemia detection in suspected CAD.

4.1. Positron emission tomography

4.1.1. Background

PET MPI has superior temporal and spatial resolution, greater count sensitivity, and accurate attenuation correction compared with SPECT. These features translate into greater diagnostic image quality with fewer equivocal results, especially in obese subjects for example [49, 50]. The latest generation of PET cameras are combined with CT usually with ≥16 slices, and provide 3-dimensional imaging. Integrated PET (emission scan)/CT (transmission scan) systems facilitate sequential scanning, faster acquisition of transmission images, and enable functional and anatomic assessments in a single study [51–53]. These features make PET a useful clinical choice, but widespread utilization is limited by cost.

4.1.2. Principles

PET imaging is based on the detection of positron emission from radionuclide decay. After emission, the positron travels a short distance before it collides with an electron, resulting in mutual annihilation. This annihilation results in the production of 2 Y photons of 511 keV that travel in nearly opposite directions. The simultaneous detection of both photons by the detector of a PET camera is called coincidence detection [51–53].

Examples of cardiac PET radiotracers include rubidium-82 (^{82}Rb; $t_{½}$ = 76 s), nitrogen-13 ammonia (^{13}N- Ammonia; $t_{½}$ = 9.96 min), and oxygen-15 water ($^{15}O\text{-}H_2O$; $t_{½}$ = 2 min). A shorter $t_{½}$ allows a lower radiation dose per test. Radiotracers are produced by a cyclotron, except for ^{82}Rb, which is eluted from a strontium-82 (^{82}Sr)/^{82}Rb generator.

Ischemia is detected in the same way as for SPECT MPI. The fundamental difference in uptake kinetics of radiotracers used in SPECT and PET explain the superior sensitivity of PET for the detection of CAD. The ideal radiotracer is $^{15}O\text{-}H_2O$, which has linear uptake by myocardial tissue with increasing blood flow and "no roll-off" phenomenon. ^{99m}Tc- labeled tracers have a much lower extraction fraction. At high MBF, ^{99m}Tc- labeled tracers are characterized by a roll-off phenomenon to a greater degree, unlike PET radiotracers [54]. At high MBF levels during stress, the relative difference in myocardial tracer uptake may be reduced leading to an underestimation of the regional flow heterogeneity between normal and diseased coronary arteries. With dynamic imaging of the tracer kinetics in PET MPI, it is feasible to measure the myocardial flow reserve (MFR), which is defined as the ratio of absolute MBF during stress compared to MBF at rest. An abnormal global MFR is indicative of diffuse atherosclerosis or microvascular dysfunction.

4.1.3. Diagnostic and prognostic accuracy

PET MPI showed superior sensitivity and diagnostic accuracy, compared to SPECT [55, 56]. A meta-analysis of three different stress perfusion modalities determined the pooled sensitivity, specificity, and area under the curve of SPECT (88%, 61%, and 0.86, respectively), CMR (89%, 76%, and 0.90, respectively) and PET (84%, 81%, and 0.92, respectively) for the detection of CAD [57].

PET MPI can be used to determine prognosis, revealing annual event rates for cardiac death and nonfatal MI of 0.4%, 2.3%, and 7.0% for SSS values of <4 (normal), 4–7, and >8, respectively [58]. A similar trend was noted when subjects were stratified according to the percentage of ischemic LV myocardium, with a relative hazard for cardiac death of 2.3%, 4.2%, and 4.9% for the strata of 0.1–9.9%, 10–19.9%, and ≥ 20%, respectively [59]. Parameters that measure the extent of ischemia have been shown to guide the decisions regarding revascularization [60]. An abnormal global MFR (<2.0) was associated with an increased incidence of MACE compared with a normal MFR (1.3% vs. 4.7%, p = 0.03), independent of a normal perfusion and a CS of 0 [61].

4.1.4. Strengths and limitations

The strengths and limitations of PET MPI are shown in Table 7.

Strengths	Limitations
High spatial resolution	Expensive
Robust attenuation correction	Not widely available
Improved diagnostic accuracy in the obese	Radiation exposure
Alternative for an equivocal SPECT study	Unable to assess exercise capacity
Short half life of tracers	Pharmacological stress
Absolute MBF	
Assessment of calcium on CT	

Table 7. Strengths and limitations of PET MPI

4.1.5. Case example 4

A 68-year-old female with obesity, hypertension and an ex-smoker presented with chest pain. Noncontrast CT showed a CS of 715. CCTA was not performed. A persantine ^{82}Rb PET MPI was performed (Figure 4A) and gated images were acquired at stress and rest (Figure 4B). Coronary calcium was visualised on CT and MBF was abnormal (Figure 4C).

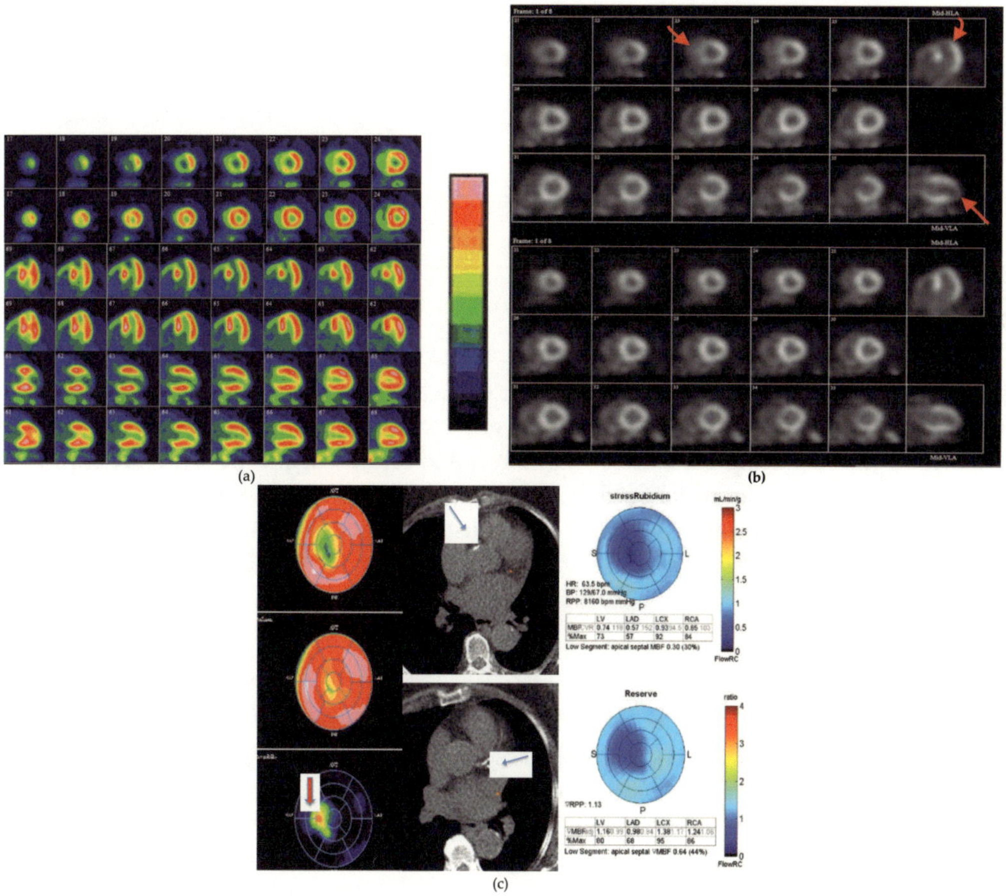

Figure 4. (a) Following stress, there is mild to moderate reduction in tracer uptake in the apical (distal) segments of the septum and anterior wall, and apex, which predominantly improves at the rest. This is consistent with a moderate sized area of moderate ischemia in the distal LAD territory. Stress images (rows 1, 3, and 5) and rest images (rows 2, 4, and 6). (b) Gated stress (top 3 rows) and gated rest (bottom 3 rows) during PET MPI. Normal LVEF and wall motion at rest. Following stress, there is mild hypokinesis in the apical (distal) septum and apex consistent with stress induced ischemia (red arrows). Stress acquisition during PET MPI is acquired at peak stress, and hence presence of regional wall motion is specific for ischemia. This differs from post-stress acquisition during SPECT which is delayed by 30 to 45 minutes. (c) Polar map shows the extent of reversible ischemia in the LAD territory (red arrow). CT shows presence of coronary calcification in the RCA (top, blue arrow), LCX and LAD (bottom, blue arrow). MBF demonstrate marked reduction in stress flow in the areas of reduced perfusion (global MBF= 0.74 ml/min/g), as depicted by the polar map which is labelled as stress Rubidium. Global MFR is reduced at 1.16, and 0.99 (after correction for RPP). There is reduced regional MFR in all three coronary artery territories (LAD= 0.98, LCX= 1.38, and RCA= 1.24), as seen on the polar map labelled as Reserve. The MFR finding is suggestive of underlying triple vessel disease. Measurement of MBF is corrected for rate-pressure product (RPP), and depicted in the shade of gray, next to the uncorrected values.

4.1.6. Clinical pearls

1. PET imaging is based on positron annihilation and coincidence detection of paired 511 keV Y photons.

2. PET has higher diagnostic accuracy compared to SPECT in the assessment of obstructive CAD.

3. PET is an excellent choice for imaging in the obese and those with an equivocal SPECT.

4. Abnormal global MFR suggest diffuse atherosclerosis or microvascular dysfunction.

5. Patient motion can result in significant misregistration artifact between the emission and transmission scans.

6. Normal PET perfusion and MFR confer an excellent prognosis.

4.2. Stress echocardiography

4.2.1. Background

SE is a robust, versatile imaging modality for CAD assessment. Advances in digital image acquisition, strain imaging, tissue harmonics, and contrast agents have increased the use of SE. In particular, the advances in tissue harmonics and contrast agents have greatly improved the visualization of endocardial borders, and diagnostic accuracy of SE for the detection of wall motion abnormalities (WMA) [62–64]. Because SE is highly operator- dependent, those who perform the test should have adequate training and experience to meet the level of competency required for performing and interpreting this test [65].

4.2.2. Principles

The fundamental principle for the detection of myocardial ischemia is the development of new or worsening WMA during stress [65, 66]. Based on the ischemic cascade, WMA appear after perfusion abnormalities and precede the manifestation of ECG changes and symptoms. Thus, SE has decreased sensitivity and superior specificity compared to perfusion-based imaging for the detection of CAD. Images are acquired at rest and stress. The images are compared on a four-screen setup side-by-side for WMA, LV cavity size and LVEF.

The stress component may be exercise (treadmill or bicycle) or pharmacologically (dobutamine or dipyridamole). An adequate level of stress using exercise requires a minimum target of 85% of the age-predicted HR, and is preferably symptom-limiting, considering the additional prognostic value of the subject's exercise capacity. Bicycle SE (supine or upright ergometry) allows simultaneous image acquisition during peak stress, and the measurement of Doppler information. During treadmill exercise SE, the stress images are acquired within 60–90 seconds post stress. The contraindications and indications for terminating an exercise SE are similar to those of exercise ECG.

Pharmacological SE using dobutamine is preferred over dipyridamole for wall motion assessment [65], although either stressor can be used [67]. The dose for dipyridamole in SE is higher at 0.84 mg/kg over 10 minutes, compared to the dose used in nuclear perfusion imaging at 0.14 mg/kg/min over 4 minutes. A typical dobutamine infusion rate is at 5 micrograms/kg/min and increasing at a 3-minute interval to 10, 20, 30, and 40 micrograms/kg/min, aiming to achieve 85% of the age-predicted target HR. Atropine can be used to achieve the desired target HR. The induction of ischemia is due to an increase in myocardial oxygen demand. Deformation analysis using the tissue velocity index (TVI) and two-dimensional speckle tracking (ST)-based strain imaging have been proposed using dobutamine SE [68, 69]. However, TVI- and ST-based analysis conferred no additional diagnostic value over WMA for detection of ischemia [70].

Indications for terminating the test include the de novo or worsening of WMA, significant arrhythmias, hypotension, severe hypertension, and intolerable symptoms. For image interpretation, normal wall motion is defined as normal wall thickening and endocardial excursion. Visual assessment of wall motion can be categorized and scored as follows: 1 = normal, 2 = hypokinetic, 3 = akinetic, 4 = dyskinetic or aneursymal. Please note that a score of "5" is no longer applicable. Each segment using the 16 segment LV model (i.e., apical cap not included) is scored and the wall motion score index (WMSI) is calculated. A normal WMSI equals to "1". WMSI = Total wall motion score/ Total number segments visualised. Unlike in MPI that utilizes the 17 segment model, for WMA assessment the 16 segment model is preferred. A WMSI of >1.7 corresponds to a perfusion defect of >20% on MPI. If feasible, the right ventricular wall motion should be assessed and presence of WMA suggest greater extent of CAD.

Normal: normal at rest; hyperdynamic at stress

Ischemia: normal at rest; inducible new or worsening WMA (hypokinesis, akinesis or dyskinesis) at stress

Infarction: fixed abnormality at rest and stress

4.2.3. Diagnostic and prognostic accuracy

The development of WMA depends on the extent of stenosis detected by ICA, and occurs at a cut-off relative diameter of 54% for exercise SE, 58% for dobutamine SE, and 60% for dipyridamole SE [71]. The sensitivities and specificities for the detection of CAD were 85% and 77%, respectively, for exercise SE, 80% and 86%, respectively for dobutamine SE, and 78% and 91%, respectively, for dipyridamole SE [71, 72]. SE had a similar diagnostic accuracy to that of SPECT MPI for the detection of CAD [73, 74]. However, because of its greater specificity, SE showed a better discriminatory capacity for the diagnosis of LM and TVD [75]. For patients presenting at an emergency department with chest pain, nondiagnostic ECG, and negative cardiac biomarkers, the overall sensitivity, specificity, positive predictive value (PPV), and negative predictive value (NPV) of SE for the diagnosis of CAD were 90%, 92%, 78% and 97%, respectively. Moreover, exercise SE had a better specificity than dobutamine SE [76].

A normal exercise SE result is associated with an excellent prognosis with an annual event rate of cardiac events of 0.54% [77]. The best discriminator of increased risk of cardiac events was WMSI ≥ 1.25 and ≤ 6 METs in both genders [78]. There was no difference in the prognostic value of dobutamine SE and dipyridamole SE [79, 80]. Therefore, the choice between these techniques may depend on institutional practices. With regards to LV cavity size, an abnormal stress LV end-systolic volume (LVESV) (i.e., no change or an increase) was associated with an increase risk of cardiac events compared with a decrease in the LVESV (2.9% vs. 1.6%) [81].

4.2.4. Strengths and limitations

The strengths and limitations of SE are shown in TABLE 8.

Strengths	Limitations
Cheap	Poor echo window (obese,
	COPD)
Widely available	Reduced sensitivity in
	detection of posterior wall
	ischemia
No radiation	Foreshortened LV apex
Portable	Operator dependent
Contrast echo improves	
endocardial definition	
Exercise and pharmacological	
stress	
Medium procedural time	

Table 8. Strengths and limitations of stress echocardiography

4.2.5. Case example 5

65-year-old woman with rheumatoid arthritis and hypertension presented with heartburn and indigestion of increasing severity for 1 month. An exercise SE with contrast was performed at rest. She experienced a similar episode of heartburn and nausea at 2 minutes into exercise. The test was stopped and stress images were acquired immediately (Figure 5A). Rest and stress images are shown as still frames captured at end-systole (Figure 5B i-iv). The patient was admitted in view of a positive SE at low workload. ICA showed ostial LAD 70%, mid LAD 90%, proximal LCX 80%, and mid RCA 100%. She was referred for CABG.

4.2.6. Clinical pearls

1. Normal wall motion at rest does not rule out the presence of obstructive CAD.
2. Abnormal regional wall motion can be seen in the presence of ischemic or nonischemic etiology.

http://dx.doi.org/10.5772/61502

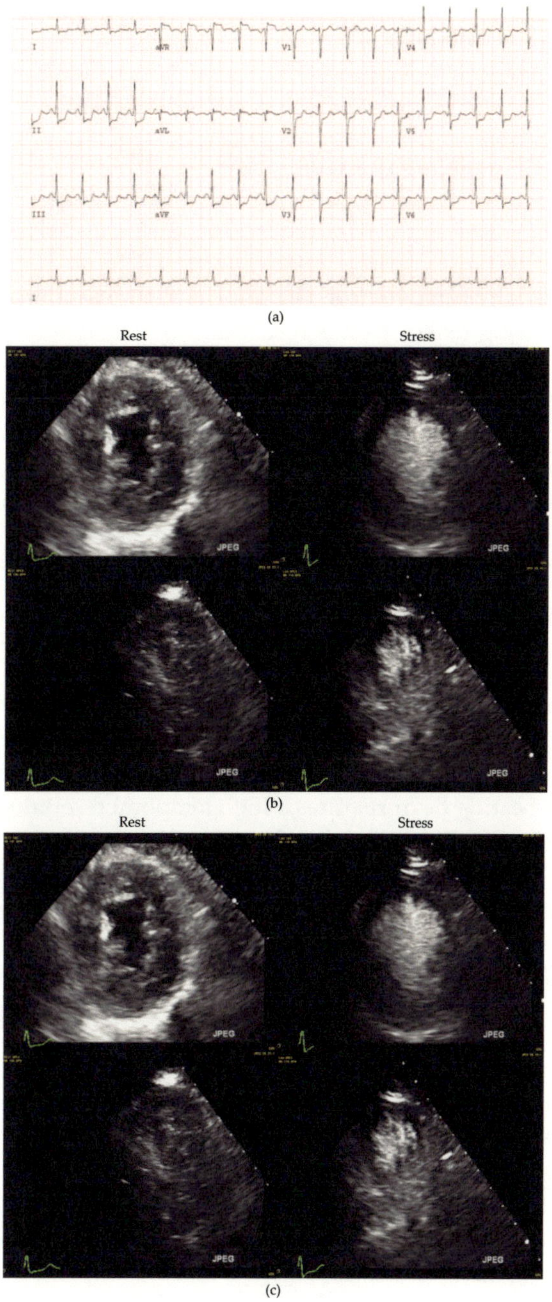

Figure 5. (a) ECG during episode of chest pain demonstrated diffuse 2 mm ST segment depression in leads II, III, aVF, V2 to V6 and ST elevation in aVR. (b) SE using contrast showing images captured at end-systole during rest and stress. The LV in different views are illustrated in the following sequence from top to bottom (i) parasternal long axis, (ii) 2-chamber, (iii) short axis, (iv) apical, demonstrate regional WMA in the anterior, anteroseptum, apex and lateral walls. Note the stress induced LV cavity dilatation, at peak stress which is suggestive of underlying triple vessel disease.

3. The absence of radial motion of the mitral valve annulus can result in a reduction in motion of the basal inferior or inferoseptal segments resulting in a false-positive study.

4. A common cause of a false negative test is a suboptimal stress level.

4.3. Coronary computed tomography angiography

4.3.1. Background

CCTA has come a long way from electron beam CT to the present multidetector CT system, with continually increasing detector rows (i.e., = slices) from 4-slices to 320-slices in some systems. A 64-slice CT system is the minimum requirement for coronary imaging. Other developments include iterative reconstruction, dual-source CT, prospective scanning, tube current modulation, and a z-flying focal spot [82]. These innovations have led to significant improvements in spatial and temporal resolution, radiation dosimetry, and image quality, which are prerequisites for coronary imaging. The ability to visualize subclinical atherosclerosis and characterize plaques has led to techniques for quantifying the extent of the atherosclerotic burden [83].

4.3.2. Principles

CCTA can determine the extent of coronary atherosclerosis and estimate the severity of coronary artery stenosis. The major components of a CT scanner include the table, X-ray tube, detector array and the gantry that rotates the X-ray tube and detector array around the patient. The ability to image a beating heart requires a high temporal resolution, which is defined as the time taken to obtain a complete data set for image reconstruction. The typical temporal resolution of CT is 280–420 ms. Data covering 180° are needed to construct one image, termed "half scan reconstruction". Accordingly, the temporal resolution of a single-source CT system is half the time required for the gantry to rotate 360°. For a dual-source CT (DSCT), the temporal resolution is one-quarter of the gantry rotation time, because data covering 90° are sufficient for image acquisition. A DSCT has a temporal resolution of 75 ms (compared to 20–30 ms for ICA) [84].

The ability for CT to discriminate two structures is called the spatial resolution, which is measured in line pairs per centimeter (lp/cm). The typical spatial resolution of CT is 10 lp/cm, which is equivalent to 0.5 mm (compared to 0.1 mm for ICA). CT data are acquired as isotropic voxels enabling the images to be viewed in multiple planes with similar spatial resolutions [85]. The spatial resolution of CT is less than ideal to accurately quantitate the degree of stenosis, hence a grading method is used [86]:

Normal: 0%; Minimal: <25%; Mild: 25–49%; Moderate: 50–69%; Severe: 70–99%; Occluded: 100%.

ECG gating is essential to minimize cardiac motion by synchronizing image acquisition to the cardiac cycle. There are two types of scanning modes. In prospective ECG-triggered scanning, data acquisition is triggered by the R waves on the ECG. Its advantage is the low radiation

http://dx.doi.org/10.5772/61502

dose, typically 3–5 mSv. Disadvantages include image reconstruction limited to the desired phase and functional evaluation is not possible. In retrospective ECG-gated scanning, data acquisition are acquired throughout the cardiac cycle and the ECG signal is simultaneously recorded with the raw data. Advantages include image reconstruction can be performed at any point in the cardiac cycle and it is useful in patients with arrhythmias. Its main disadvantage is the high radiation dose, typically 10–12 mSv because the tube current remains "on" throughout image acquisition. The application of tube current modulation can reduce the radiation dose. The best phase for image acquisition is mid-diastole, when the heart is moving the least.

The images to be acquired are the initial scout image, which defines the scan length, followed by a non-contrast calcium scan and finally the contrast-enhanced CT images. The average scan length for native coronary artery imaging is 12–14 cm. Using a 64-slice scanner, images are acquired over a few cardiac cycles, as opposed to a 320-slice scanner where one cardiac cycle is sufficient because of the larger volume covered. Data can be reconstructed in two or three dimensions, although the two-dimensional axial views should serve as a reference for image interpretation.

Contrast enhancement in the ascending aorta can be tracked using a test bolus or automated bolus tracking. Both methods are acceptable and the choice between them may depend on the institutional protocol. About 80–100 ml of iodinated contrast is typically used. The target HR of 50–65 bpm can be achieved by oral or intravenous β-adrenoceptor blockers. Nitroglycerin spray is recommended to improve image quality by inducing coronary vasodilatation.

Calcium is measured using the Agatston score (i.e., CS), which correlates with the extent of the atherosclerotic plaque burden. Screening for CS are recommended in two groups of asymptomatic patients: (1) patients with low global coronary heart disease (CHD) risk and a family history of premature CAD and (2) patients with intermediate global CHD risk [87]. CT perfusion is still research-based, and will not be discussed in this review.

4.3.3. Diagnostic and prognostic accuracy

There is extensive literature describing the diagnostic and prognostic value of CCTA. The main advantage of CCTA is the ability to exclude disease from the differential diagnosis since CCTA has an excellent NPV. The ACCURACY trial demonstrated sensitivity, specificity, PPV, and NPV of 95%, 83%, 64%, and 99%, respectively, for the detection of ≥ 50% stenosis, and 94%, 83%, 48%, and 99%, respectively, for the detection of ≥70% stenosis. The NPV was high in patient- and vessel-level analyses [88]. The low PPV is due to its tendency to overestimate stenosis, while the presence of artefacts lead may lead to a false positive test. CCTA is considered appropriate for patients with low or intermediate pre-test probabilities of CAD, and a negative scan reliably indicates the absence of significant CAD. However, CCTA is of limited clinical value and functional imaging tests are more appropriate in patients with a high pre-test probability [89]. The presence of severe coronary calcification (CS >400) can reduce the diagnostic accuracy by overestimating the severity of stenosis owing to blooming artefacts [88]. Although there is no specific cut-off level to cancel a CCTA, CS of > 600–1000 is typically used for this purpose, considering the high likelihood of a nondiagnostic study.

The use of CCTA in the emergency department resulted in a shorter hospital stay, increased discharge rate [90, 91], and reduced time to CAD diagnosis [90], while patients with a negative scan had an excellent prognosis [92]. The all-cause mortality rate was 0.65% for normal CCTA, 1.99% for <50% stenosis, 2.9% for ≥50% stenosis, and 4.95% for LM ≥50%, TVD ≥70%, or two vessel disease with proximal LAD disease [93]. The excellent prognosis of a negative CCTA result was seen in other large series of patients [94]. The "warranty period" of a normal CCTA is ~7 years [95]. Coronary calcium has prognostic value beyond traditional risk factors with a hazard ratio of 3.89, 7.08, and 6.84 for CS of 1–100, 101–300, and ≥300, respectively, for coronary events [96].

4.3.4. Strengths and limitations

The strengths and limitations of CCTA are shown in Table 9.

Strengths	Limitations
Excellent negative predictive	High calcium limits accuracy
value	of assessing stenosis
High temporal resolution	Radiation exposure
High spatial resolution	Morbidly obese
Visualize coronary anatomy	Arrhythmias
Short procedural time	Allergy to iodinated contrast
Assessment of calcium score	Heart rate control
	Follow breath hold instruction
	Renal impairment (>2.0 mg/dl)
	No functional assessment

Table 9. Strengths and limitations of CCTA

4.3.5. Case example 6

A 71-year-old female with hypertension, hyperlipidemia, and an ex- smoker presented with atypical chest pain and LBBB. CCTA was performed. Findings included a CS of 269, and ≥70% stenosis (calcified and noncalcified plaque) with positive remodeling in the mid LAD (Figure 6). There was mild disease in ostium of the RCA. She was referred for ICA.

4.3.6. Case example 7

A 57-year-old man with hypertension. CCTA showed a CS of 524 with an occluded proximal RCA. He was referred for ICA and underwent percutaneous coronary intervention to the RCA (Figure 7 A-E).

http://dx.doi.org/10.5772/61502

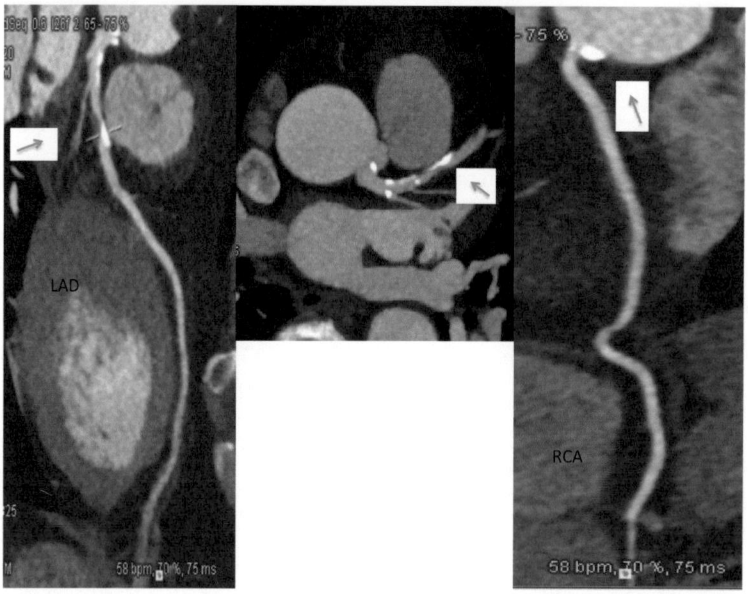

Figure 6. First two images of the curved multiplanar reformatted (MPR) and 2D-axial views demonstrate ≥70% stenosis of the LAD (blue arrows). The third image (curved MPR) of the RCA showing a calcified plaque with minimal stenosis at the ostium (blue arrow).

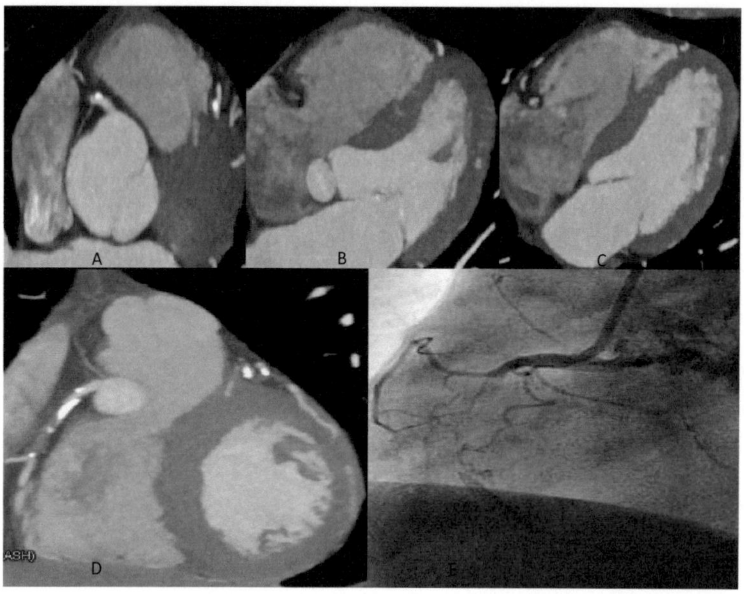

Figure 7. Axial slices from cranial to caudal demonstrate (A) contrast enhanced lumen in the proximal RCA, (B) absent of contrast enhancement and (C) reappearance of the contrast in the RCA. (D) Axial maximum intensity projection of the RCA demonstrate an occluded vessel and correlates with ICA (E).

4.3.7. Clinical pearls

1. An asymptomatic patient with a CS of 0 has a very low event rate of 0.1% per year [97].
2. Prospective ECG-triggered acquisition is preferred in view of the lower radiation dose.
3. Regular, low HR and obeying breath-hold instructions are essential for diagnostic image quality.
4. Appropriate timing of contrast injection is crucial for optimal enhancement as contrast non-uniformity in the distal coronary vessels can simulate stenoses.
5. Volume coverage in the z-axis for a 64-slice CT (0.625 mm detector width) is 4 cm (64 x 0.625), and a 320-slice CT (0.5 mm detector width) is 16 cm.

4.4. Stress cardiac magnetic resonance

4.4.1. Background

CMR has recently emerged clinically as a highly versatile technique with superior spatial and temporal resolution. The development of high field strength magnets (3T) and rapid imaging techniques such as gradient echo, echo-planar, and balanced steady-state free precession, have contributed to the feasibility of MR perfusion. The type of pulse sequence or hybrid sequences affect the contrast-to-noise ratio and the suspectibility to artifacts, which can affect image quality. In the context of MPI, CMR is a promising tool in parallel with well-established and validated modalities such as SPECT and PET MPI. The advantage of MR is its superior sensitivity for the detection of subendocardial perfusion defects without radiation exposure. The paramagnetic property of gadolinium (Gd)-based contrast agents can alter the local magnetic field in the tissue, which enables differentiation between normally and abnormally perfused myocardium. Arterial spin labeling and blood oxygen level-dependent techniques are new advances in perfusion imaging, but are still research-based. The use of coronary magnetic resonance angiography is not well established, except in some highly specialized centers, and will not be discussed here.

4.4.2. Principles

The fundamental basis of CMR perfusion imaging is the first-pass imaging of contrast transit through the LV myocardium. This exploits the effect of Gd on the T1 relaxation time of myocardial tissue [98]. Gd-based contrast agents are paramagnetic, extracellular agents that are rapidly taken up and rapidly washed out of the normal myocardium, but accumulate in damaged tissues with slower washout kinetics. Gd is highly toxic in its native state. Therefore, Gd chelators (e.g., Gd-DTPA) are used clinically. These agents shorten the T1 and T2 relaxation time constants that represent the decay of the MR signal. However, at low doses, T1 shortening is predominant. During first-pass perfusion, the normal myocardium (i.e., normal perfusion) shows substantial Gd uptake, and appears bright (i.e., hyperintense) owing to a short T1.

Ischemic myocardium (i.e., reduced perfusion) shows diminished Gd uptake and appears dark (i.e., hypointense) owing to a long T1 [98].

Similar to pharmacological stress SPECT or PET MPI, stress CMR requires the use of a pharmacological stressor, such as a vasodilator (e.g., adenosine, dipyridamole, and regadenoson) or dobutamine. Diseased coronary arteries, exhibit a lower peak myocardial signal intensity and increases in myocardial contrast transit time (e.g., signal upslope, arrival time, time-to-peak signal, and mean transit time)[99]. The difference in signal intensity can be quantitatively, semiquantitatively, or visually evaluated to identify possible perfusion defects. The use of adenosine and visual interpretation are common, and these approaches are discussed in further detail.

Historically, inducible ischemia was only assessed using stress and rest perfusion cine images. This method demonstrated a sensitivity, specificity, and diagnostic accuracy of 88%, 90%, and 89%, respectively, for the detection of significant CAD [100]. The caveat being, in patients with prior MI, the resultant perfusion deficit may include areas of prior infarct and may not reflect true inducible ischemia. Imaging with late Gd-enhancement (LGE) was used to detect prior infarction. A method combining first-pass stress and rest imaging with LGE demonstrated an overall accuracy of 0.88, or 0.96 for one-vessel disease, 0.75 for two-vessel disease, and 0.9 for prior coronary artery bypass graft, in the detection of significant stenosis [101].

A stress CMR study can be interpreted using the following algorithm [99]:

Step 1. Assess for LGE

Negative: Move to step 2.

Positive: CAD present.

Step 2. Assess stress perfusion

Negative: No CAD

Positive: Move to step 3.

Step 3. Assess rest perfusion

Negative: Inducible ischemia suggestive of CAD.

Positive: Likely artifact*

* Common being the Gibbs artifact, which is more pronounced on a 3T scanner. This usually occurs in the phase encoding direction and tends to be transient. If the segment of perfusion defect is also positive for LGE, then inducible ischemia cannot be assessed in the same segment.

An abbreviated adenosine stress CMR protocol [102]:

1. **LV structure and function module** – scout and cine imaging for cardiac structure and systolic function at rest.
2. **First pass stress perfusion module** – infusion of adenosine (140 mcg/kg/min over 4 minutes), followed by intravenous Gd (0.05 to 0.1 mmol/kg) and saline flush. Once the

contrast bolus has transited the LV myocardium, adenosine is stopped. Stress images are acquired for 40 to 50 heart beats.

3. **Rest perfusion module**– performed after 10 minutes to ensure sufficient clearing of Gd from the blood pool. Reinjection of a second dose of Gd. Rest images are acquired. Slice geometry, scan setting, and Gd dose should be similar to step (2).

4. **LGE module**– performed after 5 minutes of completion of step (3).

5. **Analysis**– visual interpretation using the 17 segment LV model. The stress and rest cine images are viewed side-by-side using equivalent slices, in addition to the LGE images.

(Some centers omit the rest perfusion module, if the first pass stress perfusion study is normal).

Adenosine ($t_{½}$ = 10 s) is safe and well-tolerated. The potential adverse effects include flushing, chest pain, palpitations, breathlessness, transient episodes of heart block, hypotension, sinus bradycardia, and bronchospasm [102]. The contraindication to adenosine stress CMR (in addition to the general contraindication of any MR study) include known hypersensitivity to adenosine, known or suspected bronchoconstrictive or bronchospastic disease, 2nd or 3rd degree AV block, sinus bradycardia (HR <45 bpm), and systolic BP <90 mmHg [102].

4.4.3. Diagnostic and prognostic accuracy

Diagnostic accuracy of stress CMR in a population with high prevalence of CAD (57%) showed on an overall sensitivity of 89% and specificity of 80% for the diagnosis of significant obstructive CAD. Adenosine-based stress demonstrated better sensitivity than dipyridamole (90% vs. 86%), but with similar specificity (81% vs. 77%) [103]. Adenosine and dobutamine stress CMR have similar sensitivity and specificity [104]. Stress CMR showed no difference in diagnostic accuracy when compared to SPECT MPI for CAD detection [105]. The concordance and accuracy of stress CMR with 320-detector row CT, showed an excellent agreement (92%, kappa value = 0.81) in an intermediate risk cohort [106]. Adenosine perfusion was the most accurate component of the stress CMR study in predicting which patients had significant CAD, compared with resting WMA and LGE [107].

Negative findings on stress CMR are reassuring and associated with annualized event rates of 0.4% for MI and 0.3% for cardiovascular death. In patients with inducible ischemia, the annual event rates for MI and cardiovascular death were 2.6% and 2.8%, respectively. The concomitant presence of LGE was associated with a worse prognosis [108]. Other predictors of cardiac events were resting WMA, inducible WMA and LGE. Patients with inducible WMA (i.e., ischemia) experienced significant benefits from revascularization, compared with patients without inducible WMA (i.e., without ischemia) [109].

4.4.4. Strengths and limitations

The strengths and limitations of stress CMR are shown in Table 10.

http://dx.doi.org/10.5772/61502

Strengths	Limitations
Good contrast resolution	Expensive
No radiation exposure	Not widely available
Visualization of subendocardial	Cardiac device/metallic
ischemia and scar	implant
Transmurality	Glomerular filtration rate
of scar	<30 mls/min
Procedural time (~45 minutes)	Allergy to gadolinium
	Breath hold instructions
	Pharmacological stress
	Claustrophobia

Table 10. Strengths and limitations of stress CMR

4.4.5. Case example 8

A 65-year-old man with prior coronary artery bypass surgery presents with chest pain. An adenosine stress CMR was performed. For study interpretation, follow the steps as described in the text starting with LGE, stress and rest images. There is inducible inferior wall perfusion defect with no LGE (Figure 8).

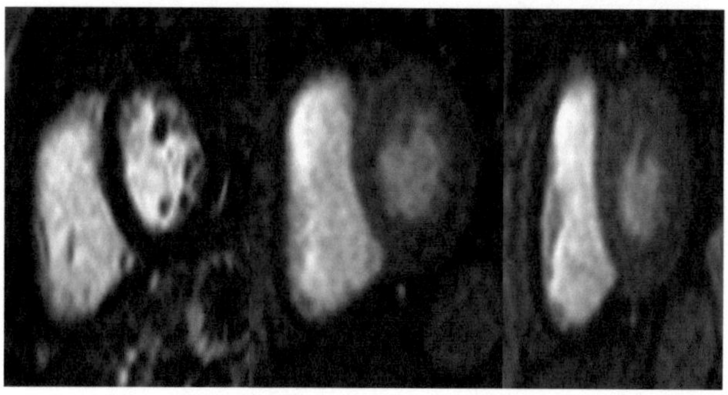

Figure 8. Left to right: 1st image: LV short axis LGE image show no evidence of scar. 2nd image: Stress first pass perfusion image demonstrate an inducible inferior wall perfusion defect. 3rd image: The corresponding rest image demonstrate no perfusion defect in the inferior wall.

4.4.6. Clinical pearls

1. Avoid caffeinated food and beverages, theophylline, and dipyridamole for 24 hours prior to stress CMR.

2. Stress CMR should be avoided in patients with a glomerular filtration rate (GFR) < 30 mls/min.

3. The presence of infarction on LGE (subendocardial or transmural in a coronary artery distribution) favors CAD, irrespective of perfusion findings.

4. Criteria for a perfusion defect is a persistent delay in enhancement pattern during first pass observed in at least 3 consecutive temporal images.

5. Perfusion defects should be graded according to transmurality.

6. Dark-rim artifact typically appear as dark lines at the blood pool-myocardium interface, and can mimic a perfusion defect (typically Gibbs artifact).

We have come to the end of our review on the essentials of noninvasive imaging modalities for the assessment of CAD. A proposed algorithm for test selection in suspected CAD is included (Figure 9). The following are four clinical scenarios commonly encountered in clinical practice and the suggested answers:

1. Would you perform a test in an asymptomatic 35-year-old woman who plans to participate in a marathon next month? She has a normal resting ECG with no cardiovascular risk factor.

Answer: No. Asymptomatic patients generally do not warrant cardiac testing. Her pretest probability of CAD is very low (<5%).

2. What is the next suitable test in a 60-year-old woman with morbid obesity who presents with chest pain? She completed 4 METs and achieved 70% of the maximum age-predicted HR following an exercise ECG.

Answer: Inability to achieve an adequate stress level reduces the sensitivity of an exercise ECG. Her pretest probability of CAD is intermediate. In the presence of morbid obesity, PET MPI or CCTA would be considered a suitable alternative.

3. What test would you perform in a 75-year-old man with a sedentary lifestyle who presents with chest pain on exertion that is relieved with nitroglycerin spray? He has underlying COPD, diabetes, and hypertension. Baseline creatinine is 300 micromol/l.

Answer: Pretest probability for CAD is high (≥90%) and the diagnosis of CAD is not in question. He has stable angina. First step would be to inititate medications such as aspirin, beta-blockers, calcium channel blockers, and statin therapy. Pharmacological SPECT or PET MPI for risk stratification is reasonable. Pharmacological SE can be performed if a good echo window can be obtained. In the presence of moderate ischemic burden, high risk variables on MPI, or worsening of symptom despite on optimal medical therapy, ICA is warranted.

4. Would you repeat another CCTA in a 50-year-old man with an active lifestyle presenting with atypical chest pain? He had a calcium score of 0 and a normal CCTA a year ago.

Answer: No. No testing is required. If symptoms persist, consider an exercise ECG.

http://dx.doi.org/10.5772/61502

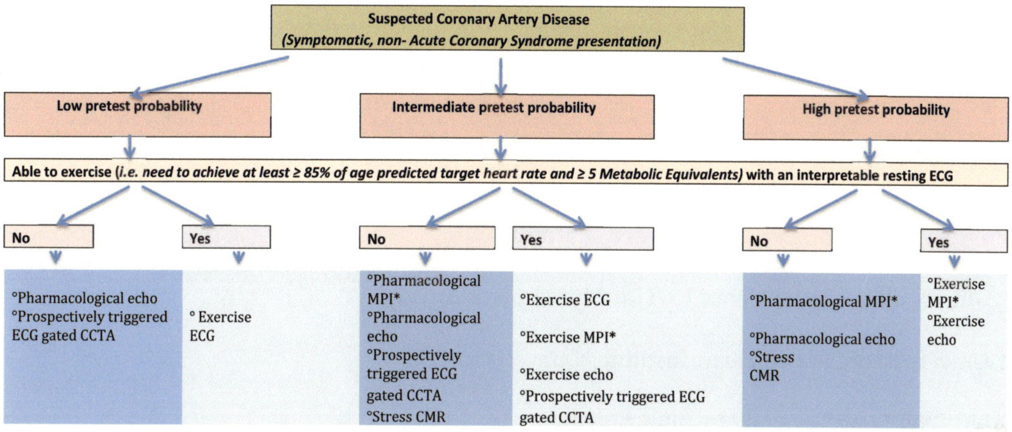

ECG= electrocardiography; CCTA= coronary computed tomography angiography; MPI= myocardial perfusion imaging; CMR= cardiac magnetic resonance; BMI= body mass index. * BMI ≥30 kg/m^2: PET MPI is preferred; BMI <30 kg/m^2: SPECT or PET MPI, depending on resource.

Patients with renal impairment (Creatinine >2.0 mg/dl, avoid CCTA; if GFR <30 mls/min, stress CMR is contraindicated.

For pharmacological MPI, use of low level exercise (1.7 mph, grade 0) is an option, in the absence of LBBB.

Figure 9. Proposed algorithm for test selection in suspected coronary artery disease.

5. Conclusion

Understanding the merits and limitations of each noninvasive imaging modality, together with local expertise and resources, will increase the clinician's confidence in selecting imaging tests for the assessment of CAD. This is crucial to avoid layered testing, unnecessary radiation exposure, and maintain a cost-effective approach. Functional and anatomical noninvasive tests are associated with similar cardiovascular outcomes in patients with low to intermediate risk [110]. The use of stress MPI to serve as a gatekeeper for ICA is well validated [111]. A detailed history and physical examination with sound clinical judgement and the integration of evidence-based guidelines are vital for selecting the right test. In summary, noninvasive tests are the cornerstone of CAD assessment. Although not covered in this chapter, such tests also serve as a guide for ischemia-driven ICA strategies.

6. Conflict of interest

The authors have no conflict of interest to disclose pertaining to the contents of this book chapter.

Acknowledgements

All images used in this chapter were obtained from the University of Ottawa Heart Institute.

Author details

Punitha Arasaratnam[1,2] and Terrence D. Ruddy[1*]

*Address all correspondence to: TRuddy@ottawaheart.ca

1 University of Ottawa Heart Institute, Ottawa, Canada

2 Ng Teng Fong General Hospital, Singapore

References

[1] Shaw L, Marwick T, et al. Why all the focus on cardiac imaging? J Am Coll Cardiol Img. 2010;3(7):789-794.

[2] Wolk, et al. ACCF/AHA/ASE/ASNC/HFSA/HRS/SCAI/ SCCT/ SCMR/ STS, 2013 Multimodality appropriate use criteria for the detection and risk assessment of stable ischemic heart disease. A Report of the American College of Cardiology Foundation Appropriate Use Criteria Task Force, American Heart Association, American Society of Echocardiography, American Society of Nuclear Cardiology, Heart Failure Society of America, Heart Rhythm Society, Society for Cardiovascular Angiography and Interventions, Society of Cardiovascular Computed Tomography, Society for Cardiovascular Magnetic Resonance, and Society of Thoracic Surgeons. JACC 2014; Vol. 63, No. 4, 2014.

[3] Diamond GA. A clinically relevant classification of chest discomfort. J Am Coll Cardiol. 1983;1:574-5.

[4] Weintraub WS, Madeira SW, et al. Critical analysis of the application of Bayes' theorem to sequential testing in the noninvasive diagnosis of coronary artery disease. Am J Cardiol. 1984;54(1):43-9.

[5] Diamond GA, Forrester JS. Analysis of probability as an aid in the clinical diagnosis of coronary artery disease. N Engl J Med. 1979:300:1350-8.

[6] Shaw L, Mieres J, Hendel R, et al. Effectiveness of exercise electrocardiography with or without myocardial perfusion single photon emission computed tomography in women with suspected coronary artery disease. Results form the What Is the Opti-

http://dx.doi.org/10.5772/61502

mal Method for Ischemia Evaluation in Women (WOMEN) trial. Circulation. 2011;124:1239-1249.

[7] Kohli P, Gulati M. Exercise stress testing in women, going back to the basics. Circulation. 2010;122:2570-2580.

[8] Okin PM, Bergman G, Kligfield P. Effect of ST segment measurement point on performance of standard and heart rate-adjusted ST segment criteria for the identification of coronary artery disease. Circulation. 1991;84:57-66.

[9] Fletcher G, Ades P, Kligfield P, et al. Exercise standards for testing and training; A scientific statement from the American Heart Association. Circulation. 2013;128:873-934.

[10] Desai MY, Crugnale S, Mondeau J, Helin K, Mannting F. Slow upsloping ST-segment depression during exercise: Does it really signify a positive stress test? Am Heart J. 2002;143:482-487.

[11] Goldschlager N, Selzer A, Cohn K. Treadmill stress tests as indicators of presence and severity of coronary artery disease. Ann Intern Med. 1976;85:277-286.

[12] Beinart R, Matetzky S, Shechter M, Fefer P, Rozen E, Beinart T, Hod H, Chouraqui P. Stress-induced ST-segment elevation in patients without prior Q-wave myocardial infarction. J Electrocardiol. 2008;41:312-317.

[13] Sullivan ID, Davies DW, Sowton E. Submaximal exercise testing early after myocardial infarction. Difficulty of predicting coronary anatomy and left ventricular performance. Br Heart J. 1985;53:180-185.

[14] Orsini E, Lattanzi F, Reisenhofer B, Tartarini G. Time-domain analysis of exercise-induced ST-segment elevation in Q-wave myocardial infarction: A useful tool for the screening of myocardial viability. Ital Heart J. 2001;2:529-538.

[15] Bruce RA, Kusumi F, Hosmer D. Maximal oxygen intake and nomographic assessment of functional aerobic impairment in cardiovascular disease. Am Heart J. 1973; 85:546-562.

[16] Bourque JM, Holland BH, Watson DD, et al. Achieving an exercise workload of ≥ 10 metabolic equivalents predicts a very low risk of inducible ischemia: Does myocardial perfusion imaging have a role? J Am Coll Cardiol. 2009;54:538-545.

[17] Lauer MS, Francis GS, Okin PM, et al. Impaired chronotropic response to exercise stress testing as a predictor of mortality. JAMA. 1999;281:524-529.

[18] Vivekananthan DP, Blackstone EH, Pothier CE, et. al. Heart rate recovery after exercise is a predictor of mortality, independent of the angiographic severity of coronary disease. J Am Coll Cardiol. 2003;42:83-838.

[19] Sanmarco ME, Pontius S, Selvester RH. Abnormal blood pressure response and marked ischemic ST-segment depression as predictors of severe coronary artery disease. Circulation. 1980;61:572-578.

[20] Mark DB, Shaw L, Harrell FE Jr, et al. Prognostic value of a treadmill exercise score in outpatients with suspected coronary artery disease. N Eng J Med. 1991;325(12): 849-53.

[21] Gianrossi R, Detrano R, Mulvihill D, et al. Exercise-induced ST depression in the diagnosis of coronary artery disease. A meta-analysis. Circulation. 1989;80:87-98.

[22] Gibbons RJ, Balady GJ, Bricker JT, et al. ACC/AHA 2002 guideline update for exercise testing: summary article: A report of the American College of Cardiology/American Heart Association Task Force on Practice Guidelines (Committee to Update the 1997 Exercise Testing Guidelines). Circulation. 2002;106:1883-1892.

[23] Alexander KP, Shaw LJ, Shaw LK, et al. Value of exercise treadmill testing in women. J Am Coll Cardiol. 1998;32:1657-1664.

[24] Mark DB, Hlatky MA, Harrell FE Jr, et al. Exercise treadmill score for predicting prognosis in coronary artery disease. Ann Intern Med. 1987;106(6):793-800.

[25] Ahmed H, Al-Mallah M, McEvoy J, et al. Maximal exercise testing variables and 10-year survival: Fitness risk score derivation from the FIT project. Mayo Clin Proc. 2015;90(3):346-55.

[26] Chang SM, Nabi F, Xu J, et al. Value of CACS compared with ett and myocardial perfusion imaging for predicting long-term cardiac outcome in asymptomatic and symptomatic patients at low risk for coronary disease: Clinical implications in a multimodality imaging world. J Am Coll Cardiol Img. 2015;8(2):134-44.

[27] Klocke FJ, Baird MG, et al. ACC/AHA/ASNC guidelines for the clinical use of cardiac radionuclide imaging- executive summary: A report of the American College of Cardiology/ American Heart Association Task Force on practice guidelines (ACC/AHA/ ASNC Committee to revise the 1995 guidelines for the clinical use of cardiac radionuclide imaging). J Am Coll Cardiol. 2003;42:1318-33.

[28] Patton J, Sandler M, et al. D-SPECT: A new solid state camera for high speed molecular imaging. J Nucl Med. 2006;47:189.

[29] Patton J, Slomka PJ, et al. Recent technologic advances in nuclear cardiology. J Nucl Cardiol. 2007;14:501-13.

[30] Marcassa C, Campini R, et al. Wide beam reconstruction for half-dose or half-time gated SPECT acquisitions: Optimization of resources and reduction in radiation exposure. Eur J Nucl Med Mol Imaging. 2011;38:499-508.

[31] Envoldsen LH, Menashi CAK, et al. Effects of acquisition time and reconstruction algorithm on image quality, quantitative parameters, and clinical interpretation of myocardial perfusion imaging. J Nucl Cardiol 2013. doi:10.1007/s12350-013-97752.

[32] Patil H, Bateman T, et al. Diagnostic accuracy of high-resolution attenuation-corrected Anger camera SPECT in the detection of coronary artery disease. J Nucl Cardiol. 2014;21:127-34.

[33] Henzlova M, Cerqueira M, Christopher L, et al. Stress protocols and tracer. ASNC imaging guidelines for nuclear cardiology procedures. J Nucl Cardiol. 2010;17:646-54.

[34] Loscalzo J, Vita JA. Ischemia, hyperemia, exercise, and nitric oxide: Complex physiology and complex molecular adaptations. Circulation. 1994;90:2556-2559.

[35] Leppo JA. Comparison of pharmacologic stress agents. J Nucl Cardiol. 1996;3:S22-S26.

[36] Thomas GS, Tammelin BR, Schiffman GL, et al. Safety of regadenoson, a selective adenosine A2A agonist, in patients with chronic obstructive pulmonary disease: A randomized, double-blind, placebo-controlled trial (RegCOPD trial). J Nucl Cardiol. 2008 May-Jun;15(3):319-28.

[37] Prenner BM, Bukofzer S, Behm S, et al. A randomized, double-blind, placebo-controlled study assessing the safety and tolerability of regadenoson in subjects with asthma or chronic obstructive pulmonary disease. J Nucl Cardiol. 2012 Aug;19(4):681-92.

[38] Beller G, Zaret B. Contribution of nuclear cardiology to the diagnosis and prognosis of coronary artery disease. Circulation. 2000;101:1465-1478.

[39] Begg CB, Greenes RA. Assessment of diagnostic tests when disease verification is subject to selection bias. Biometrics. 1983;39:207-15.

[40] Iskandrian AE. Exercise MPI. In: Iskandrian AE, Verani MS, eds. Nuclear Cardiac Imaging: Principles and Applications, 3rd ed. New York; Oxford University Press, 2003 pp. 151-163.

[41] Klocke FJ, Baird MG, Lorell BH, et al. ACC/AHA/ASNC guidelines for the clinical use of cardiac radionuclide imaging–executive summary: A report of the American College of Cardiology/American Heart Association Task Force on Practice Guidelines (ACC/AHA/ASNC Committee to Revise the 1995 Guidelines for the Clinical Use of Cardiac Radionuclide Imaging). Circulation. 2003;108:1404 -1418.

[42] Duvall WL, Guma KA, Kamen J, Croft LB, Parides M, George T, et al. Reduction in occupational and patient radiation exposure from myocardial perfusion imaging: impact of stress-only imaging and high-efficiency SPECT camera technology. J Nucl Med. 2013 Aug;54(8):1251-7.

[43] Chang SM, Nabi F, Xu J, Raza U, Mahmarian JJ. Normal stress only versus standard stress/rest myocardial perfusion imaging: Similar patient mortality with reduced radiation exposure. J Am Coll Cardiol. 2010 Jan 19;55(3):221-30.

[44] Duvall WL, Wijetunga MN, Klein TM, Razzouk L, Godbold J, Croft LB, et al. The prognosis of a normal stress-only Tc-99m myocardial perfusion imaging study. J Nucl Cardiol. 2010 Jun;17(3):370-7.

[45] Shaw LJ, Hendel R, Borges-Neto S, et al. Prognostic value of normal exercise and adenosine (99m)Tc-tetrofosmin SPECT imaging: Results from the multicenter registry of 4,728 patients. J Nucl Med. 2003 Feb;44(2):134-9.

[46] Shaw LJ, Iskandrian AE. Prognostic value of gated myocardial perfusion SPECT. J Nucl Cardiol. 2004;11:171-185.

[47] Acampa W, Petretta M, et al. Warranty period of normal stress myocardial perfusion imaging in diabetic patients: A propensity score analysis. J Nucl Cardiol. 2014;21:50-6.

[48] Hachamovitch R, Berman DS, Kiat H, et al. Exercise myocardial perfusion SPECT in patients without known coronary artery disease: Incremental prognostic value and use in risk stratification. Circulation. 1996;93:905-914.

[49] Arasaratnam P, Ayoub C, et al. Positron emission tomography myocardial perfusion imaging for diagnosis and risk stratification in obese patients. Curr Cardiovasc Imaging Re. 2015;8:9304.

[50] Lim SP, Arasaratnam P, et al. Obesity and the challenges of noninvasive imaging for the detection of coronary artery disease. Canadian Journal of Cardiology. 2015;31:223-226.

[51] Machac J. Cardiac positron emission tomography imaging. Sem Nucl Med. 2005;35:17-36.

[52] Machac J, Bacharach S, et al. Quality assurance committee of the american society of nuclear cardiology. Positron emission tomography myocardial perfusion and glucose metabolism imaging. J Nucl Cardiol. 2006;13:e121-51.

[53] Dilsizian V, Bacharach S, Beanlands R, et al. PET myocardial perfusion and metabolism clinical imaging. J Nucl Cardiol. 2009;16:651.

[54] Baggish AL, Boucher CA. Radiopharmaceutical agents for myocardial perfusion imaging. Circulation. 2008;118:1668-1674.

[55] Parker M, Iskander A, et al. Diagnostic accuracy of cardiac positron emission tomography versus single photon emission computed tomography for coronary artery disease, a bivariate meta-analysis. Circ Cardiovasc Imaging. 2012;5:700-707.

[56] McArdle B, Dowsley T, et al. Does Rubidium-82 PET have superior accuracy to SPECT perfusion imaging for the diagnosis of obstructive coronary artery disease? A systematic review and met-analysis. J Am Coll Cardiol. 2012;60(18):1828-1837.

[57] Jaarsma C, Leiner T, et al. Diagnostic performance of noninvasive myocardial perfusion imaging using single-photon emission computed tomography, cardiac magnetic resonance, and positron emission tomography imaging for the detection of obstructive coronary artery disease: A meta-analysis. J Am Coll Cardiol. 2012;59:1719-28.

[58] Yoshinaga K, Chow BJ, Williams K, et al. What is the prognostic value of myocardial perfusion imaging using rubidium-82 positron emission tomography? J Am Coll Cardiol. 2006;48:1029-39.

[59] Dorbala S, Hachamovitch R, Curillova Z, et al. Incremental prognostic value of gated Rb-82 positron emission tomography myocardial perfusion imaging over clinical variables and rest LVEF. JACC Cardiovasc Imaging. 2009;2:846-54.

[60] Hachamovitch R, Hayes SW, Friedman JD, et al. Comparison of the short-term survival benefit associated with revascularization compared with medical therapies in patients with no prior coronary artery disease undergoing stress myocardial perfusion single photon emission computed tomography. Circulation. 2003;107:2900-2907.

[61] Naya M, Murthy V, et al. Prognostic interplay of coronary artery calcification and underlying vascular dysfunction in patients with suspected coronary artery disease. J Am Coll Cardiol. 2013;61:2098-106.

[62] Franke A, Hoffman R, Kuhl H. Non-contrast second harmonic imaging improves interobserver agreement and accuracy of dobutamine stress echocardiography in patients with impaired image quality. Heart. 2000;83:133-40.

[63] Sozi F, Poldermans D, Bax J. Second harmonic imaging improves sensitivity of dobutamine stress echocardiography for the diagnosis of coronary artery disease. Am Heart J. 2001;142:153-9.

[64] Kasprzak JD, Paelinck B, Ten Cate FJ, et al. Comparison of native and contrast-enhanced harmonic echocardiography for visualization of left ventricular endocardial border. Am J Cardiol. 1999;83:211-217.

[65] Pellikka P, Nagueh S, Elhendy A, et al. American Society of Echocardiography Recommendations for Performance, Interpretation, and Application of Stress Echocardiography. J Am Soc Echocardiogr. 2007;20(9):1021-41.

[66] Sicari R, Nihoyannopoulos P, Evangeslista A, et al. Stress echocardiography expert consensus statement-executive summary: European Association of Echocardiography (EAE) (a registered branch of the ESC). Eur Heart Journal. 2009;30(3):278-89.

[67] Fox K, Garcia MA, Ardissino D, et al. Task Force on the Management of Stable Angina Pectoris of the European Society of Cardiology; ESC Committee for Practice Guidelines (CPG): Guidelines on the management of stable angina pectoris: Execu-

tive summary: The Task Force on the Management of Stable Angina Pectoris of the European Society of Cardiology. Eur Heart J. 2006;27:1341-81.

[68] Bjork Ingul C, Rozis E, Slordahl SA, et.al. Incremental value of strain rate imaging to wall motion analysis for prediction of outcome in patients undergoing dobutamine stress echocardiography. Circulation. 2007;115:1252-9.

[69] Ingul CB, Stoylen A, Slodahl SA, et al. Automated analysis of myocardial deformation at dobutamine stress echocardiography: An angiographic validation. J Am Coll Cardiol. 2007;49:1651-9.

[70] Nagy AI, Sahlen A, Manouras A, et al. Combination of constrast-enhanced wall motion analysis and myocardial deformation imaging using dobutamine stress echocardiography. Eur Heart J. 2015;16:88-95.

[71] Beleslin BD, Osojic M, Djordjevic-Dikie A, et al. Integrated evaluation of relation between coronary lesion features and stress echocardiography results: The importance of coronary lesion morphology. J Am Coll Cardiol. 1999;33:717-26.

[72] Marwick TH. Stress echocardiography. Heart. 2003;89:113-8.

[73] Picano E, Bedetti G, Varga A, et al. The comparable diagnostic accuracies of dobutamine stress and dipyridamole-stress echocardiographies: a meta-analysis. Coron Artery Dis. 2000;11:151e9.

[74] Ho FM, Huang PJ, Liau CS, et al. Dobutamine stress echocardiography compared with dipyridamole thallium-201 single-photon emission computed tomography in detecting coronary artery disease. Eur Heart J. 1995;16:570e5.

[75] Mahajan N, Polavaram N, Vankalaya et al. Diagnostic accuracy of myocardial perfusion imaging and stress echocardiography for the diagnosis of left main and triple vessel coronary artery disease: A comparative meta-analysis. Heart. 2010;96:956-966.

[76] Innocenti F, Lazzeretti D, Conti A, et al. Stress echocardiography in the ED: Diagnostic performance in high-risk subgroups. Am J Emerg Med. 2013;31:1309-1314.

[77] Metz LD, Beattie M, Hom R, et al. The prognostic value of normal exercise myocardial perfusion imaging and exercise echocardiography: A meta- analysis. J Am Coll Cardiol. 2007;49(2):227-37.

[78] Arruda-Olson AM, Juracan EM, Mahoney DW, et al. Prognostic value of exercise echocardiography in 5, 798 patients: Is there a gender difference: J Am Coll Cardiol. 2002;39(4):625-31.

[79] Schroder K, Wieckhorst A, Voller H. Comparison of the prognostic value of dipyridamole and dobutamine stress echocardiography in patients with known or suspected coronary artery disease. Am J Cardiol. 1997;79:1516-8.

[80] Pingitore A, Picano E, Varga A, et al. Prognostic value of pharmacological stress echocardiography in patients with known or suspected coronary artery disease: A

prospective, large-scale, multicenter, head-to-head comparison between dipyridamole and dobutamine test. Echo-Per- santine International Cooperative (EPIC) and Echo- Dobutamine International Cooperative (EDIC) Study Groups. J Am Coll Cardiol. 1999;34:1769-7.

[81] McCully Rb, Roger VL, Mahoney DW, et al. Outcome after abnormal exercise echocardiography for patients with good exercise capacity: Prognostic importance of the extent and severity of exercise related left ventricular dysfunction. J Am Coll Cardiol. 2002;39(8):1345-52.

[82] Flohr TG, Stierstorfer K, Ulzheimer S, et al. Image reconstruction and image quality evaluation for a 64-slice CT scanner with z-flying focal spot. Med Phys. 2005 Aug; 32(8):2536-47.

[83] Achenbach S, Raggi P. Imaging of coronary atherosclerosis by computed tomography. Eur H Journal. 2010;31:1442-48.

[84] Flohr TG, Mc Collough CH, Bruder H, et al. First performance evaluation of a dual-source CT (DSCT) system. Eur Radiol. 2006;16:256-268.

[85] Tsukagoshi S, Ota T, Fujii M, et al. Improvement of spatial resolution in the longitudinal direction for isotropic imaging in helical CT. Phys Med Biol. 2007:52(3):791-801.

[86] Arbab Zadeh A, Hoe J. Multidetector CT angiography in comparison with conventional angiography. Methods, caveats and implications. J Am Coll Cardiol Imag. 2011:4(2):191-202.

[87] Taylor A, Cerqueira M, Hodgson J, et al. ACCF/SCCT/ACR /AHA /ASE / ASNC/ NASCI/SCAI/SCMR 2010 Appropriate Use Criteria for Cardiac Computed Tomography. A Report of the American College of Cardiology Foundation Appropriate Use Criteria Task Force, the Society of Cardiovascular Computed Tomography, the American College of Radiology, the American Heart Association, the American Society of Echocardiography, the American Society of Nuclear Cardiology, the North American Society for Cardiovascular Imaging, the Society for Cardiovascular Angiography and Interventions, and the Society for Cardiovascular Magnetic Resonance. J Am Coll Cardiol. 2010;56(22):1864-1894.

[88] Budoff M, Dowe D, Jollis J, et al. Diagnostic performance of 64-multidetector row coronary computed tomographic angiography for evaluation of coronary artery stenosis in individuals without known coronary artery disease-results from the prospective multicenter accuracy (Assessment by Coronary Computed Tomographic Angiography of Individuals Undergoing Invasive Coronary Angiography) trial. J Am Coll Cardiol. 2008;52:1724-32.

[89] Meijboom WB, Meighem CA, Mollete NR, et al. 64-slice computed tomography coronary angiography in patients with high, intermediate, or low pretest probability of significant coronary artery disease. J Am Coll Cardiol. 2007;50:1469-75.

[90] Litt HI, Gatsonis C, Snyder B, et al. CT angiography for safe discharge of patients with possible acute coronary syndromes. N Engl J Med. 2012;366:1393-403.

[91] Hoffmann U, Truong QA, Schoenfeld DA, et al. Coronary CT angiography versus standard evaluation in acute chest pain. N Engl J Med. 2012;367:299-308.

[92] Goldstein JA, Chinnaiyan KM, Abidov A, et al. The CT-STAT (coronary computed tomographic angiography for systematic triage of acute chest pain patients to treatment) trial. J Am Coll Cardiol. 2011;58:1414-22.

[93] Chow BJ, Small G, Yam Y, et al. Incremental prognostic value of cardiac computed tomography in coronary artery disease using CONFIRM: COroNary computed tomography angiography evaluation for clinical outcomes: an InteRnational Multicenter registry. Circ Cardiovasc Imaging. 2011;4:463-72.

[94] Habib PJ, Green J, Butterfield RCA, et al. Association of cardiac events with coronary artery disease detected by 64-slice or greater coronary CT angiography: A systematic review and meta-analysis. Int J Cardiol. 2013; 169:112-120.

[95] Ostrom MP, Gopal A, Ahmadi N, et al. Mortality incidence and the severity of coronary atherosclerosis assessed by computed tomography angiography. J Am Coll Cardiol. 2008;52:1335-43.

[96] Detrano R, Guerci AD, Carr JJ, et al. Coronary calcium as a predictor of coronary events in four racial or ethnic groups. N Engl J Med. 2008;358:1336-1345.

[97] P. Greenland, J. S. Alpert, G. A. Beller, et al. ACCF/AHA guideline for assessment of cardiovascular risk in asymptomatic adults: A report of the American College of Cardiology Foundation/American Heart Association task force on practice guidelines. Circulation. 2010;122:584-636.

[98] Shehata ML, Basha TA, Hayeri MR, et al. MR myocardial perfusion imaging: Insights on techniques, analysis, interpretation, and findings. RadioGraphics. 2014;34:1636-57.

[99] Kim HW, Klem I, Kim R. Detection of myocardial ischemia by stress perfusion cardiovascular magnetic resonance. Cardiol Clin. 2007:25:57-70.

[100] Nagel E, Klein C, Paetsch I, et al. Magnetic resonance perfusion measurements for the noninvasive detection of CAD. Circulation. 2003;108:432-437.

[101] Cury RC, Cattani CA, Gabure LA, et al. Diagnostic performance of stress perfusion and delayed enhancement MR imaging in patients with coronary artery disease. Radiology. 2006;240:39-45.

[102] Kramer C, Barkhausen J, Flamm S, et al. Standardized cardiovascular magnetic resonance imaging (CMR) protocols, society for cardiovascular magnetic resonance: Board of trustees task force on standardized protocols. J Cardiovasc Magn Resonance. 2008;10:35. doi:10.1186/1532-429X-10-35.

[103] Hamon M, Fau G, Nee G, et al. Meta-analysis of the diagnostic performance of stress perfusion cardiovascular magnetic resonance for detection of coronary artery disease. J Cardiovasc Magn Reson. 2010;12:29.

[104] Manka R, Jahnke C, Gebker R, et al. Head-to-head comparison of first-pass MR perfusion imaging during adenosine and high-dose dobutamine/atropine stress. Int J Cardiovasc Imaging, 2011;27:995-1002.

[105] Schwitter J, Wacker C, van Rossum A, et al. MR-IMPACT: Comparison of perfusion-cardiac magnetic resonance with single-photon emission computed tomography for the detection of coronary artery disease in a multicenter, multivendor, randomized trial. Eur Heart J. 2008;29:480-489.

[106] Chen M, Bandettini W, Shanbhag S, et al. Concordance and diagnostic accuracy of vasodilator stress cardiac MRI and 320-detector row coronary CTA. Int J Cardiovasc Imaging. 2014;30:109-119.

[107] Ingkanisorn W, Kwong R, Bohme N, et al. Prognosis of negative adenosine stress magnetic resonance in patients presenting to an emergency department with chest pain. J Am Coll Cardiol. 2006;47:1427-32.

[108] Lipinski M, McVey C, Berger J, et al. Prognostic value of stress cardiac magnetic resonance imaging in patients with known or suspected coronary artery disease. A Systematic review and meta-analysis. J Am Coll Cardiol. 2013;62:826-38.

[109] Kelle S, Nagel E, Voss A, et al. A bi-center cardiovascular magnetic resonance prognosis study focusing on dobutamine wall motion and late gadolinium enhancement in 3, 138 consecutive patients. J Am Coll Cardiol. 2013;61:2310-12.

[110] Douglas P, Hoffmann U, Patel M, et al. Outcomes of anatomical versus functional testing for coronary artery disease. N Engl J Med. 2015;10.1056/NEJMoa1415516.

[111] Takx R, Blomberg B, Aidi H, et al. Diagnostic accuracy of stres myocardial perfusion imaging to invasive coronary angiography with fractional flow reserve meta-analysis. Circ Cardiovasc Imaging. 2015;8:e002666. doi:10:1161/CIRCIMAGING.114.002666.

Chapter 3

Non-Invasive Imaging of Coronary Artery Disease — The Expanding Role of Coronary Computed Tomographic Angiography in the Management of Low- to Intermediate-Risk Patients and Dealing with Intermediate Stenosis

Michael Campbell, Stephen Lyen, Jonathan Rodrigues, Mark Hamilton and Nathan Manghat

Additional information is available at the end of the chapter

http://dx.doi.org/10.5772/61837

Abstract

Non-invasive anatomic imaging modalities play a crucial role in the diagnosis of coronary artery disease (CAD), particularly in the case of the symptomatic patient presenting in the emergency department.

Some of the key issues of discussion will be the appropriate use of coronary computed tomography (CT) in the anatomical assessment of CAD, the prognostic information that this assessment holds and how the role of CT may evolve in the coming years.

The aim of this chapter is to summarise and evaluate the current best non-invasive anatomical strategies of CAD imaging, notably in those with a low to intermediate pre-test risk of CAD and those with an intermediate luminal stenosis.

Keywords: Coronary artery disease, computed tomography, imaging, intermediate stenosis

1. Introduction

The British physician William Harvey described the heart as, "the household of Divinity which, discharging its function, nourishes, cherishes, quickens the whole book and is indeed the foundation of life."[1] In Harvey's words, together with his wider body of work, he encapsulates three simple truths; it is the heart's role to pump the blood that it is the role of the blood vessels to circulate the blood and it is the blood that sustains living tissue. These assertions may seem obvious, but they are just as pertinent now as when they were first penned in the 17th century. The reason for this is clear, the leading cause of mortality in the developed world is coronary artery disease(CAD). CAD is a narrowing of the lumen of the arteries that supply blood to the heart resulting in a 'failure' of the circulation to deliver blood to the heart.[2] Modern medical imaging allows the physician to accurately assess the extent to which the coronary arteries are narrowed (anatomical imaging), and to what extent this narrowing results in a 'failure' to circulate the blood (functional imaging).

It is an undisputed fact that the current best method for imaging the burden of CAD is invasive coronary angiography (ICA). This fact is reflected in its ubiquitous use in clinical practice today; figures from 2004 show that 201,000 of these procedures were undertaken in the United Kingdom, an increase of 7% from the previous year. Whilst the risks may be small – a mortality of 0.07% and a radiation exposure risk lower than other imaging procedures [3] – it would not be safe, practical or cost effective to offer every patient with symptoms of CAD to ICA. Furthermore, up to 40% of the patients who do go on to have elective ICA are found to have sub-clinical stenosis in all coronary arteries.[4,5] This highlights the inadequate and inaccurate information provided by orthodox first-/second-line investigations in the assessment of symptomatic patients with suspected CAD.

There is an increasing body of evidence which suggests that non-invasive anatomical imaging modalities have a crucial role to play in the diagnosis of CAD, particularly, in the case of the symptomatic patient presenting in the emergency department. That is, not to say that non-invasive imaging will completely supplant ICA, but it may, and in some instances already has been proven to be clinically useful in the right patient group, at the right stage of the patient pathway [6, 7, 8]. One such promising imaging modality, which will be evaluated in explicit detail in the course of this review, is CT. Some of the key issues of discussion will be the appropriate use in anatomic assessment of CAD, the prognostic information that this assessment holds and how the role of CT may evolve in the coming years.

The aim of this chapter is to summarise and evaluate the current best non-invasive anatomical strategies of imaging CAD. The main focus will be to unveil the best to approach the two less well understood (and sometimes overlapping) cohorts of CAD symptomatic patients: those with a low to intermediate pre-test risk (10–29%) of CAD and those with CAD, who have an intermediate amount of luminal stenosis (40–69% of the luminal cross-sectional area).

2. What is CAD? Blood haemodynamics and myocardial demand

Coronary artery disease has one main consequence: it limits blood flow to the myocardium. When this happens, CAD can cause an imbalance between the myocardial oxygen demand and the rate of delivery of oxygen by the blood, leading to tissue hypoxia. The overall process is a broad spectrum of conditions known as ischaemic heart disease. In 1772, when William Heberden described an 'uncomfortable sensation' while walking and called it angina, he was describing a manifestation of ischaemic heart disease (Figures 1 and 2).[2]

- The flow of the blood to heart is summarised by Darcy's law: *flow=pressure/resistance* [9]
- In coronary artery disease (CAD) the reduction in flow is as a result of an increase in resistance.
- The resistance in blood vessels is frequently described by a mathematical law called Poiseuille's law.
- Poiseuille's law demonstrates that the resistance to a fluid flowing through a tube, assuming laminar flow, is inversely proportional to the radius to the power of four. [2][1]
- However, the relationship between the amount of vessel occlusion, resistance and flow, is a great deal more complicated than this when applied to CAD.
- It is of paramount importance that a more nuanced physiological account of blood hemodynamics in CAD is understood when interpreting imaging of suspect lesions.

Figure 1. Darcy's law and Poiseuille's law

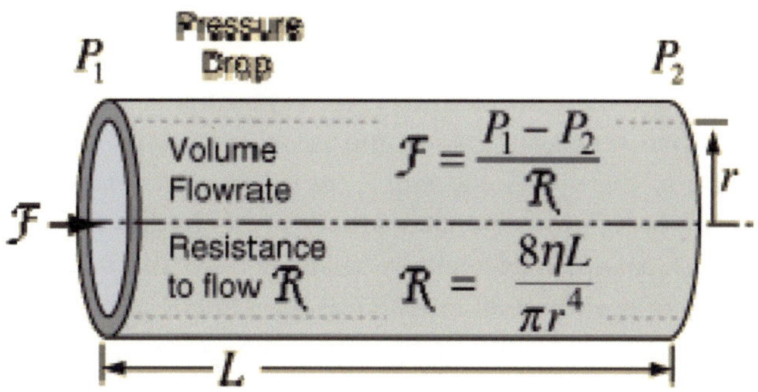

Figure 2. Schematic representation to show Darcy's law (volume flow rate) and Poiseuille's law (resistance to flow) in a rigid tube, assuming laminar flow. *adapted without permission*[42]

The situation presented by traditional thinking, derived from animal experimental models in the 1970s, is that CAD is not deemed to be flow limiting at all, when 60% of the lumen cross-sectional area is occluded and is only deemed to be obstructive to flow during stress when 70% of the luminal cross-sectional area is blocked (Figure 3).[10] The relationship between the percentage of obstruction and flow forms the basis for much of the findings in anatomical imaging, such as CT coronary angiography (CTCA). For example, it is a well-reported fact that sub-clinical stenosis (<50%). CAD is associated with a very low myocardial infarction event rate.[7]

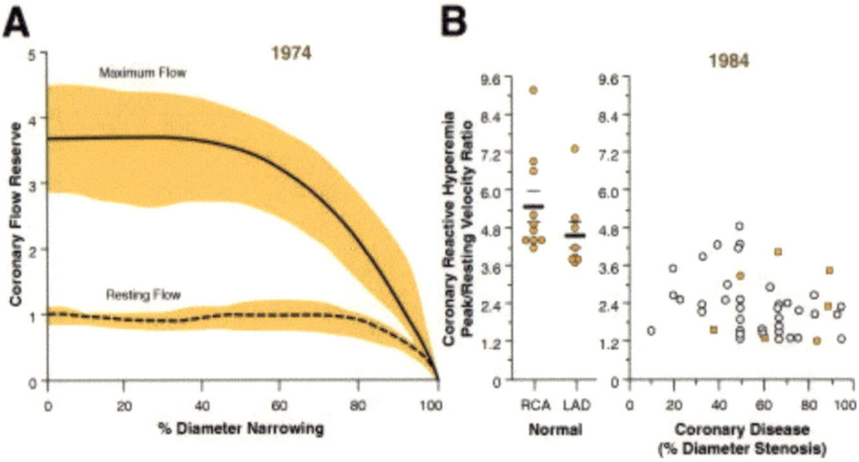

Figure 3. A graph derived from animal experiments in the 1970s, showing the relationship between the amount of vessel occlusion and flow at rest and during stress. It can be seen that flow is affected at a lower threshold of diameter narrowing during exercise than during stress. This was originally cited as the cause of angina described by Heberden in the 18th century. However, it is now known that the relationship between percentage of vessel narrowing and coronary flow is a more complicated process than this experiment implied [10] *graph adapted without permission*

The problem with the traditional thinking and the experimental models, from which it was derived, is that the animal experiments were done on healthy coronary arteries, which were externally compressed at one point along the coronary artery. Equating the flow demonstrated in an externally compressed coronary artery to that in an equally stenosed, diseased coronary is wrong for two main reasons. Firstly, the pathophysiological process that causes CAD does far more than physically 'block' the vessel. Secondly, CAD can exist 'diffusely' along a great portion of the vessel and still have profound haemodynamic consequences. For example, one can use ICA to demonstrate that diffuse disease with narrowing as little as 38% can cause as much as a 65% decrease in coronary flow reserve (Figure 4). The implications of this for imaging are clear; an anatomical assessment of coronary artery stenosis is useful information, however, this test alone cannot comprehensively assess the extent or be the best approach to tackle CAD.[11]

3. Atherosclerosis (Figures 5–7)

As highlighted earlier, CAD results in a narrowing of the coronary arteries. The narrowing of these coronary arteries can cause a limitation of blood flow and therefore oxygen supply

http://dx.doi.org/10.5772/61837

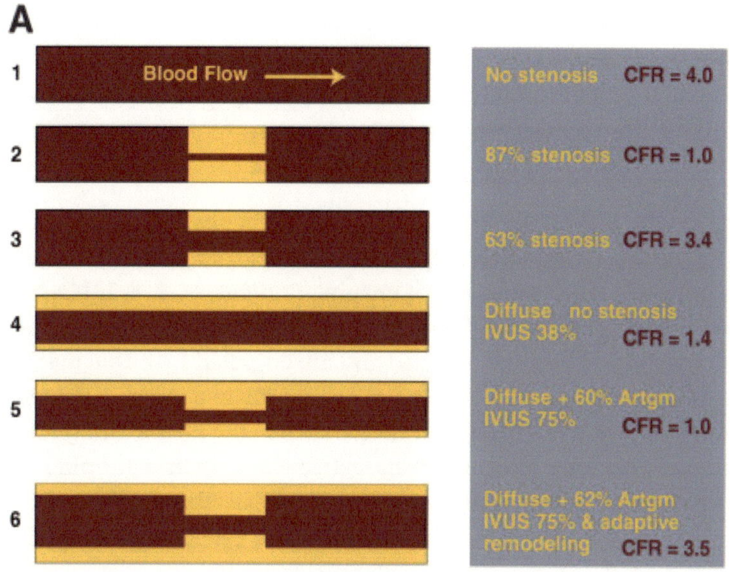

Figure 4. A schematic representation that illustrates the limitations of anatomic imaging by Artgm (arteriogram) and IVUS (intravascular ultrasound) during invasive coronary angiography. The recorded value of blood flow, measured by CFR, is severely at odds with the findings using only anatomic measurements. *Adapted without permission*[11]

(ischaemia) to the myocardium. The cause of this 'narrowing' is a poorly understood chronic inflammatory process called atherosclerosis.[2]. Atherosclerosis, literally meaning 'hard gruel', is a more complicated process than the development of an atherosclerotic plaque, which thickens the vessel wall, intruding and obstructing the vessel lumen. The reason for this atherosclerosis is that the healthy coronary artery cannot be thought of as simply an inert tube through which blood flows. [2, 9] In fact, the healthy artery must be thought of as three layers of differing function: the tunica intima, tunica media and tunica adventitia.

The intima must be recognised as more than simply a mechanical barrier which encloses the blood; it is involved in metabolism, signalling and through a combination of both, and it plays a crucial role in haemodynamics of blood flow. The way it does this is twofold:

1. The intima plays a role in producing anti-thrombotic molecules, lowering the tendency of blood to clot, therefore lowering its viscosity and the resistance to flow.

2. The intima produces signalling molecules, which alters the contractility on smooth muscle cells and therefore controls the size of the coronary artery lumen. In health, the intima triggers vasodilatation of the arterial lumen during exercise and therefore increases the myocardial blood flow to meet the demand.

During the process of atherosclerosis, for reasons beyond the scope of this chapter, the intima lining cells fail to perform their normal role in regulating the flow of blood at a local level. As a result, endothelial cell dysfunction arising from atherosclerosis causes both inappropriate vasoconstriction and loss of normal anti-thrombotic properties (thus increasing blood viscosity).[2] This is relevant to imaging because the relationship between how much of the luminal cross-sectional area of a coronary artery is occluded is not always directly proportional to flow limitation. Therefore, imaging modalities that merely acquire anatomical information cannot provide haemodynamic information specific to the individual.

Another reason why a good understanding of the pathophysiology of atherosclerosis is important is because the composition of the atherosclerotic plaque itself is having an incremental role in interpreting the significance of imaging findings. [4, 7, 8, 12] During the process of atherosclerosis, 'bad' cholesterol, low-density lipoproteins, accumulate under the intimal wall; these lipids quickly become oxidised and are engulfed by tissue macrophages forming 'foam cells'. Another thing that happens, not necessarily in a sequential order, is that smooth muscle cells are moved away from their native sites in the media and these migrate into the intima. These smooth muscle cells secrete extracellular matrix forming a fibrous plaque, which often have high calcium concentrations.[2] Misleadingly, this calcium does not always concentrate at the site of maximal stenosis and calcified plaque only represents approximately 20% of the total coronary atherosclerotic burden. Therefore, calcium can be considered a good marker of CAD and its absence is an excellent marker of no CAD [13], but it cannot diagnose obstructive CAD. [6] [12] The relative proportions of fibrous tissue to lipid also determine the vulnerability of the plaque to rupture. This is crucial in risk stratification when assessing CAD.

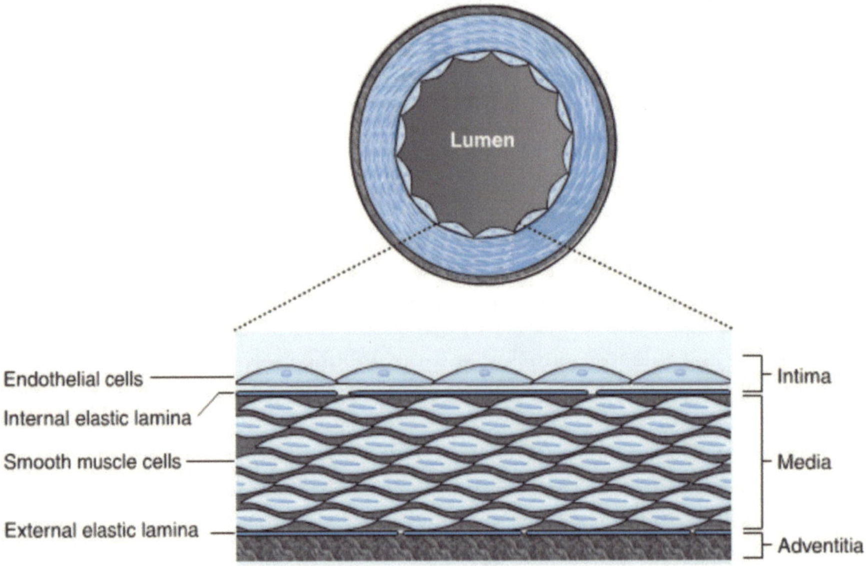

Figure 5. The three layers of artery wall: tunica intima, media and adventitia. The media contains smooth muscle cells. During the process of atherosclerosis, these can migrate into the intima and elaborate fibrous ECM. The adventitia is composed of connective tissue, nerves and lymph. *adapted without permission*[2]

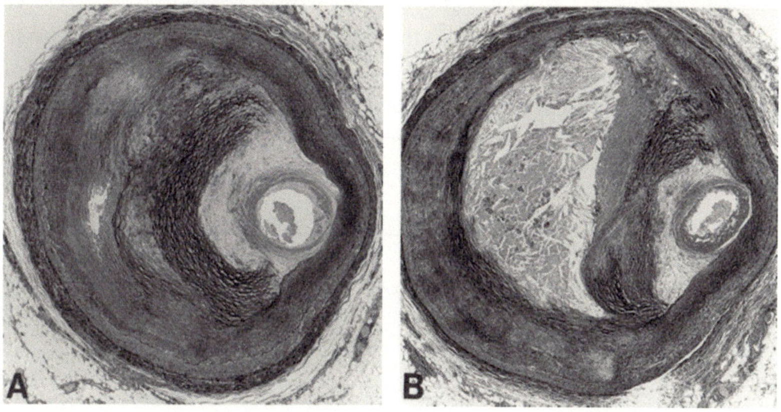

Figure 6. A micrograph showing that atherosclerotic plaques are not homogeneous in their composition. The figure illustrates two stenotic plaques of differing morphology a) plaque consisting of hard, collagen rich sclerotic tissue b) A plaque many comprised lipid-rich atheromatous core, separated from the vessel lumen by a thin fibrous cap. *Adapted without permission*[45]

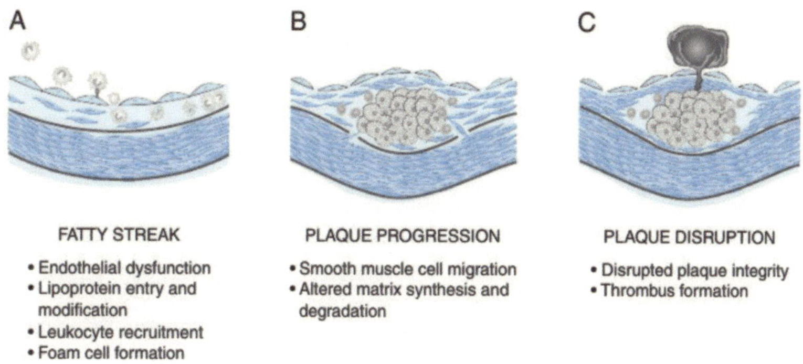

Figure 7. Schematic showing the pathological development of Atherosclerosis and the factors that contribute during each phase. One of the key aims going forward in anatomic imaging is to identify plaques which are at high risk of rupture as seen in C *adapted without permission*[2]

4. Anatomic imaging: The evolving role of coronary CT in the management of chest pain (Figures 8–12)

CT has come a long way since the first clinical scans in 1971. It is now estimated that over 4 million scans are performed annually in the UK and one of the recent successful applications of CT has been the emergence of CT coronary angiography (CTCA) in the management of chest pain.[4] A moving object, such as the heart, was thought impossible to image by CT as the discrete nature of the imaging process meant early scanners had poor temporal resolution. However, with the advancement in CT technology, particularly the development of greater number of detector row and more rapid gantry rotation, CT can now accurately evaluate structures in constant motion like the heart and coronary arteries due to its superior spatial and temporal resolution. [4, 14] CTCA involves visualising the coronary arteries directly with sub-millimetre isotropic spatial resolution and using this anatomic information on stenosis severity to determine the true extent of CAD.

- CT became possible in 1917 when the mathematician, J.H. Radon proved that the 2D distribution of an object can be determined exactly, if the integral values along any number of lines passing through the same layer are known.
- It was realised that the same principle was true of 3D objects.
- The practical implications of this in medicine were not realised until the English engineer, Hounsfield showed that by measuring attenuation x-rays fired from different angles in a plane perpendicular to the scanning subject (although theoretically any arbitrary plane can be used) one can gather the line integrals necessary to reconstruct an image in 3D.
- He called this technique CT.
- CT visualises the body as composed of a series of finite slices.
- Modern CT scanners use multiple x-ray beam collimators, which convert the x-ray beam into a 'fan' beam, covering the individual body section or slice.
- Multiple detectors measure the difference between the known primary intensity of the x-ray sheets and their attenuated intensity having passed through different tissues. [14]
- X-ray beam generators and detectors spin 360 degrees around the scanning subject collecting many thousands of attenuation intensities from different angles within the same plane.
- These attenuation intensities are used to create a discrete number of cubic volume elements or voxel. Each individual voxel is described by its individual CT number or Hounsfield unit.
- [15] The intensity of radiation recorded at all the detectors during the scan is equal to the integration of all the CT numbers of the voxels.
- This is called the ray sums. The ray sums can be solved simultaneously to obtain the co-ordinates of each voxel in three dimensions and pair it to its exact attenuation properties, thus eliminating the superimposition that occurs in conventional radiography.
- Each individual voxel is then combined to produce a thin sliced, three-dimensional image.

Figure 8. A brief summary of the Physics of CT

$$HU = 1000 \times \frac{\mu_X - \mu_{water}}{\mu_{water}}$$

Figure 9. CT number (Hounsfield) equation – the equation used to calculate the voxel intensity

5. A Mandate for CTCA (Figure 13)

Traditionally, a patient presenting with chest pain in the emergency department with a clinical history indicating CAD, but with no ECG changes or troponin-plasma irregularities, would be sent for an exercise treadmill test (ETT). The weaknesses of ETT are encapsulated

http://dx.doi.org/10.5772/61837

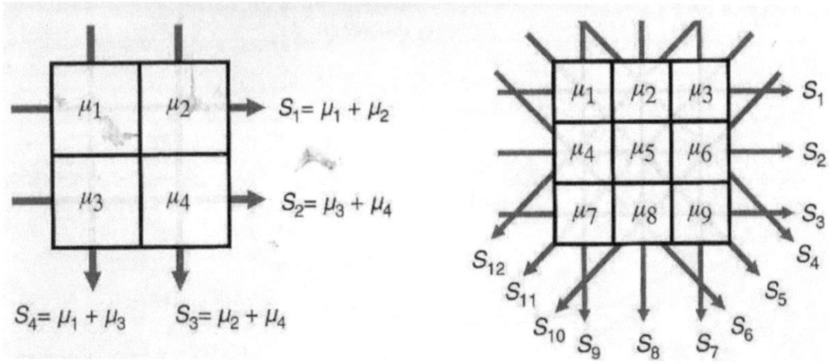

Figure 10. Schematic demonstrating how the ray sums are acquired in the simplest image matrices possible (2 × 2 and 3 × 3). There are N squared unknown values of attenuation for an N × N image matrix. The ray sums can then be solved as simultaneous linear equations to find the attenuation values of each voxel. *Image adapted without consent*[14]

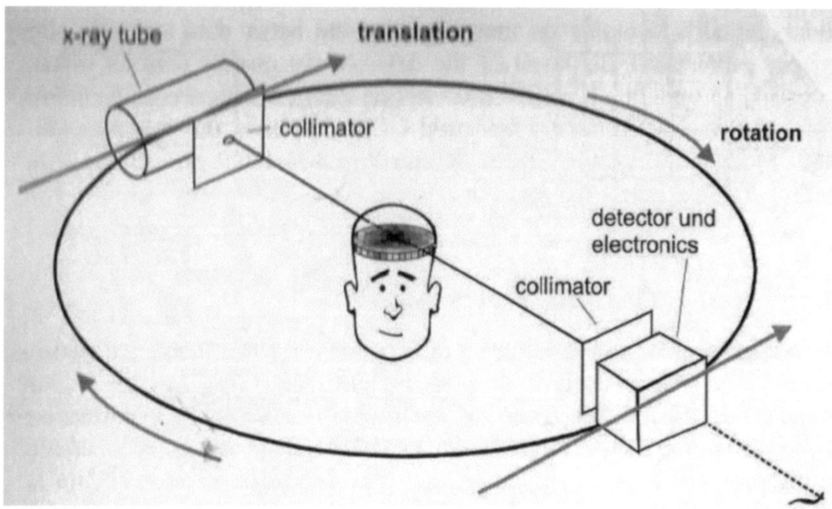

Figure 11. In a single plane, perpendicular to the scanning subject, the x-ray tube, and detector acquire attenuation values 360 degrees around the scanning subject (thus the scanning subject is the axis of rotation). This allows a single 'volume' slice to be obtained. Slices can be combined to form a 3D image visualised from any angle. *image adapted without consent*[14]

in a meta-analysis conducted by Patel et al, reviewing a sample of 398,978 cases of chest pain admissions with unknown CAD. The results show that 59% of the positive tests had no obstructive CAD and 28% were false negatives when ICA was performed. This level of inaccuracy is unacceptable, regardless of the fact that ETT is inexpensive and readily available; it is no better than flipping a coin at positively predicting flow-limiting CAD. The findings of Patel et al also illustrate that in the established patient pathway only 37.6% of patients referred to ICA were found to have obstructive CAD. The overall conclusion of the study was that "better strategies for risk stratification...to increase diagnostic yield of cardiac catheterisation in routine practice" are necessary [17]

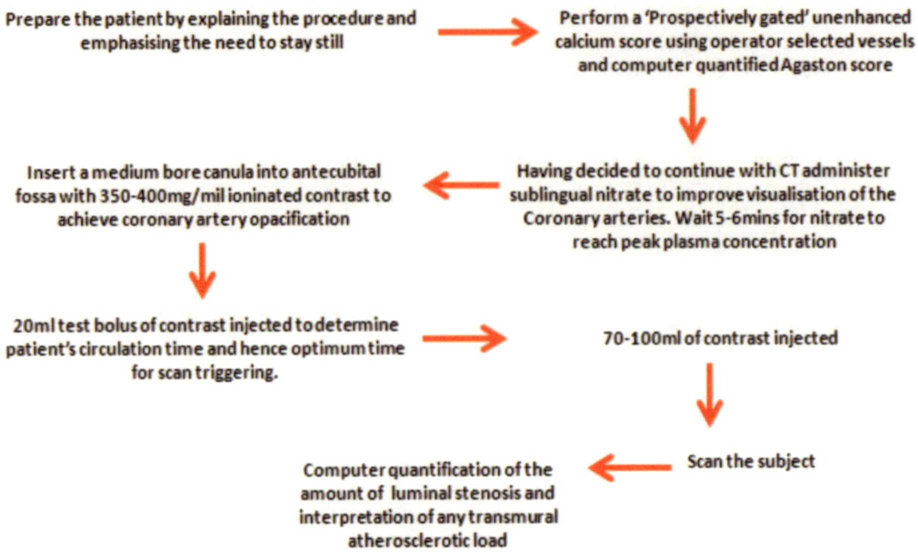

Figure 12. A flow diagram to show the procedure of calcium scoring and full-blown, contrast-enhanced CTCA. *Original figure: information adapted*[7]

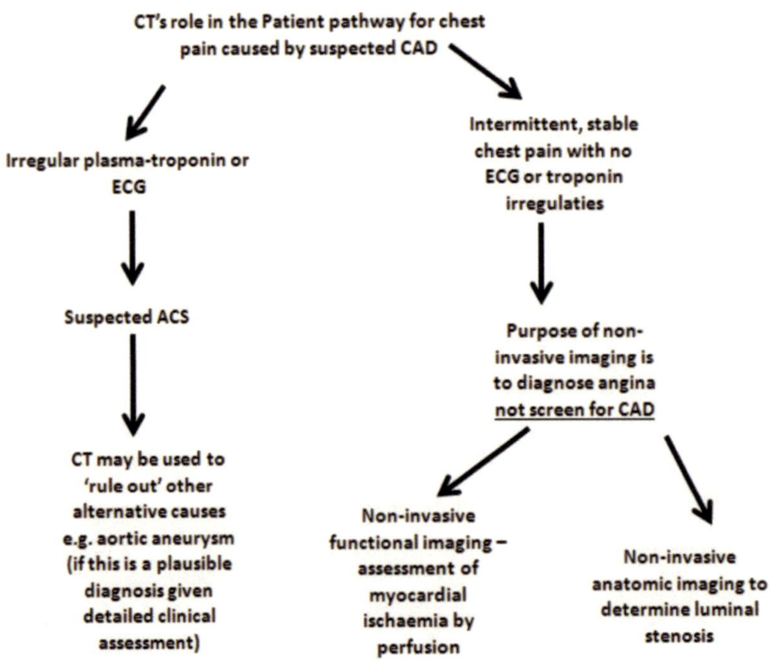

Figure 13. Flow diagram illustrating CT's current role in the management of chest pain in the UK does not extend beyond a 'rule out' in the intermediate stenosis group. It currently has no role in suspected ACS in the UK. *original figure, information adapted*[7]

http://dx.doi.org/10.5772/61837

The mandate for CT, if proven to work, is clear; too many patients, who do not need it are being sent for ICA. This is expensive and unnecessarily increases the patient's risk of complication. ICA has a serious complication rate of about 1/1,000[12]. Importantly, indecisive testing also increases the amount of time a patient spends in the waiting room. The CT coronary angiography for systematic triage of acute chest pain patients to treatment (CT-STAT) and randomised controlled trial (RCT) showed that as compared with the conventional pathway, a patient evaluated with CTCA can expect to wait on average less than 4 h at a cost, which is on average $1,500 cheaper compared with the healthcare provider.[18] Another large-scale RCT (n = 1,365), which compared the traditional care group with that who received CTCA after first line tests, found that there were 26.8% fewer (95% CI 21.4–32.2) unnecessary admissions in the CCTA group. In addition, there were fewer negative invasive angiograms and a greater number of patients who were correctly identified as having obstructive CAD. [19] In fact, the health economic model, using ICA as the reference standard, shows that at a pre-test probability of 50% or lower, CTCA results in a lower cost per patient with a true positive diagnosis.[15] Annually, there are 6 million presentations for chest pain, only 20% of these receive a diagnosis of CAD, and a large number are hospitalised unnecessarily. In 2006, the bill for non-specific chest pain in the UK came to £11.2 billion.[8] On the issue of assessing chest pain for patients in the emergency department, medicine can and should do better than ETT. The evidence shows CTCA is far superior on the basis of time and expense [18].

6. How can CTCA be used and does it work?

CTCA has advanced to the stage that it is now advocated by 'National Institute for Clinical Excellence (NICE) Guidance 95' for patients with a low–intermediate risk of CAD (10–29%). [7] The main reason CTCA has taken on this new role is because of its high negative predictive value and thus the exceptional ability to rule out CAD (Figures 14–16). [20, 8, 4, 6, 21]

- Pre-test probability is calculated using an algorithm, which involves 12 lead ECG, typicality of symptoms, age, sex and risk factors.
- It should also be noted that the RCT evidence out there is based on the use of at least 64 MDCT scanners and therefore the result findings are not applicable to centres that do not have this facility available. There is a lack of RCT evidence on the accuracy of the newer 320 MDCT scanners, exclusively.
- Accuracy of CTCA varies according to the level of disease prevalence and the level at which anatomic imaging defines luminal obstruction as haemodynamically significant.

Figure 14. A note on methodology of the trials

- A key strength of EVASCAN, which is not seen in many other studies of this kind, is that non evaluable segments were not excluded from the analysis, or as they are in other studies, assumed to be stenosed; falsely elevating the negative predictive value (NPV) and specificity.
- One of the EVASCAN study limitations was that currently, stenosis analysis is more often performed by more crude qualitative assessment in clinical practice rather than the quantitative approach taken in research.[20] For this reason, the findings of EVASCAN should be evaluated with caution when applied to the clinical setting.
- A weakness of CTCA pointed out by all major RCT study findings is that diagnostic accuracy of CTCA is limited in distal vessels or in vessels that are narrower than 1.5 mm due to its limited spatial resolution (0.5 mm) which is still by far inferior to that of the invasive angiograph (0.2 mm)[27].
- All studies pointed toward the need for further study on the 'real life' management of patients with chest pain. It is hoped that this could help to define a precise role for CCTA in symptomatic patients with CAD and determine exactly what benefit it can provide to specific patient groups rather than using ICA

Figure 15. Strengths and weaknesses of the EVASCAN study methodology

Study Name	Degree of stenosis severity assessed	Disease Prevalence	Study Number	Sensitivity	Specificity	Positive Predictive Value	Negative Predictive value
CORE 64[22]	>50%	51%	N=291	85	90	91	83
ACCURACY [25]	>70%	13.9%	N=231	91	84	51	99
ACCURACY OF 64 SLICE CTCA [26]	>50%	68%	N=360	99	64	86	97

Figure 16. A table summarising the data concerning the accuracy of 64 MDCT at various disease prevalence and degrees of stenoses, considered flow limiting

One of the most definitive RCTs conducted to evaluate the accuracy of CTCA at detecting or ruling out >50% stenosis is the EVAluation of CT SCANner (EVASCAN) study, which included the largest sample of intermediate–high risk stable symptomatic patients, to date. Considering the low–intermediate group forms, the greatest proportion of individuals presenting with symptomatic CAD in the emergency department (ED) is 50–70% [19], EVASCAN's study sheds light on a previously under-investigated and crucial patient group. EVASCAN examined population with a prevalence of CAD of 54%, in a study sample of 757, using a 64 slice multi-detector row CT scanner. The sensitivity, specificity, positive predictive value (PPV) and negative predictive value (NPV) compared with ICA as the reference standard were 91%, 50%, 68% and 83%, respectively.[20] At 83%, EVASCAN's negative predictive value concords with the CORE 64 RCT [22], which also examines CTCA's effectiveness at detecting CAD severity compared with the gold standard of ICA. At a lowly 68%, the positive predictive value (PPV) of CTCA is badly affected by CT's facility to systematically over-estimate stenosis severity due to local accumulation of non-obstructive local foci of calcium.

The results of EVASCAN and CORE 64 must be contextualised. Both look at the ability of CT to determine haemodynamically obstructive CAD, based on a 'binary', > or <50% stenosis severity. For reasons highlighted earlier, 50% stenosis is quite a low boundary to be considered flow limiting across the board. Whilst the inability to account for other physiological factors in flow limitation is an inherent weakness of anatomical CTCA, ruling out CAD exclusively on the basis of a 50% stenosis severity is bound to be less accurate than using the 70% threshold. For this reason, NICE guidance advocates the use of the >70% threshold in the assessment of flow limitation.[23]

The challenging question of, "what extent of luminal obstruction should be assumed to be flow limiting?" has recently been tackled by a few small-scale RCTs. These RCTs call for a re-evaluation of the binary classification of stenosis severity as flow limiting/not flow limiting according to a single cut-off threshold. These studies demonstrate the potential clinical usefulness of a more quantitative, tiered approach to evaluating stenosis severity. These studies also illustrate that stenosis severity can be accurately 'graded' by CTCA and this 'grading' shows excellent correlation with flow limitation (r = 0.82), assessed by ICA.[24] Further large-scale RCTs are needed to evaluate the usefulness of this graded approach in risk stratification and prognostic outcome. More evidence is also needed to determine the exact effectiveness of anatomical CTCA in assessing flow limitation in the intermediately stenosed group (40–69%).

The ACCURACY RCT illustrates CTCA's excellent ability to rule out CAD in populations of low prevalence of CAD with a negative predictive value of 99%.[25] At the other end of the spectrum, ACCURACY of 64 shows that CTCA can accurately rule out CAD in populations with a high prevalence of CAD with an NPV of 98%.[26] These results demonstrate that it is feasible to use CTCA in populations at high and low risk of the disease. Something that needs to be considered from a research perspective is that 99% rule out is extremely impressive and far more encouraging than ETT. However, from a clinical perspective 1 mistake in every 100, given the high turnover of chest pain patients in the ED, could prove to be very costly in terms of lives lost. Therefore, while it is feasible to use CTCA in the rule out of obstructive CAD in both of these patient populations, it does not necessarily provide clear clinical benefit over ICA, the gold standard to which CTCA is being compared with, in terms of accuracy of the 'rule out'.

The overall findings of EVASCAN, and associated RCTs, illustrate that in populations with a low prevalence of disease and using a 70% stenosis as a threshold for flow limitation, CTCA can be used to a great effect to rule out flow-limiting CAD. This is why EVASCAN and other studies call for clinicians to recognise the importance of the pre-test probability. In low to intermediate pre-test probability of CAD (10–29%), where the disease prevalence of obstructive CAD will be low, it is more cost effective, safer than and almost equally as accurate as the gold standard ICA at ruling out CAD. The reason CTCA's use cannot be extended to high pre-test risk population (>61%) is because in spite of the high NPV, a patient will receive no benefit from receiving CTCA.[7] In this high-risk group, a rule-in test is required, and CCTA's unimpressive PPV and ICA's added benefit of being able to revascularise straight away, if the culprit lesion is shown to be flow limiting, makes it more cost effective than CCTA in this patient group.

7. Prognostic value of CTCA

The focus thus far has been to assess to what extent CT can accurately identify obstructive CAD and the monetary and time-saving benefit CT can offer. It is also crucial to follow up patients after diagnosis by CTCA and record their outcomes that is. given a negative finding on CT, what proportion of patients still go on to have major adverse coronary event (MACE)?

A recent meta-analysis (n = 9,592), with a median 20-month follow-up, showed that the risk of MACE following a negative test on CTCA is 0.17% per year, a figure that is comparable with the baseline rate (0.15% per year). In patients with abnormal findings on CTCA, there is a risk of MACE of 8.8%, 40 times more than the risk in the general population.[27] Another meta-analysis (n = 3,670), which performed similar analysis over a longer mean follow-up period (21.6 months), found a tenfold higher risk in patients with "any detectable coronary stenosis by CTCA compared with subjects without coronary stenosis".[28]

A recent case–control study went into more detailed analysis at the potential for CT to stratify risk. It was found that, by grading coronary stenosis using a segmental stenosis score, and following up after 52 months, those with a score up to 5 (less severe stenosis) had an event-free survival of 85%, whereas those who had a score >5 had an event-free survival of just 20%. The same study also found that those with an intermediate degree of the stenosis (40–69% ruled out as flow limiting) showed an event-free survival between those with normal coronary arteries and those with obstructive CAD.[29] This study conceded that it could not be sure that the higher number of deaths in this group was because of the non-obstructive CAD, developing into obstructive CAD, or because of non-obstructive CAD plaque rupture, and highlighted, "early identification of non-obstructive CAD with CTCA is clinically important because it may lead to a more aggressive strategy of cardiovascular risk factor control and modification of clinical follow-up."[29] It is for exactly this reason that prognostic information obtained by CTCA is so useful; rather than widespread distribution of primary and secondary interventions, targeted aggressive treatment can be handed to the patients who need it the most.

8. Prognostic value of CTCA: Calcium scoring

Calcium scoring is a tool available for cardiac CT (Figures 17 and 18), which can be performed immediately, without the use of contrast and without the use of high doses of radia-

http://dx.doi.org/10.5772/61837

tion, in order to stratify for cardiac risk. It works on the basis that coronary artery calcium (CAC) has excellent x-ray attenuation properties and is a quantifiable marker of atherosclerotic plaque. However, the quantity of CAC is poorly correlated with the degree of stenosis, so its presence should not be extrapolated to be a good predictor of flow limitation.[8]

- A calcium score of zero is indicative of no detectable calcium
- NICE recommend that symptomatic low-intermediate (10–29%) risk patients should be offered CAC scoring
- In a score between **1** and **400**, the recommendation is to proceed to formal CTCA
- In a score that exceeds **400**, with no alternative explanation, the recommendation is to proceed to ICA[7] as CTCA is less effective in patients with significant calcification [30]

Figure 17. NICE Recommendations on the calcium score

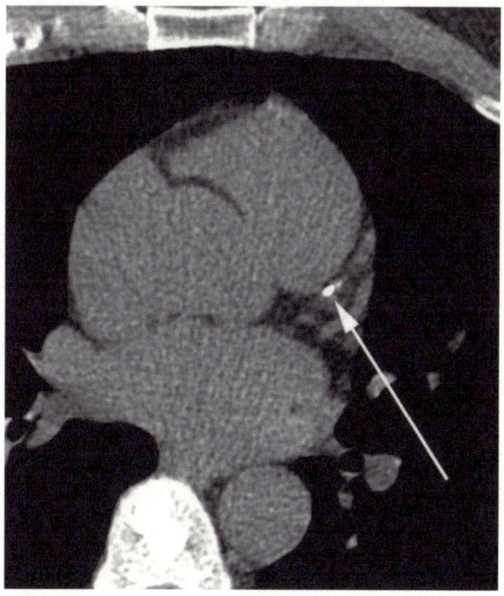

Figure 18. An unenhanced calcium score showing low degree calcification in proximal left anterior, descending artery. The patient was thus referred to CTCA. *Figure adapted without consent*[7]

A calcium score of zero has a 12-year-survival of 99.4% and a score of 100–400 Agatston units has a lifetime risk ratio of myocardial infarction of 4.3 compared with those with a calcium score of zero. Despite the excellent prognosis of a CAC score of zero, its use is not indicated for the purpose of screening as the likelihood of finding stenosis in low-risk patients (using the Framingham score) is too low to warrant imaging.[12] The CAC score is best deployed in the intermediate-risk population.[7] A serious consideration which requires the physician's meticulous attention is the calcific distribution; a relatively low overall calcium score may be taken more seriously if it is found in the 'spotty distribution' of calcium.[30]

Another aspect of the calcium score in risk stratification is the patient's age. Whilst no coronary calcium is an excellent marker of prognosis, the true false negative rate is not really known and controversy surrounds the ability of CAC to rule out non-calcified fibrolipid plaque.[7] In a meta-analysis of 10,355 symptomatic patients, testing the ability of CAC scoring to detect significant CAD compared with ICA, results showed as high as 2% of the patients had significant CAD with no detectable calcium and CAC scoring had a poor overall specificity of just 40%.[31] These individuals (significant CAD with no CAC) tend to be younger than 50 years of age and particular diligence must be taken with patients in this age group. Worryingly, the presence of this non-calcified plaque is higher in patients with serious acute coronary syndrome (ACS) rather than stable angina.[12]

9. Prognostic value of CTCA: Plaque composition

An advantage of CTCA, and an area of great promise, is the ability to provide more information about the coronary artery than just the luminal information offered by ICA. CTCA can offer insight into the degree of mural plaque burden and the plaque sub-type, which is beyond ICA without the use of intravascular ultrasound.[4]

Broadly speaking, CTCA can identify three types of plaque: calcified, non-calcified and mixed. Comparison with intravascular ultrasound during ICA shows that CTCA can correctly identify 95% of the calcified plaque, 83% of the non-calcified plaque and 84% of the mixed plaque. The accuracy for the identification of non-calcified plaque is lower for the same reason; CAC scoring is a poor predictor of obstructive CAD: CTCA systematically overestimates CAC due to the high attenuation properties of calcium and the partial volume effect. However, it is hoped that one day CTCA will be able to unlock useful prognostic information about the chance of CAD plaque rupture, and therefore detect and direct medical intervention.[12]

It has already been highlighted that 90% of the ACS is caused by plaque rupture [2] and up to two-thirds of MIs occur from disruption of plaque that causes less than 50% stenosis. [12] Currently, CTCA would result in the discharge a patient with chest pain at this intermediate degree of stenosis and any further functional testing that would be performed (stress testing or ICA) is unlikely to show any signs of ischaemia. [12]

Plaques at the risk of rupture have a specific morphology called 'thin-capped fibroatheroma'. These have a lipid-rich, necrotic core with a thin fibrous cap. The most important property in the risk of rupture of plaques is the thickness of the fibrous cap; the thinner the fibrous cap, the greater the risk of rupture. Currently, the spatial resolution of CT is limited to 330 μm and, by definition, the fibrous cap is less than 65 μm in thickness. The current limits of CT suggest that being able to visualise 'at risk' fibrous caps is impossible. However, these 'fibroatheromas' have slightly different attenuation properties to more stable, fibrous lesions. Although there is still much progress to be made, promise remains in the ability of CTCA to distinguish the attenuation properties of the lipid-rich core in the hope of recognising and quantifying the risk of rupture in vulnerable plaque. [30, 12]

10. CT in the assessment of Fractional Flow Reserve(FFR): The future

ICA has been referred to many times throughout the course of this chapter as the 'gold standard' in the assessment of CAD (Figure 19). In order to define a precise role for anatomic CTCA, in the assessment of CAD, one must first understand the process of ICA, what useful information it gathers and whether it is within the capability of CTCA to gather similar, useful information.

- ICA, or, as it is more simplistically known, coronary angiography involves 'cardiac catheterisation'
- Cardiac catheterisation is the process where the femoral or brachial artery (most commonly on the left side) is punctured and a long, thin, flexible, hollow, tube-like device (a catheter) is fed in a retrograde fashion through the circulatory system to the heart and coronary arteries
- The movement of the catheter tip is guided by an x-ray machine and injections of contrast are used to enhance visualisation of the vasculature. [33] This allows the physician to directly visualise the degree of coronary artery stenosis in real time
- FFR is calculated by measuring the ratio of pressure proximal to and distal to a stenotic lesion during vasodilator induced hyperaemia

Figure 19. The procedure of ICA

One of the major advantages of ICA is the ability to perform percutaneous coronary intervention (PCI) in an attempt to restore normal flow to the obstructed coronary artery. This assumption was called into question by the COURAGE RCT trial, which compared the outcomes of elective, stable angina patients with those who received optimised medical therapy (anti-platelet therapy and statins) when compared with PCI. The findings of this study were that, "as an initial management strategy in patients with stable coronary artery disease, PCI did not reduce the risk of death, myocardial infarction or other major cardiovascular events when added to optimal medical therapy."[32]

The COURAGE trial was followed up by the COURAGE nuclear substudy, which took into account the extent of ischaemia on perfusion imaging, using the same two treatment allocations. The substudy found that revascularisation did lead to a decrease in ischaemia and a decrease in adverse cardiac events.[27] The results of the two trials were not incongruent. When taken together, they imply that there is a lack of revascularisation benefit, identified on anatomical grounds exclusively. In order to effectively identify patients who require revascularisation, some other test, which directly measures haemodynamic consequences of stenosis, is required. The test that has been developed and proven to be clinically useful is the fractional flow reserve (FFR). It has been found that if FFR > 0.75, PCI can be deferred without increased patient risk, despite an angiographic appearance of significant stenosis. Moreover, the cardiac event rates were lower in patients with FFR > 0.75 who did not have PCI than patients who did have PCI. [27, 33, 34]Finally, the evidence supports the fact that there is no benefit in revascularising, unless the haemodynamic consequences of stenosis are known.

The relevance to CTCA is that with modern 320 detector row CT scanners, one can also measure FFR (Figure 20) by applying fluid mechanical modelling to CCTA images, with no extra radiation exposure and no change to the normal CCTA procedure.[35]

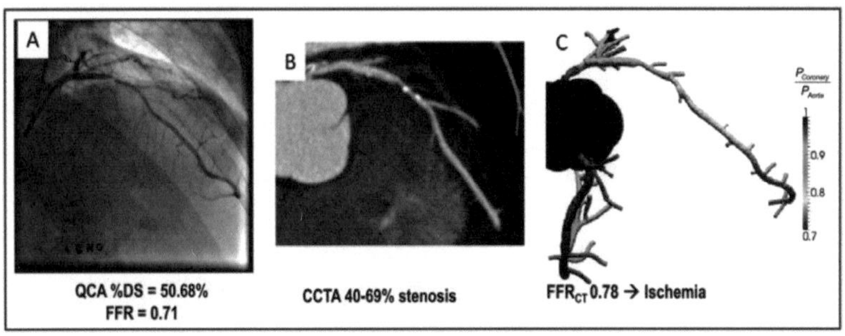

Figure 20. A) An invasive coronary angiogram of LAD artery. QCA – Quantified coronary angiography (maximal quantified stenosis) is 50.68% showing it is an intermediately stenosed lesion. Invasively measured fractional flow reserve (FFR) is 0.71, which indicates this lesion is causal of ischaemia B) Conventional CCTA concurs with the findings on ICA that the lesion is in the intermediately stenosed group and C) Combined function and anatomical image of LAD artery. The shading corresponds with the FFR at that point along the coronary artery. FFR measured by CCTA is 0.78, which by this study's definition (ischaemia if FFR<0.8) is an ischaemia causing lesion. This highlights the combined ability of anatomic and, new, functional CCTA to diagnose a lesion as flow limiting despite the fact it is only modestly stenosed (50.68% by QCA) [35]

How best could we use the anatomical information obtained by CCTA and apply it to the haemodynamic consequences of CAD on blood flow? The group of patients this has posed a particular problem for is the intermediate stenosis group (40–69%). Within this group CTCA has, as yet, been unable to unlock the haemodynamic consequences of CAD through an anatomical approach.

Recent evidence has shown early promising signs; using CTCA measured FFR can produce a diagnosis of ischaemia in lesions of intermediate stenosis severity with a PPV (compared with ICA measured FFR) of 82.4% and a NPV of 90.6%.[35] CTCA measured FFR, in combination with anatomical imaging, has been shown to increase the accuracy of the diagnosis of ischaemia in lesions of all types by 25%. Another potential benefit is that in instances of multi-segment stenoses, the culprit lesion(s) can be correctly identified. [35] The findings of these studies are based on a very small cohort ($n = 60$) and need to be shown to be reproducible on a larger scale. Furthermore, the potential to use CCTA measured FFR should not be seen as a challenge to ICA and its potential benefits, compared or in conjunction with stress-testing modalities, need to be fully evaluated before its precise role can be defined.

11. Conclusion

This chapter has aimed to show that the process and manifestations of CAD are nuanced; therefore, what is required is a far more detailed analysis than the current diagnosis of, or the 'ruling out' of, the ACS.

CTCA has been shown to be a cost effective, quick and accurate means of managing patients with acute chest pain, and it has been established that for CTCA to be used effectively, it must be targeted at the right patient group (10–29% pre-test probability). The prognostic information that can be garnered by CTCA is useful; however, the role of the prognostics in the direction of primary and secondary intervention requires further study in order for its precise use in risk stratification and direction of primary, secondary and tertiary interventions.

The findings demonstrate that the role of CTCA is not to supplant ICA as the gold standard in the investigation of CAD in a similar way that CT pulmonary angiography has its invasive counterpart. The current role of CTCA must be viewed as a means to avoiding unnecessary invasive angiography and the associated risks that come with it in the right patient population. There is no longer a role or a need for ETT in the assessment of patients with acute chest pain.[36]

Whilst the focus of this chapter is purely upon the merits of anatomical assessment of CAD, it must be noted that the role of cardiac CT in the management of chest pain in the ED is evolving.[37] Growing evidence is emerging about the possibility of a 'one-stop shop' approach where the anatomy, physiology and perfusion of the heart and coronary arteries, as well as assessment of pulmonary embolism and aortic aneurysm, are all used to diagnose the cause of chest pain in one study.[38] This has been reflected by a readiness of centres in the USA to use the modern 320 MDCT scanners in the emergency department assessment of chest pain.

The potential of using CTCA to determine FFR in the diagnosis of ischaemic heart disease is also an exciting development and has the potential to expand the role of CTCA further by elucidating the haemodynamic significance of the intermediate stenosis. Another avenue of much research lies in the attempt to increase the accuracy of CAD assessment of stable, symptomatic, intermediate-risk patients, by combining the anatomical approach of CTCA alongside myocardial perfusion imaging by CT.[27] What is clear is that CTCA, and CT more broadly, has and will continue to have an expanding role in safeguarding the function of the heart that William Harvey breathlessly outlined for the first time.

Author details

Michael Campbell[1], Stephen Lyen[2,3], Jonathan Rodrigues[2,3], Mark Hamilton[2,3] and Nathan Manghat[2,3*]

*Address all correspondence to: nathan.manghat@uhbristol.nhs.uk

1 University of Bristol, UK

2 Bristol Heart Institute, University Hospitals Bristol NHS Foundation Trust, Bristol Royal Infirmary, Bristol, UK

3 National Institute for Health Research, Bristol Cardiovascular Biomedical Research Unit, Bristol Royal Infirmary, Bristol, UK

References

[1] V. Fuster, R. A. O'Rourke, R. Walsh and P. Poole-Wilson, Hurst's the Heart, 12th Edition, McGraw-Hill Medical, 2007.

[2] Leonard S. Lilly, Pathophysiology of Heart Disease:A collaborative project of medical students and faculty. 4th Edition, Lipincott William and Wilkins, 2007.

[3] A. H. Gershlick et al, "Role of non-invasive imaging in the management of coronary artery disease: An assessment of likely change over the next 10 years. A report from the British Cardiovascular Society Working Group," Heart, vol. 93, pp. 423-431, 2007.

[4] M. C. Williams, J. H. Reid, G. McKillop, N. W. Weir, E. J. van Beek, N. G. Uren and D. E. Newby, "Cardiac and coronary CT comprehensive imaging approach in the assessment of coronary heart disease," Heart, vol. 97, pp. 1198-1205, 2011.

[5] M. R. Patel, E. D. Peterson, D. Dai, J. M. Brennan, R. F. Redberg, R. G. Brindis and P. S. Douglas, "Low diagnostic yield of elective coronary angiography", The New England Journal of Medicine, vol. 362, pp. 886-895, 2010.

[6] M. Michail, "Feasibility of using coronary computed tomography angiography (CCTA) in patients with acute low-to-intermediate likelihood chest pain," British Journal of Cardiology, vol. 20, 2013.

[7] A. Wallis, N. Manghat and M. Hamilton, "The role of coronary CT in the assessment and diagnosis of patients with chest pain," Clinical Medicine, vol. 12, pp. 222-229, 2012.

[8] G. Bastarrika, C. Thilo, G. F. Headden, P. L. Zwerner, P. Costello and U. J. Schoepf, "Cardiac CT in the assessment of acute chest pain in the emergency department," American Journal of Roentgenology, vol. 2, pp. 397-409, 2009.

http://dx.doi.org/10.5772/61837

[9] E. P. Widmaier, H. Raff and K. T. Strang, Vander's Human Physiology: The Mechanisms of Body Function, New York: McGraw-Hill, 2008.

[10] K. L. Gould and K. Lipscomb, "Effects of coronary stenoses on coronary flow reserve and resistance," American Journal of Cardiology, vol. 34, pp. 48-55, 1974.

[11] K. L. Gould, "Does coronary flow trump coronary anatomy?," American Journal of Cardiovascular Imaging, vol. 2, no. 9, p. 1146, 2009.

[12] D. R. Obaid, "Contemporary coronary imaging from patient to plaque: Part 3 cardiac computed tomography," British Journal of Cardiology, vol. 17, pp. 235-239, 2010.

[13] J. Schuijf, "Cardiac imaging in CAD: differing modalities," Heart, vol. 91, no. 8, pp. 1110-1117, 2005.

[14] W. A. Kalender, Computed Tomography: Fundamentals, System Technology, Image quality, Applications, Munich: Publicis MCD Verlag, 2000.

[15] V. Gorenoi, M. P. Schonermark and A. Hagen, CT coronary angiography vs invasive coronary angiography in CHD," GMS Health Technol Assess, vol. 8, Doc 02, 2012.

[16] T. Flohr and B Ohnesorge, "Developments in CT," Imaging, vol. 18, pp. 45-61, 2006.

[17] M. R. Patel, D. P. Enc, D. Dai, J. M. Brennan, V. Anderson, R. G. Brindis and P. S. Douglas, "Low diagnostic yield of elective coronary angiography," The New England Journal of Medicine, vol. 362, pp. 886-895, 2010.

[18] James A. Goldstein, Kavitha M. Chinnaiyan, Aiden Abidov, Stephan Achenbach, Daniel S. Berman, Sean W. Hayes, Udo Hoffmann, John R. Lesser, Issam A. Mikati, Brian J. O'Neil, P. Leslee J. Shaw and Michael Y. H Shen, The CT-STAT (Coronary Computed Tomographic Angiography for Systematic Triage of Acute Chest Pain Patients to Treatment)," Journal of the American College of Cardiology, vol. 58, no. 14, pp. 1414-1422, 2011.

[19] H. I. Litt, C. Gatsonis, B. Snyder, H. Singh, C. D. Miller, D. W. Entrikin, J. M. Leaming, L. J. Gavin, C. B. Pacella and J. E. Hollander, "CT angiography for the safe discharge of patients with possible acute coronary syndromes," The New England Journal of Medicine, vol. 366, pp. 1393-1403, 2012.

[20] P. Gueret, J. Deux, L. Bonello, A. Sarran, C. Tron, L. Christiaens, J. Dacher, D. Bertrand, L. Leborgne, C. Renard, C. Caussin, P. Cluzel, G. Helft, D. Crochet, H. Vernhet-Kovacsik, V. Chabbert, E. Ferrari, M. Gilard, S. Willoteaux, A. Furber, G. Barone-Rochette, A. Jankowski, P. Douek, E. Mousseaux, M. Sirol, R. Niarra, G. Chatellier and J. Laissy, "Diagnostic performance of computed tomography coronary angiography (from the prospective National Multicentre Multivendor EVASCAN study)," The American Journal of Cardiology, vol. 111, no. 4, pp. 471-478, 2013.

[21] E. A. Hulten, S. Carbonaro, S. P. Petrillo, J. D. Mitchel and T. C. Villines, "Prognostic value of cardiac computed tomography angiography: A systematic review and meta-analysis," American Journal of Cardiology, vol. 10, no. 57, pp. 1237-1247, 2011.

[22] J. M. Miller, C. E. Rochitte, M. Dewey, A. Arbab-Zadeh, H. Niinuma, I. Gottlieb, N. Paul, M. E. Clouse, E. P. Shapiro, J. Hoe, A. C. Lardo, D. E. Bush, A. de Roos, C. Cox, J. Brinker and J. A. Lima, "Diagnostic performance of coronary angiography by 64-row CT,"The New England Journal of Medicine, vol. 359, pp. 2324-2336, 2008.

[23] N. I. f. H. a. C. Excellence, "Chest pain of recent onset:Assessment and diagnosis of recent onset chest pain or discomfort of suspected cardiac origin (NICE guidance 95)," National Institute for Health and Clinical Excellence, London, 2010.

[24] C. V, A. Gutstein, A. Wolak, Y. Suzuki, D. Dey, H. Gransar, L. Thomson, S. Hayes, J. Friedman and D. Berman, "Moving beyond binary grading of coronary arterial stenoses on coronary computed tomographic angiography. Insights for the imager and referring clinician.," JACC Cardiovascular Imaging, pp. 460-471, 2008.

[25] Matthew J. Budoff, David Dowe,. James G. Jollis, Michael Gitter, John Sutherland, Edward Halamert, Markus Scherer, RayeBellinger, Arthur Martin, Robert Benton, Augustin Delago and James K. Min, "Diagnostic performance of 64-multidetector row coronary computed tomographic angiography for evaluation of coronary artery stenosis in individuals without known coronary artery disease," Journal of the American College of Cardiologists, vol. 52, no. 21, pp. 1724-1732, 2008.

[26] Meijboom WB, Meijs MF, Schuijf JD, Cramer MJ, Mollet NR, van Mieghem CA, Nieman K, van Werkhoven JM, Pundziute G, Weustink AC, de Vos AM, Pugliese F, Rensing B, Jukema JW, Bax JJ, Prokop M, Doevendans PA, Hunink MG, Krestin GP, de Feyter PJ"Diagnostic accuracy of 64-slice computed tomography coronary angiography: a prospective, multicenter, multivendor study," Journal of the Journal American College of Cardiology, vol. 52, no. 25, pp. 2135-2144, 2008.

[27] B. Tamarappoo and R. Hachamovitch, "Myocardial perfusion imaging vs computed tomography coronary angiography: When to use which?," Journal of Nuclear Medicine, vol. 52, no. 7, pp. 1079-1086, 2011.

[28] F. Bamberg, W. H. Sommer, V. Hoffman, S. Achenbach, K. Nikolaou, D. Conen, M. F. Reiser, U. Hoffman and C. R. Becker, "Meta-analysis and systematic review of long-term predictive value of assessment of coronary atherosclerosis by contrast enhanced coronary computed tomography angiography," Journal American College of Cardiology, vol. 24, no. 57, pp. 2426-2436, 2011.

[29] D. Andreini, G. Pontone, S. Mushtaq, A. L. Bartorelli, E. Bertella, L. Antonioli, A. Formenti, S. Cortinovis, F. Veglia, A. Annoni, P. Agostoni, P. Montorsi, G. Ballerini, C. Fiorentini and M. Pepi, "A long-term prognostic value of coronary CT angiography in suspected coronary artery disease," JACC: Cardiovascular Imaging, vol. 5, no. 7, p. 690–701, 2012.

[30] J. Sun, Z. Zhang, B. Lu, W. Yu, Y. Yang, Y. Zhou, Y. Weng and Z. Fan, "Identification and quantification of coronary atherosclerotic plaques: A comparison of 64 MDCT and intravascular ultrasound," American journal of Roentgenology, no. 190, pp. 748-754, 2008.

[31] A. Sarwar, L. J. Shaw, M. D. Shapiro, R. Blankstein, U. Hoffman, R. C. Cury, S. Abbara, T. J. Brady, M. J. Budoff, R. S. Blumenthal and K. Nasir, "Diagnostic and prognostic value of absence of coronary artery calcification," American Journal of Cardiological Imaging, vol. 2, no. 6, pp. 675-688, 2009.

[32] W. E. Boden, R. A. O'Rourke, K. K. Teo, P. M. Hartigan, D. J. Maron, W. J. Kostuk, M. Knudtson, M. Dada, P. Casperson, C. L. Harris, G. Gau, A. S. Blaustein, D. C. Booth, E. R. Bates, J. A. Spertus, D. S. Berman, J. Mancini and W. S. Weintraub, "Optimal medical therapy with or without PCI for stable coronary disease," New England Journal of Medicine, vol. 356, pp. 1503-1516, 2007.

[33] P. A. Tonino, B. De Bruyne, N. H. Pijls, U. Siebert, F. Ikeno, M. van `t Veer, V. Klauss, G. Manoharan and T. Engstrøm, "fractional flow reserve versus angiography for guiding percutaneous coronary intervention," The New England Journal of Medicine, vol. 360, pp. 213-223, 2009.

[34] R. Ascione, "Debates on myocardial revascularisation," in European Society of Cardiology: Congress - http://www.escardio.org/congresses/esc-2012/congress-reports/Pages/911-Ascione.aspx, 2012.

[35] J. K. Min, B. Koo, A. Erglis, J. Doh, D. Daniels, S. Jegere, H. Kim, A. Dunning, T. Defrance, A. Lansky and J. Leipsic, "Usefulness of non invasive fractional flow reserve computed from coronary computed tomographic angiograms for intermediate stenoses confirmed by quantitative coronary angiography," American Journal of Cardiology, vol. 110, no. 7, pp. 971-976, 2012.

[36] A. C. McCulloch, "Correspondence: Coronary angiography by 64-row CT," New England Journal of Medicine, vol. 360, pp. 2027-2031, 2009.

[37] R. Rubinshtein, D. A. Halon, T. Gaspar, J. E. Schliamser, N. Yaniv, R. Ammar, M. Y. Flugelman, N. Peledand B. S. Lewis, "Usefulness of 64-slice multidetector computed tomography in diagnostic triage of patients with chest pain and negative or non diagnostic exercise treadmill test result," American Journal of Cardiology, vol. Volume 99, no. 7, p. 925–929, 2007.

[38] J. Gruettner, C. Fink, T. Walter, M. Meyer, P. Apfaltrer, U. Schoepf, J. Saur, T. Sueselbeck, D. Traunwieser, R. Takx, S. Kralev, M. Borggrefe, S. Schoenberg and T. Henzler, "Coronary computed tomography and triple rule out CT in patients with acute chest pain and an intermediate cardiac risk profile. Part 1: impact on patient management," European Journal of Radiology, vol. 82, no. 1, pp. 100-105, 2013.

[39] D. R. Nave, "HyperPhysics," [Online]. Available: http://hyperphysics.phy-astr.gsu.edu/%E2%80%8Chbase/ppois.html. [Accessed 9th March 2013]

[40] B. Tamerappoo and R. Hachemovitch. Myocardial perfusion imaging versus CT coronary angiography: when to use which?. J Nucl Med. 2011 Jul;52(7):1079-86.

[41] R. F. Farr and P. J. Allisy-Roberts, Physics for medical imaging, Elsevier, 2002.

[42] N. Herring and D. J. Patterson, "ECG diagnosis of acute Ischaemia and infarction: Past, present, future," QJM: An international Journal of Medicine, vol. 4, no. 99, pp. 219-230, 2006.

[43] S. Achenbach, "Quantification of coronary artery stenosis by computed tomography," American College of Cardiology Imaging, vol. 1, no. 4, pp. 472-474, 2008.

[44] W. E. Brant, Fundamentals of Diagnostic Imaging, 2nd Edition, Lippincott Williams and Wilkins, 1999.

[45] A. Arbab-Zadeh, J. M. Miller, C. E. Rochitte, M. Dewey, H. Niinuma, I. Gottlieb, N. Paul, M. E. Clouse, E. P. Shapiro, J. Hoe, A. C. Lardo, D. E. Bush, A. de Roos, C. Cox, J. Brinker and J. A. Lima, "Diagnostic accuracy of computed tomography coronary angiography according to pre-test probability of coronary artery disease and severity of coronary artery calcification," Journal of the American College of Cardiology, vol. 59, no. 4, pp. 379-387, 2012.

[46] S. D. Kristensen, H. B. Ravn and E. Falk, "Insights into the pathophysiology of unstable coronary artery disease," The American Journal of Cardiology, vol. 80, no. 5, pp. 5E-9E, 1997.

[47] M. Poon, "North American Society for Cardiovascular Imaging Conference 2010: Advanced application of cardiac CT in the emergency department using a 320 Detector row CT scanner," 7 July 2011. [Online]. Available: http://www.youtube.com/watch?v=NiDFJI8ECiI. [Accessed 2nd February 2013]

[48] J. Qin, L. Y.Liu, X. C. Meng, J. S. Zhang, Y. X. Dong, Y. Fang and H. Shan, "Prospective versus retrospective ECG gating for 320-detector CT of the coronary arteries: comparison of image quality and patient radiation dose," Clinical Imaging, vol. 35, no. 3, pp. 193-197, 2011.

Chapter 4

Optical Coherence Tomography for the Assessment of Coronary Plaque Vulnerability

Takao Hasegawa and Kenei Shimada

Additional information is available at the end of the chapter

http://dx.doi.org/10.5772/61615

Abstract

Optical coherence tomography (OCT) is a high-resolution imaging technology, which can provide detailed observation of the vulnerable coronary atherosclerotic plaques in clinical settings. The current understanding of the major cause of acute coronary syndrome is that it results from plaque rupture of a vulnerable plaque. OCT can provide detailed observation of the vulnerable coronary plaque. The main findings of vulnerable plaque by OCT are considered to be a lipid-rich plaque, a thin-cap fibroatheroma, microchannel structure, spotty calcification, macrophage infiltration, and cholesterol crystal. These features observed by OCT can provide cardiologists to consider pathological mechanisms of coronary atherosclerosis and suitable medical and interventional treatments for vulnerable patients. In this review, we will discuss the characteristics of OCT assessment for coronary atherosclerosis and the clinical impacts of OCT imaging for the treatment of coronary artery disease.

Keywords: Optical coherence tomography, Coronary artery disease, Vulnerable plaque

1. Introduction

Optical coherence tomography (OCT) is an optical analog of intravascular ultrasound (IVUS) that allows physicians to visualize various morphological features of coronary atherosclerotic plaques *in vivo*. Recently, several vulnerable features of coronary atherosclerosis have been suggested in both histopathological and clinical studies with the emerging use of OCT. The main findings of vulnerable plaque by OCT are considered to be a lipid-rich plaque, a thin-cap fibroatheroma (TCFA), microchannel structure, spotty calcification, macrophage infiltration, and cholesterol crystal. We describe the features of vulnerable plaques by OCT and the impact of OCT findings for diagnosis and clinical treatment.

OCT is a high-resolution intracoronary imaging technology with near-infrared light to produce cross-sectional images of coronary artery disease. The spatial resolution of OCT, nearly 10 μm on the lateral axis, is almost 10 times greater than that of IVUS. OCT could provide detailed plaque morphology near to pathological assessment. More than 70% of acute coronary syndrome (ACS) was caused by plaque rupture, and nonruptured type (plaque erosion or calcified nodules) was shown in 30% of ACS. OCT is able to visualize vulnerable plaque which was prone to plaque rupture possibly agree with autopsy findings. Vulnerable feature by OCT were a lipid-rich plaque, a TCFA, vasa vasorum, spotty calcification, macrophage infiltration, cholesterol crystal. We describe the natural history of vulnerable plaques and the clinical impact of each vulnerable feature detected by OCT images.

Recent studies have shown that vulnerable plaques could develop not only in native coronary arteries but also in the neointima after coronary stent implantation. OCT studies have reported the development of neoatherosclerosis changes within both bare-metal stents and drug-eluting stents after stent implantation. Neoatherosclerosis includes lipid accumulation, calcium deposition, macrophage infiltration, and development of neovascularization within neointima area of the stent. These changes after stent implantation could play an important role in the development of late stent failure (late stent restenosis and late stent thrombosis).

Primary percutaneous coronary intervention (PCI) is widely performed for patients with coronary artery disease. Sometimes, no-reflow phenomenon occurred during PCI, and no-reflow is associated with poor functional and clinical patient outcomes when compared with patients with adequate reflow. Recent studies have shown that some vulnerable findings (lipid-rich plaque, TCFA, and spotty calcification) are predictors of no-reflow phenomenon. We describe how to treat vulnerable plaques during PCI with OCT.

Optimal medical therapy (OMT) is regarded as one of the effective treatments for the stabilization of coronary artery plaques, and it reduces the risk for coronary events and mortality. However, cardiovascular events occur in some patients even with OMT; the residual risk has become a problem. OCT detects and follows vulnerable plaque serially. Dyslipidemia is a strong risk for coronary artery disease and promotes coronary atherosclerosis. We describe the impact of oral lipid-lowering agents on stabilizing vulnerable plaques with OCT.

2. Optical coherence tomography technology

OCT is a new high-resolution intracoronary imaging technology based on near-infrared interferometry. As near-infrared light is unable to penetrate red blood cells (RBCs), OCT imaging is needed to remove RBCs in the coronary artery with a bolus injection of contrast medium. The high pull-back speed of OCT enables cardiologists to assess the long coronary plaque components in a few seconds. At present, 2 types of OCT systems, Frequency Domain OCT (St. Jude Medical, ST. Paul, Minnesota, USA) and Frequency Domain Optical Imaging (Terumo, Tokyo, Japan) are available for clinical use. The spatial resolution of OCT, nearly 10 μm on the lateral axis, is almost 10 times greater than that of IVUS. As shown

http://dx.doi.org/10.5772/61615

in Figure 1, OCT visualizes 3-layer structures of coronary artery. OCT-imaging technology allows cardiologists to examine tissue characterization of coronary atherosclerotic lesions *in vivo*.

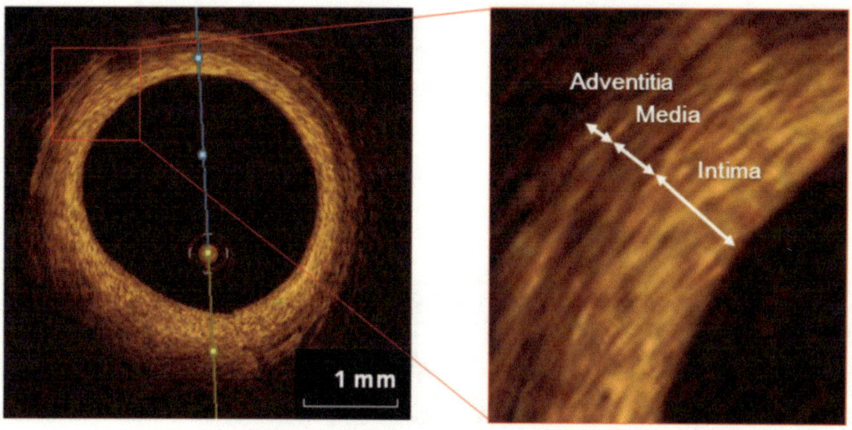

Figure 1. Representative optical coherence tomography images of the three layers of the vascular wall. Optical coherence tomography could identify the three layers of the vascular wall.

3. Coronary plaque vulnerability by OCT

Recently, several vulnerable features of coronary atherosclerosis have been suggested in both histopathological and clinical studies with the emerging use of OCT [1-3]. The ability of OCT in tissue characterization of coronary atherosclerotic lesions has been well-validated in clinicopathological studies [4-6]. OCT could provide detailed plaque morphology near to pathological assessment. OCT can provide three morphological features of coronary atherosclerosis: fibrous plaques, calcified plaques, and lipid-rich plaques (Figure 2). Fibrous plaque is defined as homogeneous, signal-rich regions with low attenuation. Calcified plaque is defined as well-delineated, signal-poor regions with sharp borders. Lipid-rich plaque is defined as signal-poor regions with diffuse borders.

The current understanding of the major cause of ACS is that it results from rupture of a vulnerable plaque. OCT is a high-resolution imaging technology that can provide detailed observation of the vulnerable coronary plaque. The main findings of vulnerable plaque by OCT are considered to be a TCFA, ruptured plaque, intracoronary thrombus, vasa vasorum, spotty calcification, macrophage infiltration, and cholesterol crystal (Figure 3).

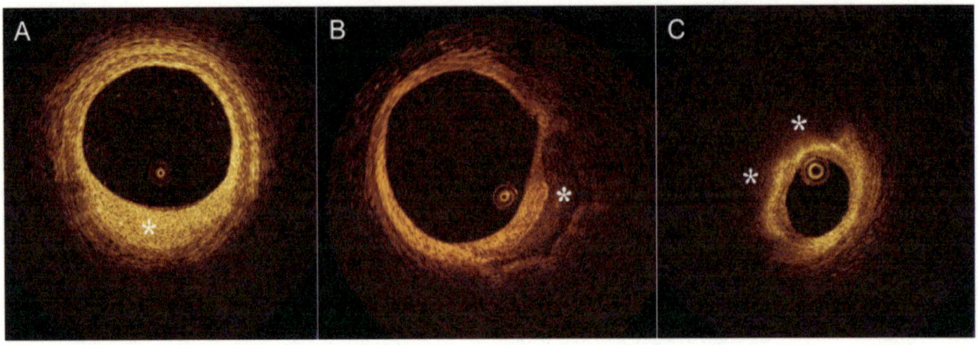

Figure 2. Plaque morphology by optical coherence tomography. (A) Fibrous plaque is defined as homogeneous, signal-rich regions with low attenuation. (B) Calcified plaque is defined as well-delineated, signal-poor regions with sharp borders. (C) Lipid-rich plaque is defined as signal-poor regions with diffuse borders.

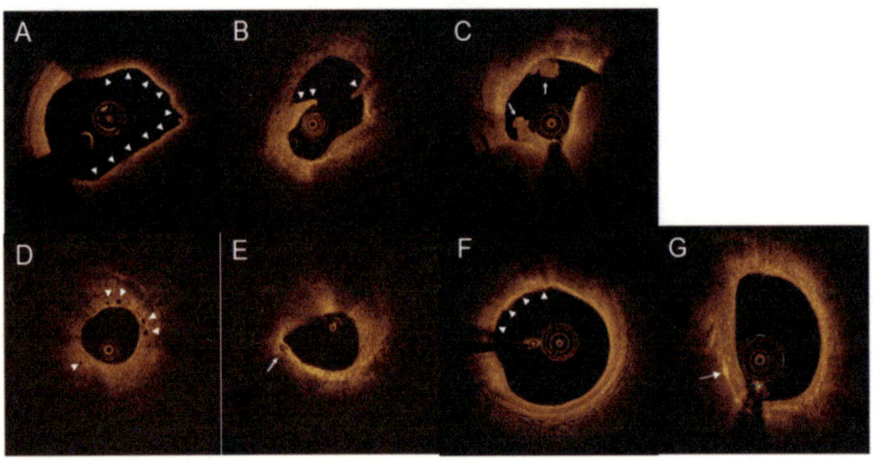

Figure 3. Vulnerable findings of optical coherence tomography images in coronary plaques. (A) Thin-cap fibroatheroma (TCFA), (B) Ruptured plaque, (C) Intracoronary thrombus, (D) Vasa vasorum, (E) Spotty calcification, (F) Macrophage infiltration, (G) Cholesterol crystal.

3.1. Thin-cap fibroatheroma

TCFA is considered when the fibrous cap thickness is ≤65 μm in the lipid-rich plaque. OCT–TCFA has relationship with several characteristics of vulnerable plaque in the other intracoronary imagings, such as attenuated plaque by gray-scale IVUS, necrotic plaque by virtual histology IVUS, and yellow plaque by intracoronary angioscopy [7-9]. Fibrous cap thickness is associated with serum C-reactive protein, oxidized low-density lipoprotein, and insulin resistance [10-12]. OCT–TCFA is a predictor of ACS and consequent plaque progression [13, 14].

http://dx.doi.org/10.5772/61615

3.2. Ruptured plaque

Ruptured plaque is defined as an intimal interruption and cavity formation in the plaque. OCT enables detection of ruptured plaque more frequently than IVUS. OCT examination after thrombus aspiration in patients with ACS revealed that 73% of patients showed ruptured plaque, and the mean thickness of the ruptured fibrous cap was 49 μm [15]. Ruptured plaque was often observed in non-culprit lesions of ACS especially in diabetic patients, which showed development of pan-coronary atherosclerosis.

3.3. Intracoronary thrombus

Intracoronary thrombus is a major cause of ACS, which is identified as an irregular high- or low-backscattering mass protruding into the lumen. OCT can distinguish between thrombus white and red thrombus [16]. White thrombus presents with a low-backscattering structure. Red thrombus presents with a high-backscattering structure with signal-free shadowing.

3.4. Vasa vasorum

Vasa vasorum plays a pivotal role in coronary plaque growth by increasing red blood cells, thereby supplying inflammatory cells and cytokines into the plaque. Sluimer et al. revealed that vasa vasorum was increased in advanced plaques compared with early plaques in a human histological study [17]. OCT has been proposed as a high-resolution imaging modality that can identify vasa vasorum as microchannels with tiny black holes (50-100 μm). The proliferation of vasa vasorum has been identified recently as a common feature of vulnerable plaque [18]. Kitabata et al. demonstrated increase of vasa vasorum counts in TCFA [19]. An observational study of OCT revealed that the presence of vasa vasorum in the plaques was also associated with positive remodeling and elevated high-sensitive C-reactive protein levels. The OCT evaluation of vasa vasorum counts might be helpful for assessing plaque vulnerability.

3.5. Spotty calcification

Clinical observations have suggested that the culprit lesions responsible for ACS are generally less calcified than those responsible for stable angina pectoris (SAP), indicating that calcium renders plaques more, rather than less stable [20]. However, the pattern of plaque calcification may also matter; a small amount of calcium was reported as a characteristic of vulnerable plaque that contributes to plaque instability. A pathological study by Burke et al. demonstrated that plaque rupture and TCFA, considered to represent vulnerable plaque, were most frequently associated with spotty calcification [21]. Previous IVUS studies have revealed a positive relationship in patients with acute myocardial infarction (AMI) between small and discrete calcifications within an arc of less than 90°, the presence of a fibrofatty plaque, and positive remodeling of the culprit arterial segment [22]. Recently, two OCT clinical studies as for spotty calcification (with an arc of <90°) have been reported. Kataoka Y et al. showed that plaques containing spotty calcification exhibited a greater lipid plaque volume, thinner fibrous caps (89.0 ± 31.6 μm vs. 136.5 ± 32.5 μm, P = 0.002) and a higher prevalence of vasa vasorum

(45.9% vs. 17.7%, P = 0.007) in the culprit lesion of SAP patients [23]. Another study reported by Mizukoshi M et al. showed that in the ACS patients compared with SAP patients spotty calcification was more frequently observed in the ACS patients compared with SAP patients and located close to the luminal surface [24]. Thus, spotty calcification detected by OCT was positive relationship with plaque vulnerability.

3.6. Macrophage infiltration

Degradation of the fibrous cap matrix by macrophages is associated with atherosclerotic plaque instability [25]. Macrophages infiltration detected by OCT were observed as a "bright spot," with a high signal variance from the surrounding tissue. Tearney et al. [26] and MacNeill et al. [27] descried OCT was capable to evaluate cap macrophage content accurately. High degree of positive correlation was observed between OCT and histological measurements of macrophage density in fibrous cap ($r < 0.84$, $P < 0.0001$). OCT provided detection of cap macrophage density >10% with 100% sensitivity and specificity [19].

3.7. Cholesterol crystal

Previous studies demonstrated that cholesterol crystallization is higher in vulnerable pathological examination [28]. Kellner-Weibel et al. suggested that, within the lesion, macrophages may have the pivotal role in initial nucleation and subsequent growth of cholesterol crystals [29]. Meanwhile, it has been shown that phagocytosis of cholesterol crystals by macrophages causes and advances an inflammation in the atherosclerotic plaques [30, 31]. OCT-imaging system with high-resolution could visualize structures suggestive of accumulations of cholesterol crystals *in vivo* [6]. Cholesterol crystal by OCT was defined as a thin linear region of high density without attenuation [32]. Clinical OCT studies have suggested that cholesterol crystals frequently coexist with the major findings of vulnerable plaque (spotty calcification, vasa vasorum, and lipid-rich plaque), and are often seen in poorly controlled diabetic patients [32].

4. In-stent neoatherosclerosis

In-stent neoatherosclerosis has been reported several years after drug-eluting stent (DES) and bare-metal stent (BMS) implantation. Neoatherosclerosis is more frequent and occurs earlier in patients undergoing DES implantation than those treated with BMS [33]. Neoatherosclerosis includes lipid accumulation, calcium deposition, macrophage infiltration, neovascularization within neointima, and results in very late stent failure including late stent thrombosis and in-stent restenosis [34]. OCT studies have reported that in both BMS and DES, neointima in the stent often comprises lipid-laden tissue in late phase of stent implantation and that expansion of neovascularization from peri-stent to intra-intima leads to atherosclerotic progression of neointima [35, 36]. Although the causes of neoatherosclerosis are unknown, Kato et al. recently showed that predictors of neoatherosclerosis are old stent age ≥48 months, DES usage, age ≥65 years old, current smoking, and chronic kidney disease [37].

5. Relationship vulnerable plaque by OCT and no-reflow phenomenon

Primary PCI is widely performed for patients with coronary artery disease. Sometimes, no-reflow phenomenon occurred during PCI in both patients with ACS and SAP, and no-reflow after PCI is associated with poor functional and clinical patient outcomes when compared with patients with adequate reflow [38, 39]. Thus, accurately detecting high-risk lesions of no-reflow phenomenon is warranted for interventional cardiologists. Recent OCT studies have shown that some vulnerable findings (lipid-rich plaque, TCFA, and spotty calcification) are predictors of no-reflow phenomenon. Ikenaga et al. showed that length of lipid pool was longer in the ST-segment resoluton (–) group than in the ST-segment resoluton (+) group in patients with ST elevation myocardial infarction (10.1 ± 2.8 mm and 7.8 ± 3.2 mm, p = 0.02) [40]. Lee et al. showed that TCFA was associated with cardiac troponin I elevation after PCI and the presence of TCFA was an independent predictor of periprocedural myocardial infarction (odds ratio, 10.47; 95% confidence interval, 3.74–29.28; P < 0.001) [39]. Tanaka et al. showed that TCFA was more often observed in the no-reflow group than in the reflow group (50% vs. 16%, P = 0.005) and the frequency of the no-reflow phenomenon increased according to the size of the lipid arc in the culprit lesion in patients with ACS (Lipid arc 1–90°, 4.7%; 91–180°, 35%; 181–360°, 75%) [41]. Furthermore, Ueda et al. showed that colocalization of TCFA and spotty calcification was an independent predictor of PCI-related cardiac troponin T elevation (odds ratio 8.40, 95% confidence interval 1.65–52.78, P < 0.01) [42]. Thus, OCT could be a useful tool for risk stratification of PCI.

6. Considering optimal medical therapy for vulnerable plaque with OCT

Atherosclerosis has an important inflammatory component and acute cardiovascular events can be initiated by inflammatory processes occurring in vulnerable plaques. The current understanding of the major cause of ACS is that it results from rupture of a vulnerable plaque. OCT is a high-resolution imaging technology that can provide detailed observation of the vulnerable coronary plaque. TCFA is the most typical OCT findings as a vulnerable plaque. OMT is regarded as one of the effective treatments for the stabilization of coronary vulnerable plaques, and it reduces the risk of coronary events and mortality. Intensive lipid-lowering therapy with statins is regarded as one of the effective treatments for the stabilization of coronary artery plaques, and reduces the risk for coronary events and mortality [43]. Serial OCT observations could explain this efficacy of statin therapy. Takarada et al. showed that statin therapy for 9 months after the onset of AMI significantly increased the fibrous-cap thickness in patients with hyperlipidemia (151 +/- 110 μm to 280 +/- 120 μm, P < 0.01) [44]. However, cardiovascular events occur in some patients even with statin therapy, and residual risk has become a problem. Habara et al. showed the effect of ezetimibe in addition to fluvastatin on the progression of coronary vulnerable plaque evaluated by OCT. The change in the fibrous cap thickness was significantly greater in the ezetimibe and fluvastatin group than in the fluvastatin alone group (0.08 ± 0.08 mm vs 0.04 ± 0.06 mm, P < 0.001) [45]. The Japan EPA (eicosapentaenoic acid) Lipid Intervention Study, which was a large randomized clinical trial, showed that purified EPA administration along with statin therapy reduced the incidence of coronary events by 19% [46]. Hasegawa et al. showed that lower EPA/AA ratio was associated with higher vulnerability of coronary plaques by OCT examination. The low EPA/AA group had wider maximum lipid arc (114.0 ± 94.8° vs. 56.4 ± 66.0°, p = 0.0097), longer lipid length (4.8 ± 4.5 mm vs. 1.6 ± 2.6 mm, p = 0.0037), and thinner fibrous cap (69.3 ± 28.3 μm vs. 113.3 ± 46.6 μm, p = 0.005) compared with the high EPA/AA group [47]. Nishio et al. showed that the EPA and statin group had a greater increase in fibrous-cap thickness, with a greater decrease in lipid arc and lipid length compared with the statin alone group [48].

7. Conclusion

OCT is a high-resolution imaging technology that can provide detailed observation of vulnerable coronary atherosclerotic plaques in clinical settings. Since only OCT imaging of coronary artery is not able to accurately predict the future adverse events in patients with coronary artery disease (CAD), bringing together clinical data obtained by OCT with clinical data will improve future outcome of patients with CAD. Further developments in imaging technology could enable cardiologists to precisely detect vulnerable plaques in coronary artery and to improve more optimal treatments for vulnerable patients.

Author details

Takao Hasegawa and Kenei Shimada*

*Address all correspondence to: shimadak@med.osaka-cu.ac.jp

Department of Internal Medicine and Cardiology, Osaka City University Graduate School of Medicine, Abeno-ku, Osaka, Japan

References

[1] Bourantas CV, Garcia-Garcia HM, Serruys PW. Letter by Bourantas et al. regarding article, "Nonculprit plaques in patients with acute coronary syndromes have more vulnerable features compared with those with non-acute coronary syndromes: a 3-vessel optical coherence tomography study." *Circ Cardiovasc Imaging*. 2012 Nov; 5(6):e68. 23169984.

[2] Kato K, Yonetsu T, Kim SJ, Xing L, Lee H, McNulty I, et al. Nonculprit plaques in patients with acute coronary syndromes have more vulnerable features compared with those with non-acute coronary syndromes: a 3-vessel optical coherence tomography study. *Circ Cardiovasc Imaging*. 2012 Jul;5(4):433-40. 22679059.

[3] Ambrose JA. In search of the "vulnerable plaque." Can it be localized and will focal regional therapy ever be an option for cardiac prevention? *J Am Coll Cardiol.* 2008 Apr 22;51(16):1539-42. 18420095.

[4] Kume T, Akasaka T, Kawamoto T, Watanabe N, Toyota E, Neishi Y, et al. Assessment of coronary arterial plaque by optical coherence tomography. *Am J Cardiol.* 2006 Apr 15;97(8):1172-5. 16616021.

[5] Rieber J, Meissner O, Babaryka G, Reim S, Oswald M, Koenig A, et al. Diagnostic accuracy of optical coherence tomography and intravascular ultrasound for the detection and characterization of atherosclerotic plaque composition in ex-vivo coronary specimens: a comparison with histology. *Coron Artery Dis.* 2006 Aug;17(5):425-30. 16845250.

[6] Tearney GJ, Regar E, Akasaka T, Adriaenssens T, Barlis P, Bezerra HG, et al. Consensus standards for acquisition, measurement, and reporting of intravascular optical coherence tomography studies: a report from the International Working Group for Intravascular Optical Coherence Tomography Standardization and Validation. *J Am Coll Cardiol.* 2012 Mar 20;59(12):1058-72. 22421299.

[7] Takano M, Jang IK, Inami S, Yamamoto M, Murakami D, Okamatsu K, et al. In vivo comparison of optical coherence tomography and angioscopy for the evaluation of coronary plaque characteristics. *Am J Cardiol.* 2008 Feb 15;101(4):471-6. 18312760.

[8] Kubo T, Matsuo Y, Ino Y, Tanimoto T, Ishibashi K, Komukai K, et al. Optical coherence tomography analysis of attenuated plaques detected by intravascular ultrasound in patients with acute coronary syndromes. *Cardiol Res Pract.* 2011;2011:687515. 21941667. Pubmed Central PMCID: 3173965.

[9] Sukiennik A, Radomski M, Rychter M, Kubica J. Usefulness of optical coherence tomography in the assessment of atherosclerotic culprit lesions in acute coronary syndromes. Comparison with intravascular ultrasound and virtual histology. *Cardiol J.* 2008;15(6):561-3. 19039763.

[10] Takarada S, Imanishi T, Ishibashi K, Tanimoto T, Komukai K, Ino Y, et al. The effect of lipid and inflammatory profiles on the morphological changes of lipid-rich plaques in patients with non-ST-segment elevated acute coronary syndrome: follow-up study by optical coherence tomography and intravascular ultrasound. *JACC Cardiovasc Intervent.* 2010 Jul;3(7):766-72. 20650439.

[11] Matsuo Y, Kubo T, Okumoto Y, Ishibashi K, Komukai K, Tanimoto T, et al. Circulating malondialdehyde-modified low-density lipoprotein levels are associated with the presence of thin-cap fibroatheromas determined by optical coherence tomography in coronary artery disease. *Eur Heart J Cardiovasc Imaging.* 2013 Jan;14(1):43-50. 22573905.

[12] Iguchi T, Hasegawa T, Otsuka K, Matsumoto K, Yamazaki T, Nishimura S, et al. Insulin resistance is associated with coronary plaque vulnerability: insight from optical

coherence tomography analysis. *Eur Heart J Cardiovasc Imaging*. 2014 Mar;15(3): 284-91. 24022065.

[13] Bouki KP, Katsafados MG, Chatzopoulos DN, Psychari SN, Toutouzas KP, Charalampopoulos AF, et al. Inflammatory markers and plaque morphology: an optical coherence tomography study. *Int J Cardiol*. 2012 Feb 9;154(3):287-92. 20974497.

[14] Uemura S, Ishigami K, Soeda T, Okayama S, Sung JH, Nakagawa H, et al. Thin-cap fibroatheroma and microchannel findings in optical coherence tomography correlate with subsequent progression of coronary atheromatous plaques. *Eur Heart J*. 2012 Jan;33(1):78-85. 21831910.

[15] Kubo T, Imanishi T, Takarada S, Kuroi A, Ueno S, Yamano T, et al. Assessment of culprit lesion morphology in acute myocardial infarction: ability of optical coherence tomography compared with intravascular ultrasound and coronary angioscopy. *J Am Coll Cardiol*. 2007 Sep 4;50(10):933-9. 17765119.

[16] Kume T, Akasaka T, Kawamoto T, Ogasawara Y, Watanabe N, Toyota E, et al. Assessment of coronary arterial thrombus by optical coherence tomography. *Am J Cardiol*. 2006 Jun 15;97(12):1713-7. 16765119.

[17] Sluimer JC, Kolodgie FD, Bijnens AP, Maxfield K, Pacheco E, Kutys B, et al. Thin-walled microvessels in human coronary atherosclerotic plaques show incomplete endothelial junctions relevance of compromised structural integrity for intraplaque microvascular leakage. *J Am Coll Cardiol*. 2009 Apr 28;53(17):1517-27. 19389562. Pubmed Central PMCID: 2756458.

[18] Kolodgie FD, Gold HK, Burke AP, Fowler DR, Kruth HS, Weber DK, et al. Intraplaque hemorrhage and progression of coronary atheroma. *New Eng J Med*. 2003 Dec 11;349(24):2316-25. 14668457. Epub 2003/12/12. eng.

[19] Kitabata H, Tanaka A, Kubo T, Takarada S, Kashiwagi M, Tsujioka H, et al. Relation of microchannel structure identified by optical coherence tomography to plaque vulnerability in patients with coronary artery disease. *Am J Cardiol*. 2010 Jun 15;105(12): 1673-8. 20538113.

[20] Beckman JA, Ganz J, Creager MA, Ganz P, Kinlay S. Relationship of clinical presentation and calcification of culprit coronary artery stenoses. *Arterioscler Thromb Vasc Biol*. 2001 Oct;21(10):1618-22. 11597935. Epub 2001/10/13. eng.

[21] Burke AP, Weber DK, Kolodgie FD, Farb A, Taylor AJ, Virmani R. Pathophysiology of calcium deposition in coronary arteries. *Herz*. 2001 Jun;26(4):239-44. 11479935. Epub 2001/08/02. eng.

[22] Fujii K, Carlier SG, Mintz GS, Takebayashi H, Yasuda T, Costa RA, et al. Intravascular ultrasound study of patterns of calcium in ruptured coronary plaques. *Am J Cardiol*. 2005 Aug 1;96(3):352-7. 16054456. Epub 2005/08/02. eng.

[23] Kataoka Y, Puri R, Hammadah M, Duggal B, Uno K, Kapadia SR, et al. Spotty calcification and plaque vulnerability in vivo: frequency-domain optical coherence tomog-

raphy analysis. *Cardiovasc Diagn Ther*. 2014 Dec;4(6):460-9. 25610803. Pubmed Central PMCID: 4278040.

[24] Mizukoshi M, Kubo T, Takarada S, Kitabata H, Ino Y, Tanimoto T, et al. Coronary superficial and spotty calcium deposits in culprit coronary lesions of acute coronary syndrome as determined by optical coherence tomography. *Am J Cardiol*. 2013 Jul 1;112(1):34-40. 23540654.

[25] Moreno PR, Falk E, Palacios IF, Newell JB, Fuster V, Fallon JT. Macrophage infiltration in acute coronary syndromes. Implications for plaque rupture. *Circulation*. 1994 Aug;90(2):775-8. 8044947. Epub 1994/08/01. eng.

[26] Tearney GJ, Yabushita H, Houser SL, Aretz HT, Jang IK, Schlendorf KH, et al. Quantification of macrophage content in atherosclerotic plaques by optical coherence tomography. *Circulation*. 2003 Jan 7;107(1):113-9. 12515752. Epub 2003/01/08. eng.

[27] Hoffmann R, Mintz GS, Dussaillant GR, Popma JJ, Pichard AD, Satler LF, et al. Patterns and mechanisms of in-stent restenosis. A serial intravascular ultrasound study. *Circulation*. 1996 Sep 15;94(6):1247-54. 8822976. Epub 1996/09/15. eng.

[28] Abela GS, Aziz K, Vedre A, Pathak DR, Talbott JD, Dejong J. Effect of cholesterol crystals on plaques and intima in arteries of patients with acute coronary and cerebrovascular syndromes. *Am J Cardiol*. 2009 Apr 1;103(7):959-68. 19327423. Epub 2009/03/31. eng.

[29] Kellner-Weibel G, Yancey PG, Jerome WG, Walser T, Mason RP, Phillips MC, et al. Crystallization of free cholesterol in model macrophage foam cells. *Arterioscler Thromb Vasc Biol*. 1999 Aug;19(8):1891-8. 10446067. Epub 1999/08/14. eng.

[30] Rajamaki K, Lappalainen J, Oorni K, Valimaki E, Matikainen S, Kovanen PT, et al. Cholesterol crystals activate the NLRP3 inflammasome in human macrophages: a novel link between cholesterol metabolism and inflammation. *PloS One*. 2010;5(7):e11765. 20668705. Pubmed Central PMCID: PMC2909263. Epub 2010/07/30. eng.

[31] Duewell P, Kono H, Rayner KJ, Sirois CM, Vladimer G, Bauernfeind FG, et al. NLRP3 inflammasomes are required for atherogenesis and activated by cholesterol crystals. *Nature*. 2010 Apr 29;464(7293):1357-61. 20428172. Pubmed Central PMCID: PMC2946640. Epub 2010/04/30. eng.

[32] Nakamura S, Inami S, Murai K, Takano M, Takano H, Asai K, et al. Relationship between cholesterol crystals and culprit lesion characteristics in patients with stable coronary artery disease: an optical coherence tomography study. *Clin Res Cardiol*: Official Journal of the German Cardiac Society. 2014 Dec;103(12):1015-21. 25086962.

[33] Nakazawa G, Otsuka F, Nakano M, Vorpahl M, Yazdani SK, Ladich E, et al. The pathology of neoatherosclerosis in human coronary implants bare-metal and drug-

eluting stents. *J Am Coll Cardiol*. 2011 Mar 15;57(11):1314-22. 21376502. Pubmed Central PMCID: 3093310.

[34] Park SJ, Kang SJ, Virmani R, Nakano M, Ueda Y. In-stent neoatherosclerosis: a final common pathway of late stent failure. *J Am Coll Cardiol*. 2012 Jun 5;59(23):2051-7. 22651862.

[35] Takano M, Yamamoto M, Inami S, Murakami D, Ohba T, Seino Y, et al. Appearance of lipid-laden intima and neovascularization after implantation of bare-metal stents extended late-phase observation by intracoronary optical coherence tomography. *J Am Coll Cardiol*. 2009 Dec 29;55(1):26-32. 20117359.

[36] Kang SJ, Mintz GS, Akasaka T, Park DW, Lee JY, Kim WJ, et al. Optical coherence tomographic analysis of in-stent neoatherosclerosis after drug-eluting stent implantation. *Circulation*. 2011 Jun 28;123(25):2954-63. 21646494.

[37] Yonetsu T, Kato K, Kim SJ, Xing L, Jia H, McNulty I, et al. Predictors for neoatherosclerosis: a retrospective observational study from the optical coherence tomography registry. *Circ Cardiovasc Imaging*. 2012 Sep 1;5(5):660-6. 22798521.

[38] Morishima I, Sone T, Okumura K, Tsuboi H, Kondo J, Mukawa H, et al. Angiographic no-reflow phenomenon as a predictor of adverse long-term outcome in patients treated with percutaneous transluminal coronary angioplasty for first acute myocardial infarction. *J Am Coll Cardiol*. 2000 Oct;36(4):1202-9. 11028471.

[39] Lee T, Yonetsu T, Koura K, Hishikari K, Murai T, Iwai T, et al. Impact of coronary plaque morphology assessed by optical coherence tomography on cardiac troponin elevation in patients with elective stent implantation. *Circ Cardiovasc Intervent*. 2011 Aug;4(4):378-86. 21791670.

[40] Ikenaga H, Ishihara M, Inoue I, Kawagoe T, Shimatani Y, Miura F, et al. Longitudinal extent of lipid pool assessed by optical coherence tomography predicts microvascular no-reflow after primary percutaneous coronary intervention for ST-segment elevation myocardial infarction. *J Cardiol*. 2013 Aug;62(2):71-6. 23680004.

[41] Tanaka A, Imanishi T, Kitabata H, Kubo T, Takarada S, Tanimoto T, et al. Lipid-rich plaque and myocardial perfusion after successful stenting in patients with non-ST-segment elevation acute coronary syndrome: an optical coherence tomography study. *Eur Heart J*. 2009 Jun;30(11):1348-55. 19383736.

[42] Ueda T, Uemura S, Watanabe M, Sugawara Y, Soeda T, Okayama S, et al. Colocalization of thin-cap fibroatheroma and spotty calcification is a powerful predictor of procedure-related myocardial injury after elective coronary stent implantation. *Coron Artery Dis*. 2014 Aug;25(5):384-91. 24681754.

[43] LaRosa JC, Grundy SM, Waters DD, Shear C, Barter P, Fruchart JC, et al. Intensive lipid lowering with atorvastatin in patients with stable coronary disease. *New Eng J Med*. 2005 Apr 7;352(14):1425-35. 15755765.

[44] Takarada S, Imanishi T, Kubo T, Tanimoto T, Kitabata H, Nakamura N, et al. Effect of statin therapy on coronary fibrous-cap thickness in patients with acute coronary syndrome: assessment by optical coherence tomography study. *Atherosclerosis.* 2009 Feb;202(2):491-7. 18572175.

[45] Habara M, Nasu K, Terashima M, Ko E, Yokota D, Ito T, et al. Impact on optical coherence tomographic coronary findings of fluvastatin alone versus fluvastatin + ezetimibe. *Am J Cardiol.* 2014 Feb 15;113(4):580-7. 24388622.

[46] Yokoyama M, Origasa H, Matsuzaki M, Matsuzawa Y, Saito Y, Ishikawa Y, et al. Effects of eicosapentaenoic acid on major coronary events in hypercholesterolaemic patients (JELIS): a randomised open-label, blinded endpoint analysis. *Lancet.* 2007 Mar 31;369(9567):1090-8. 17398308.

[47] Hasegawa T, Otsuka K, Iguchi T, Matsumoto K, Ehara S, Nakata S, et al. Serum n-3 to n-6 polyunsaturated fatty acids ratio correlates with coronary plaque vulnerability: an optical coherence tomography study. *Heart Vess.* 2014 Sep;29(5):596-602. 24005765.

[48] Nishio R, Shinke T, Otake H, Nakagawa M, Nagoshi R, Inoue T, et al. Stabilizing effect of combined eicosapentaenoic acid and statin therapy on coronary thin-cap fibroatheroma. *Atherosclerosis.* 2014 May;234(1):114-9. 24637411.

Chapter 5

Coronary CT Angiography and the Napkin-ring Sign Indicates High-Risk Atherosclerotic Lesions

Lucia Agoston-Coldea, Carmen Cionca and Silvia Lupu

Additional information is available at the end of the chapter

http://dx.doi.org/10.5772/61393

Abstract

Coronary computed tomography angiography (CCTA) is used extensively nowadays as a non-invasive imaging method for the evaluation of patients suspected of coronary artery disease, providing data on calcium burden, the presence of coronary artery stenoses, but also, more recently, on coronary atherosclerotic plaque morphology and composition. Plaque morphology analysis by CCTA aims to accurately identify vulnerable plaques, in an attempt to reduce the number of ischemic events triggered by high-risk atherosclerotic lesions. Recent research provides CCTA descriptions of vulnerable plaques and a particular radiological sign shows promising perspectives. The napkin-ring sign refers to a rupture-prone plaque in a coronary artery, comprising a necrotic core covered by a thin cap fibro-atheroma. The napkin-ring sign is described on CCTA in cross-sectional images of coronary arteries as a central low-attenuation area surrounded by an open ring area of high attenuation, having a high specificity and positive predictive value for the presence of advanced lesions. These lesions have been designated as vulnerable plaques, indicating an increased probability of rupture, and were shown to correlate with a higher incidence of cardiovascular events. In acute coronary syndromes, the location of the napkin-ring sign was shown to correspond to the culprit lesions. The aim of the current paper is to provide an overview of the current literature on available methods for quantitative measurement of atherosclerotic plaque features from CCTA and to discuss the clinical implications of the napkin-ring sign as detected by CCTA.

Keywords: Coronary computed tomography angiography, Coronary artery plaque, Napkin-ring sign, Plaque quantification, Plaque characterization

1. Introduction

The development of atherosclerosis by lipoprotein storage, inflammation, muscle cell proliferation, necrosis, apoptosis, calcification, and fibrosis in the arterial wall triggers important changes in the coronary vessels, leading to coronary artery disease (CAD). In fact, atherosclerosis is the main etiology of CAD, and plaque rupture followed by intraluminal thrombosis is the most common cause of acute coronary events, including sudden coronary death [1, 2]. For that reason, the early and accurate characterization and quantification of atherosclerotic plaques is valuable for preventing and managing acute coronary syndrome (ACS) [3]. In everyday clinical practice, major acute ischemic cardiac events involve plaque rupture in thin-cap fibroatheromas, which are considered vulnerable plaques; these rupture-prone atherosclerotic lesions usually contain a high level of lipids and have a large necrotic core, numerous inflammatory cells, and a thin, vulnerable fibrotic cap [4]. Vulnerable atherosclerotic plaques can be characterized by several invasive and non-invasive methods that are either fully validated, pending validation, or still under scrutiny for clinical practice. Among non-invasive methods, coronary computed tomography angiography (CCTA) by multi-detector computed tomography (MDCT) is currently the preferred modality for evaluating the extent of CAD, providing the advantage of accurate assessment of coronary atherosclerotic plaque morphology and composition. In two recent multicenter trials [5, 6], CCTA was shown to have excellent sensitivity (95–99%) and negative predictive value (97–99%), although rather low specificity (64–83%) for identifying patients with at least one coronary artery stenosis among individuals at low to intermediate risk for CAD. Moreover, CCTA imaging of atherosclerotic plaques was found to correlate well with invasive assessment by intravascular ultrasound (IVUS) [7, 8, 9].

2. Role of MDCT in the detection of plaque morphology and composition

2.1. Plaque characteristics

2.1.1. Plaque morphology and composition

Pathophysiologically, a subendothelial accumulation of lipoproteins generates inflammatory responses involving macrophages and T-cells, leading to the further development of atherosclerotic lesions [10]. Initially, atherosclerotic lesions were classified as fatty streaks, fibroatheromas [11], and advanced plaques, complicated with hemorrhage, calcification, ulceration, and thrombosis [12]. Over the years, this classification became more complex and six types of atherosclerotic lesions have been defined by the American Heart Association (AHA) Consensus Group: type I - characterized by adaptive intimal thickening; type II - fatty streak; type III - transitional or intermediate lesions; type IV - advanced plaques (atheromas); type V - fibroatheroma or atheroma with thick fibrous cap; and type VI - complicated plaques with denudated surface, and/or hematoma/hemorrhage, and/or thrombosis [13]. The earliest lesions are represented by adaptive intimal thickening (AHA type I) and fatty streaks or intimal xanthoma, which are basically foam cell collections (AHA type II) [13]. AHA type III transi-

http://dx.doi.org/10.5772/61393

tional lesions, described as pathological intimal thickening, represent the earliest stage of the progressive plaques and are considered precursor lesions of more advanced fibroatheroma. This type of lesions consists of multiple layers of proliferating smooth muscle cells near the lumen, with an increased quantity of lipids on the intimal medial border. Intimal xanthomas are lesions containing a large amount of foamy macrophages but without lipid acumulation outside the cell [14]. Type IV AHA, also called fibrous cap atheromas, are the first of the advanced lesions of coronary atherosclerosis [15] and are characterized by the presence of a necrotic core with a high amount of lipids surrounded by a fibrous cap containing smooth muscle cells, collagen, and proteoglicans, as well as inflammatory cells such as macrophages and lymphocytes. This type of lesion can cause significant artery stenosis and may be submitted to complications, namely surface disruption, thrombosis, and calcification. Fibrous cap plaques may be more or less prone to complications depending on the thickness of the cap: fibroatheromas are more stable due to the rather thick fibrous cap, while thin-cap fibroatheromas characterize the typycal "vulnerable plaques" [15].

In fact, thin-cap fibroatheromas are very likely to lead to plaque rupture. Although they are not included as individual entities in the AHA consensus classification, plaque erosion and calcified nodules are also prone to coronary thrombosis. Erosions may occur on intimal thickening or fibroatheroma, whereas the notion of calcified nodules refers to eruptive fragments of calcium that protrude into the lumen, causing a thrombotic event [16]. Also, plaque ruptures may heal by wide accumulation of proteoglycans, having more reduced necrotic cores and more extensive areas of calcification. In their study on early coronary lesion progression near branch points, Nakashima et al. provided evidence endorsing the hypothesis that intimal thickening lesions with macrophages are more advanced [17].

Macrophage infiltration in lipid pools rich in cholesterol and the deterioration of the extracellular matrix believed to be induced by matrix metalloproteinase activity suggest early stages of the necrosis process and should be recognized. This particular feature, combined with macrophage destruction as a consequence of an anomalous phagocytic clearance of apoptotic cells, may contribute to the development of late plaque necrosis. In addition to that, an extended necrotic core is a strong predictor of complications [17, 18].

Thin-cap fibroatheromas are highly prone to plaque rupture due to their rather large necrotic core and thin, inflamed fibrous cap (<65 μm). The accumulation of an increased number of macrophages at the level of the cap is characteristic, although exceptions may occur. However, as a significant number of fatal coronary events are triggered by plaque rupture due to the impairment of the fibrous cap followed by thrombosis, early recognition of thin-cap fibroatheromas is crucial. The fibrous cap mainly contains type I collagen, variable numbers of macrophages and lymphocytes, and rather few alpha-actin positive smooth muscle cells. Fibrous cap disruption exposes the lipid-rich necrotic core, favoring the formation of local thrombi by platelet accumulation. Most plaque ruptures are reported in the proximal segments of the coronary arteries, near branch points, with the left anterior descending coronary artery being the most frequently affected, followed by the right and left circumflex coronary arteries [19]. Although the mechanisms behind plaque rupture are far from being fully understood, the increased activity of matrix metalloproteinases, excessive enzyme secretion by inflammatory cells, high shear stress, macrophage calcification, and iron build-up are recognized as implicated factors. Data are also beginning to pool on different gene expression in stable and unstable atherosclerotic plaques [20]. For instance, in one study, differential expression of 18 genes coding for metalloproteinase ADAMDEC1, retinoic acid receptor responser-1, cysteine protease legumain (a potential activator of matrix metalloproteinases), and cathepsins was shown to contribute to increased lesion vulnerability [20]. As previously mentioned, the extension of the necrotic core is also a main factor in plaque complication development, and intraplaque hemorrhage was shown to favor the accumulation of free cholesterol provided by red blood cells in these lesions [21]. As atherosclerotic lesions expand, more vasa vasorum infiltrate the plaque and become leaky, triggering intraplaque hemorrhage [22]. Morphologic studies have suggested that repeated ruptures are responsible for plaque progression beyond 40–50% cross-sectional luminal stenoses [23]. Three hystological types of lesions have been described in association with acute coronary events: rupture, erosion, and calcified nodule [13]. Ruptured coronary atherosclerotic plaques folowed by intraluminal thrombosis are the most common cause of acute myocardial infarction [24]. In fact, two-thirds of luminal thrombi in acute events result from ruptured atherosclerotic lesions characterized by a necrotic core covered by a thin layer of fibrous cap [4]. Ruptured plaques are characterized by a lipid-rich necrotic core (>40% of the total volume of the plaque), surrounded by a thin, fibrous cap with active inflammation (increased number of monocytes, macrophages, and sometimes even T-cells), endothelial denudation leading to superficial platelet aggregation, and the presence of hemodynamically significant coronary artery stenosis (>90%) [19]. Vulnerable plaques prone to rupture share most of the morphological characteristics with ruptured plaques, showing a large necrotic core, macrophage infiltration, and often an increased number of intraplaque vasa vasorum [4], but an intact, thin fibrous cap [13]. These lesions—called thin-cap fibroatheromas—are considered to be at high risk for rupture and subsequent ischemic events [4].

The destruction of the endothelium exposes the minimally inflammed intima containing smooth muscle cells and proteoglycans to circulating platelets, favoring thrombus formation. In a post-mortem study of 20 patients who died with acute myocardial infarction, plaque ruptures were found in 60% of lesions with thrombi, while the remainder of 40% only revealed superficial erosion [16]. Plaque erosion refers to the lack of endothelial cells on the luminal surface beneath the thrombus. Kramer et al. showed in their study that, when plaque erosion was the incriminated lesion, the thrombus was limited to the luminal portion of the plaque, and no ruptures were identified following serial sectioning of these lesions. In the same study, more than 85% of thrombi in erosions showed evidence of healing, such as acute inflammatory cell lysis, invasion by smooth muscle cells and/or endothelial cells, or organized layers of smooth muscle cells and proteoglycans with varying degrees of platelet/fibrin layering. By contrast, only half of the ruptured plaques showed signs of healing [25].

Beyond histopathological description, a clinically relevant definition of vulnerable plaques refers to the risk of developing future major cardiac events, which may also involve the presence of "vulnerable blood" (prone to hypercoagulability) or "vulnerable myocardium" (susceptible to arrhythmia), either due to acute or pre-existing ischemia and/or non-ischemic electrophysiological anomalies. The presence of one or more of these elements elevates the individual risk of the patients for cardiovascular events, turning them into "vulnerable patients".

Identifying vulnerable plaques is currently a major challenge, although recent progress in cardiovascular imaging raises new possibilities. As vulnerable plaques are prone to rupture and rapid evolution towards the development of ACS, [26, 27, 28] finding reliable imaging characteristics that could help detect unstable plaques are of the utmost importance. Early identification of such plaques could facilitate timely initiation of adequate primary prevention measures, thus diminishing the incidence of acute coronary events [29]. For this purpose, several imaging methods have been proposed, including IVUS, optical coherence tomography (OCT), magnetic resonance imaging (MRI), or MDCT (Table 1), with variable success [30, 31, 32]. However, the use of many of these methods is mainly confined to experimental studies and has not yet been validated for everyday clinical practice.

Non-invasive imaging methods	Advantages	Limitations
- MDCT	Measures local tissue attenuation to assess plaque morphology and composition Molecular imaging using new contrast agents is under study Identifies lumen narrowing accurately Can help characterize plaque morphology and composition (within limits) Has high spatial and temporal resolution	Patient exposure to ionizing radiation Implies contrast agent use May be hindered by artifacts (e.g., blooming) The attenuation spectrum of non-calcified plaque components (lipid and fibrous) can overlap
- Contrast-enhanced ultrasonography	Uses acoustically active microbubbles acting as pure intravascular tracers; when exposed to ultrasound, they produce a strong backscatter signal and specific nonlinear signal that differentiates them from surrounding tissues Molecular imaging is available There is no exposure to ionizing radiation Has high temporal and spatial resolution Allows neovasculature assessment	Spatial resolution and penetration are limited Good application for coronary arteries
- High-resolution magnetic resonace imaging	Uses different contrast weightings (T1, T2, proton-density, and time-of-flight) to evaluate plaque components Molecular imaging uses specific agents (paramagnetic nanoparticles targeting) Has high temporal and spatial resolution Has high contrast resolution	Contraindicated with many intracardiac devices Cardiac motion Poor reproducibility Contrast agent Limited spatial resolution Time consuming reconstruction techniques
Invasive imaging methods		

Non-invasive imaging methods	Advantages	Limitations
- Coronary angiography	Identifies complex plaques, with irregular surface Quantifies stenoses accurately	Invasive Limited tissue penetration and spatial resolution
- IVUS		
Standard	Quantifies plaque volume, vascular remodeling, and neovascularization Characterizes plaque morphology and composition	Invasive Limited temporal resolution Limited spatial resolution prevents thin cap fibroatheroma quantification Low accuracy for detecting plaque composition by gray scale IVUS
IVUS elastography	Measures the local strain rate of vessel wall and plaque (fibrous plaques are stiffer than lipid-rich ones); high strain regions describe more vulnerable plaques	Invasive Limited spatial resolution Artefacted by cardiac motion
Virtual histology	Identifies the necrotic core, fibro-lipidic plaques, calcified, and non-calcified plaques	Invasive Limited spatial resolution
- Optical methods		
Angioscopy	Identifies lipid plaques, plaque rupture, erosion, and thrombosis	Invasive Limited tissue penetration and spatial resolution
OCT	Provides microscopic characterization of plaque morphology Identifies macrophages presence Allows accurate quantification of the fibrous plaque Highest spatial resolution of all imaging methods Can identify thin fibrous caps <65 μm The only technique for eroded plaques detection Accurate detection of plaque composition	Invasive Limited tissue penetration; however, the most relevant morphologic findings are primarily localized within the first 500 μm under lumen surface
Spectroscopy	Identifies the lipid core and evaluates the chemical structure, temperature and inflammation of the plaque	Invasive Limited tissue penetration Cardiac motion
- Termography	Quantifies plaque temperature Detects plaque inflammation and neoangiogenesis	Invasive Limited tissue penetration and spatial resolution The cooling effect of the blood leads to underestimated temperature differences
- Intravascular cardiac MRI	Quantifies the lipid content of the plaque	Invasive Prolonged duration

http://dx.doi.org/10.5772/61393

Non-invasive imaging methods	Advantages	Limitations
		Implies the use of contrast agents
Plasma markers of plaque vulnerability	Identifies blood hypercoagulability states (augmented platelet activation and aggregation, high levels of coagulation factors, low levels of anticoagulation factors, decreased endogenous fibrinolytic activity, thrombogenic factors)	

Table 1. Methods for the Identification and Characterization of Vulnerable Plaques

A possible imaging method for coronary artery plaque assessment is IVUS, which has been used to measure lumen area, plaque burden, and vascular remodeling [33, 34]; plaque burden and positive remodeling, in particular, can identify high-risk, thin-cap fibroatheromas during follow-up [34, 35, 36]. As suggested by IVUS-based studies, a vulnerable plaque is characterized by the presence of an extensive necrotic core surrounded by a thin-cap fibrous with macrophage infiltration, a large lipid pool, and several more specific traits such as positive remodeling or spotty calcifications [37, 38]. When such characteristics occur, there is an increased risk of fibrous rupture, exposing the thrombogenic lipid core, which leads to thrombus formation and the development of ACS. A more detailed analysis of coronary plaque composition has been provided by virtual histology (VH)-IVUS studies [39, 40, 41].

Another recently developed method for the assessment of coronary artery plaques quantification is intracoronary OCT that provides the advantage of very high resolution (approximately 10 to 20 μm), which is about 10-fold higher than that of IVUS [42, 43]. Unlike some other imaging methods, including CCTA [27, 44, 45], OCT can be used for measuring fibrous cap thickness and for detecting lipid content, which makes it useful for in vivo identification of thin-cap fibroatheromas and for evaluating plaque vulnerability [46]. For the time being, the correspondence between OCT- and IVUS-derived characteristics of thin-cap fibroatheromas, as well as the angiographic stenosis severity, is yet to be established.

As advanced coronary artery plaques have a high level of complexity, basic classifications that include non-calcified plaques, calcified plaques, and mixed plaques are rather crude and of limited use for establishing the potential risk for acute ischemic clinical events of individual lesions [4, 26, 47]. For that reason, some authors have attempted to provide more detailed descriptions of vulnerable plaques and to establish correlations between CCTA imaging characteristics (Figure 1) of the lesions and the risk for acute events. Motoyama et al. suggested that vulnerable plaques are characterized by positive remodeling, low attenuation plaque and spotty, limited calcification [44]. In later research, non-calcified plaques were more extensively characterized by modern MDCT and several authors described a ring-like attenuation of the non-calcified portion of the coronary atherosclerotic lesion, which is now called the napkin-ring sign [48, 49, 50]. The description of the napkin-ring sign has changed current classifications of non-calcified plaques, which are now classified in three categories: homogenous plaques, non-napkin-ring sign heterogeneous plaques, and napkin-ring sign heterogeneous plaques [49]. The napkin-ring sign corresponds to a morphological type of vulnerable plaque described on coronary CCTA (thin-cap fibroatheromas) comprising a necrotic, low attenuation core surrounded by a thin area of higher attenuation, which some believe may represent the thin peripheral fibrous cap (Figure 2) [26, 47]. However, in vulnerable plaques, the fibrous cap has extremely reduced thickness [48, 51], which makes it indistinguishable by non-invasive imaging methods; by contrast, the necrotic core may be visualized and quantified on thin sections (<0.6 mm) on modern CCTA [52, 53]. As the presence of the napkin-ring sign was shown to have a high predictive value for future cardiac events and is considered a valuable correlate of unstable plaques [49, 27, 20, 54, 55], its detection could add specificity to the CCTA assessment of vulnerable plaques.

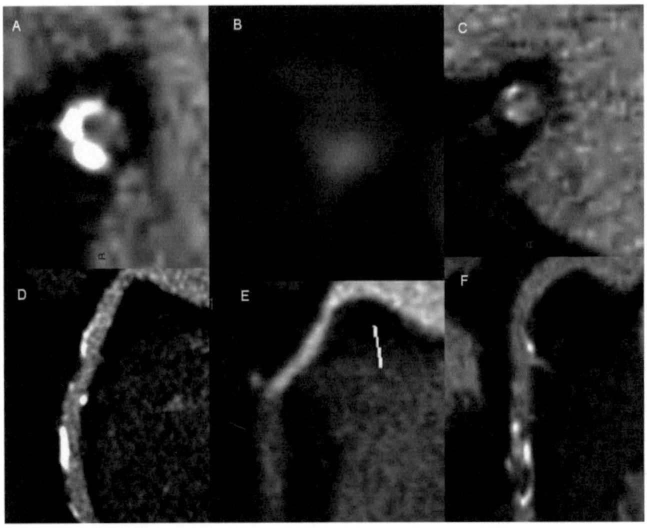

Figure 1. Different Types of Coronary Plaques by CCTA. The 3 main types of coronary plaques are shown: calcified plaques (A, D), non-calcified plaques (B, E) and partially calcified plaques (C, F), illustrated in curved planar reformatted and cross-sectional views.

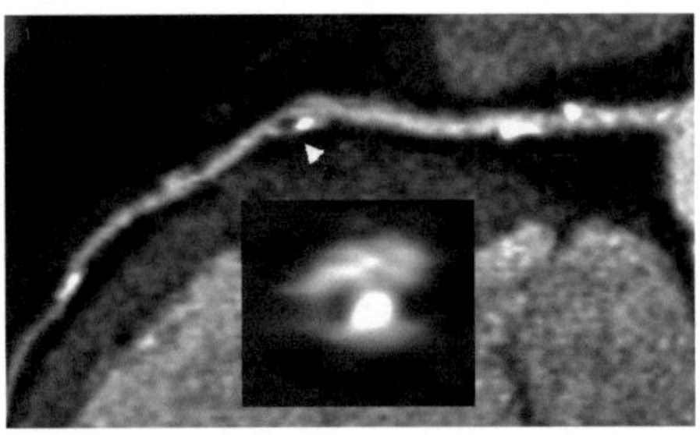

Figure 2. Representative CCTA Images with Napkin-ring Signs. An atherosclerotic plaque with positive remodeling, low attenuation plaque, and a napkin-ring sign in the proximal left anterior descending artery on computed tomography angiography. The boxed area indicates cross-sectional images of atherosclerotic plaque showing a napkin-ring sign.

However, in studies conducted over the last decade, CCTA was also shown to have excellent sensitivity for detecting, and particularly, for excluding coronary atherosclerosis in patients with symptoms suggesting either stable or acute CAD [56]. In addition to that, data from large prospective registries support the use of CAD absence/presence and extension evaluation by CCTA for prognostic purposes [53, 57, 58, 59, 60]. Recent studies conducted with more advanced scanners having 64 to 320 detector rows, and higher spatial (230 to 625 μm) and temporal (75 to 175 ms) resolution focused on identifying vulnerable coronary artery plaques and on establishing correlation between plaque characteristics and ischemic events [61]. Currently available spatial resolution of CCTA scanners approach the spatial resolution provided by invasive methods such as IVUS (100 μm) and invasive coronary angiography (200 μm). Moreover, spatial resolution reaching 0.3 mm in-plane in modern CCTA scanners allows a more accurate discrimination of the non-calcified portion of the plaques [62].

Some researchers [63, 64, 65] attempted to distinguish lipid-rich from fibrous plaque by CCTA based on attenuation criteria, as expressed by Hounsfield Units (HU), but conflicting results have been obtained. In addition to that, HU values cannot accurately discriminate between the types of plaques, mostly due to the small dimensions of the plaque, insufficient spatial resolution of CCTA, and reduced contrast difference between lipid-rich and fibrous plaques. In these studies, certified methods of coronary artery plaque quantification (such as IVUS and histology) were used for comparison to CCTA [63, 64, 65].

Despite current technical limitations, progress has been made in the non-invasive imaging assessment of coronary artery lesions by CCTA. Data from recent studies suggest that low attenuation (<30 HU) is more common to culprit lesions in acute coronary events, as well as to high-risk, vulnerable plaques [26, 27, 47, 66]. Currently, there is not enough data to support a valid assumption on the accuracy of CCTA for detecting non-calcified coronary plaques at high risk. Small studies comparing CCTA to IVUS reported sensitivities and specificities between 80 and 90% for the detection of coronary artery segments with plaque [8, 9, 67, 68]. Other studies demonstrated significant correlations between measurements of plaque cross-sectional area, volume of single plaques, and plaque volume per coronary segment on CCTA and IVUS [8, 69, 70, 71]. However, despite significant and quite high correlation coefficients, the limits of agreement were typically large in most studies, which betrays the limitations of CCTA, mainly imposed by the spatial resolution of the method. Plaque quantification is particularly challenging when plaques have low thickness. Reported interobserver variability is also unusually high (30% variability for plaque volume quantification) [9, 72, 73] and is very much influenced by image quality. In a research on 41 patients, the interobserver variability was 17±10% for the left anterior descending coronary artery, which was best, visualized with fewer artifacts, but escaladed to 29±13% for the left circumflex and 32±10% for the right coronary artery [73].

2.1.2. Low CT attenuation plaques

In CCTA studies investigating patients with ACS, several features of high-risk plaques have been described, such as low attenuation plaque, positive remodeling, and spotty calcification [74, 54]. Recent studies have also described a specific CCTA aspect of coronary artery lesions called the napkin-ring sign consisting of a low attenuation area surrounded by a rim-like area of higher CCTA attenuation [22, 47]. Speculations were made on the histological substrate of this aspect, as it was believed to be given by either a central lipid core within a fibrous cap, deep micro-calcifications, neo-vascularization, or the presence of intramural thrombus [22, 27]. Current criteria for the definition of the napkin-ring sign include the presence of a high attenuation ring around a certain coronary artery plaque and higher CCTA attenuation of the ring by comparison to the adjacent plaque, but no greater than 130 HU, in order to differentiate from calcium deposits [27, 47]. Plaques with rich necrotic core have been described as plaques of low attenuation; low attenuation areas were shown to correlate strongly with echolucent areas in IVUS [75]. In a large prospective study on more than 1000 patients, low attenuation plaques and positive remodeling were shown to correlate with the development of acute coronary events. In this group, 45 patients had both CCTA characteristics and 10 of them (22%) experienced an acute coronary event vs. only 4 (0.5%) of the patients who did not exhibit neither positive remodeling nor low attenuation plaques. Patients with normal CCTA did not have any coronary events at all ($p<0.001$). In this study, positive remodeling and/or low attenuation plaques were independent predictors of acute coronary events (hazard ratio: 23, 95% confidence interval: 7 to 75, $p<0.001$) [74].

A limitation of CCTA in quantifying atherosclerotic plaques may have its origin in the fact that intravascular attenuation significantly influences the attenuation of the plaques. Cademartiri et al. performed a phantom test that supports this hypothesis [76, 77] and Schroeder et al. also obtained similar results in their study [78]. Comparative studies between CCTA density and IVUS or histopathology suggest that lipid-rich plaques have lower CCTA density than fibrous plaques. However, low CCTA attenuation is not a constant finding in lipid-rich plaques, raising controversy over its ability to discriminate between lipid-rich and fibrous plaques. As mentioned above, some studies have reported that luminal density influences neighboring structures CCTA attenuation. Some authors reported that, when contrast medium is not used for examination, significant overlaps can occur between CCTA attenuation values of lipid-rich and fibrous plaques.

CCTA resolution is defined in terms of spatial, contrast and temporal resolution. Although significant technological progress has been made in CCTA, the spatial resolution of CCTA (0.5 mm) is still inferior to that of cardiac catheterization or IVUS. The 0.5 resolution is suboptimal, considering the fact that the average diameter of a coronary artery is 3–4 mm. CCTA density is influenced by the partial volume effect and contrast resolution has not improved despite other technological advances in MDCT [27]. CCTA attenuation values, measured in HU, are given by the amount of radiation absorbed by tissue in the voxel and density is directly proportional to the attenuation coefficient. A CCTA value of –1,000 HU corresponds to air, while 0 HU corresponds to water. Most soft tissues CCTA averages have values of 50 HU. Some tissues, such as bone, calcified tissues, or the iodine-rich tissue of the thyroid gland are >100 HU, whereas fat or fatty mixed tissue and lung tissue are <0 HU. If the value for a tissue type, with the exception of calcified or fatty tissues, deviates from the soft tissue attenuation, artifacts should be considered, particularly if contrast is used and the beam hardening effect is suspected; another element of confusion may be the presence of a near-by area of calcification or fat that may induce a partial volume effect. MIn addition to that, motion artifacts should be considered. CCTA values can also be influenced by tube voltage [27].

2.1.3. *Spotty calcium in plaques*

Besides plaque density (Figure 3), other CCTA features such as positive remodeling and spotty calcification can suggest plaque vulnerability. Positive remodeling is appreciated by referral to the remodeling index; obviously, expanded plaques have higher remodeling index, above the cut-off values, but borderline values can hamper interpretation, considering the narrow lumen of the coronary arteries, which barely averages 4 mm; a difference of 10% is less than 1 pixel on the CCTA image. Consequently, when the set cut-off value is near one, plaque expansion may be erroneously measured as positive. Also, the presence of spotty calcification can lead to overestimation of plaque expansion. As the presence of more calcium is considered to be an element of increased atherosclerotic plaque stability, low calcification plaques are regarded as more vulnerable [27].

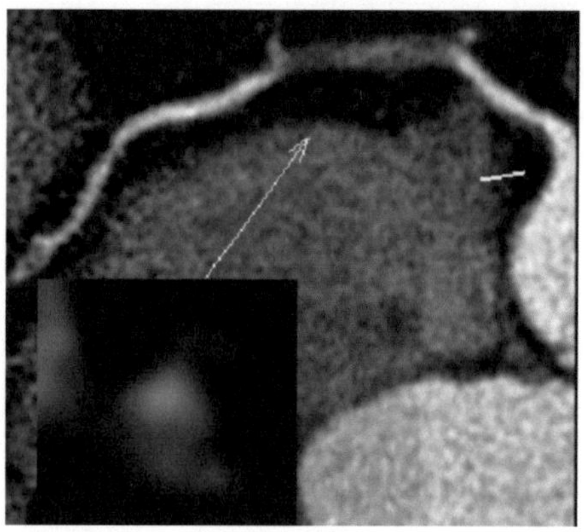

Figure 3. Curved Planar Reformation of the Coronary Artery in CCTA. The curved planar reformatted computed tomography angiography image of the right coronary artery demonstrates two large, predominantly non-calcified atherosclerotic plaques with spotty calcification (arrowheads) in the proximal segment and mild of the right coronary artery.

However, pathological studies concluded that calcium is commonly encountered in ruptured plaques causing sudden cardiac death and that a few scattered small calcium deposits are often present in the fibrous cap of fibroatheromas [79]. The development of scattered small calcium around the necrotic core is believed to be triggered by osteogenic changes under the influence of inflammatory factors and oxidized lipids [80, 81]. The presence of spotty calcifications seems to induce mechanical instability at the interface with non-calcified plaque components [82]. Clinical studies have shown that: spotty calcification has been associated with an increased incidence of ischemic cardiovascular events [83] and, more accurately, that patients with ACSs have a different pattern of calcification when compared to those with stable angina [84]; spotty calcifications are more likely to be found in culprit lesions in patients with myocardial infarction than in patients with stable angina [38]; spotty calcification are more commonly encountered in patients with accelerated disease progression [85]; ruptured coronary plaques are associated with spotty calcification, particularly in deep locations and the number of deep calcium deposits is an independent predictor of culprit plaque ruptures in patients who had ACSs [84]; and superficial spotty calcifications in IVUS are associated with very late stent thrombosis after bare-metal stent implantation [86]. A possible caveat in CCTA imaging may be the fact that microcalcifications under the detection level of CCTA seem to induce very high plaque instability. However, the presence of calcification increases CCTA values, which seems to contradict the finding that low attenuation plaques are unstable.

2.2. Plaque quantification

Currently, MDCT with at least 64 detectors allows nearly motion-free visualization of the coronary arteries and accurate detection of significant stenosis, comparing well to coronary angiography at low heart rates [8, 87]. Contrast-enhanced scans are performed by injecting intravenously 80–100 ml of contrast agent at a flow rate of 6 ml/s followed by 70 ml of saline. The delay time is previously established using the bolus tracking technique with a region of interest positioned in the ascending aorta; a manually triggered threshold of 100 HU is specified for the main scanning. All scans are performed during a single breath-hold.

Non-contrast CCTA is also useful for atherosclerotic plaque description, allowing the calculation of the coronary artery calcium (CAC) score. The CAC is validated as a good marker of atherosclerotic burden and high values are associated with increased cardiovascular risk [88], However, despite relatively easy quantification, the CAC is hindered by several disadvantages, including the inability to identify small, scattered calcifications in non-calcified plaques, which may lead to the underestimation of disease severity and cardiovascular risk. Also, plaque morphology cannot be described on native calcium scans.

Quantitative measurements of coronary plaques aim to assess global atherosclerotic burden and provide detailed and specific descriptions of plaque morphology that could accurately evaluate the risk for cardiovascular events [70, 89, 90]. However, volumetric measurements of coronary artery plaques with manual tracing contours is strenuous and time-consuming; current software, such as AUTOPLAQ (APQ; Cedars-Sinai Medical Center, Los Angeles, CA), allow semi-automated quantification of both calcified and non-calcified plaques that has reduced the examination time and was shown to correlate very well to the IVUS assessment of the coronary plaque volume

[91]. Dey et al. [92] evaluated the accuracy of APQ and compared semi-automated quantification on CCTA using APQ to IVUS with manual tracing of the coronary artery plaque. Average examination time was significantly reduced by automated quantification. Manual IVUS required the longest processing time (15 to 35 minutes), followed by manual CCTA (5 to 15 minutes), while automated plaque segmentation and quantification took less than 20 seconds. There were no significant differences in plaque volumes calculation between IVUS compared with APQ, or between manual CCTA quantification and APQ. Interestingly, APQ quantification revealed smaller absolute differences from IVUS results than CT manual quantification. APQ has also been shown to have reliable interscan reproducibility of quantitative plaque measurements. Schuhbaeck et al. evaluated total plaque volume, volume of calcified and non-calcified plaque, and maximal remodeling index by performing CCTAs

twice in consecutive patients; using APQ there were no significant differences in any of the measurements between scans [93].

Another CCTA automated software for plaque quantification, QAngio (Medis, Netherland), has been developed and compared with IVUS. In their study, Boogers et al. [90] evaluated the accuracy of CCTA automated plaque quantification using a single algorithm to co-register CT and IVUS after having previously established anatomical markers; slice-by-slice comparisons of each location along the transverse axis of the coronary arteries have been made. The compared parameters included the percent lumen area stenosis, plaque burden, the degree of remodeling at the level of minimal lumen area, and the mean plaque burden for the whole coronary plaque. The study revealed significant correlations between the two methods regarding the quantification of lumen area stenosis, plaque burden at the level of the minimal lumen area, as well as mean plaque burden. However, CCTA failed to quantify all parameters as accurately as IVUS, underestimating minimal lesion area and overestimating lumen area stenosis. Moderate correlations were established between the two methods regarding coronary plaque remodeling. Automated plaque quantification methods are expected to reduce interobserver variability by comparison with manual quantification techniques. Several studies were conducted in order to assess the reproducibility of the results. Papadopoulou et al. [94] reported little inter- and intraobserver variability for lumen and vessel areas. Also, in an additional study inter- and intraobserver relative differences for lumen, vessel, plaque area, and plaque burden did not reach statistical significance. Automated plaque quantification proved, however, less reliable for compositional measurements of plaque attenuation values, demonstrating high inter-observer variability (12%), which is an important limiting factor. Despite this drawback, automated softwares can be used for evaluating coronary artery sclerosis progression, as demonstrated by Papadopoulou et al [95]. In another study, Blackmon et al. [96] tested the accuracy and interobserver variability for volumetric measurement of non-calcified lesions of another automated postprocessing software algorithm. Very strong correlations were found between manual measurements performed by highly experienced examiners and automated plaque volumetry, and interobserver variability was reduced when using the plaque analysis algorithm. As demonstrated by the aforementioned studies, automated softwares provide the major advantage of higher reproducibility, while also allowing faster quantifications, which make them elligible for more widespread use. CCTA is very accurate for stenosis detection [97] and for the measurement of calcified plaque burden [98, 99]. The amount of coronary calcification quantified by CCTA is a strong predictor of CAD [100, 101], but fails to accurately identify the site of stenosis. Moreover, even in modern CT scanners, spatial resolution is not sufficient to provide an accurate analysis of the fibrous cap by CCTA [102]. Also, histopathologically-based studies suggest that vulnerable plaques are enlarged in all three spatial dimensions [103] and that average measurements of the necrotic core, such as length and area [104] are beyond the plaque detection threshold for CCTA [105].

2.3. Functional plaque characteristics

Recently, some techniques have been developed for the purpose of analyzing functional parameters, as well as anatomical structures. CT-based fractional flow reserve (FFR-CT) and

CT perfusion allow the non-invasive hemodynamic assessment of coronary stenoses and increase the specificity of CCTA, which may greatly influence the management of CAD patients in the future [106].

2.3.1. Endothelial Shear Stress (ESS)

ESS refers to the tangential stress that is applied on the endothelial surface of the arterial wall by flowing blood friction and is expressed in units of force/unit area [107]. ESS is influenced by blood viscosity and the spatial gradient of blood velocity at the wall. When a fluid passes through a tube, its flow is influenced by the characteristics of the tube walls such as surface irregularities or obstructions. Fluid flow may be laminar or turbulent. Laminar flows are streamlined and may be either completely smooth ("undisturbed flows") or "disturbed", with areas of reversed flow. In turbulent flow, velocities vary continuously in a certain point in space [108]. The presence of low ESS favors the formation and development of coronary artery plaques, as well as their progression to high-risk, vulnerable plaques. Local blood hemodynamics can influence atherosclerosis development for better or for worse. Therefore, an accurate in vivo quantification of plaque characteristics, local ESS, and vascular remodeling response would facilitate a better understanding of the mechanisms behind CAD progression, as well as clinical decision making regarding possible pre-emptive local interventions [109]. The evolution of each coronary artery plaque is individual and considerably influenced not only by the progression of atherosclerosis, but also by vascular remodeling. Extensive remodeling leads to the development of vulnerable plaques and is triggered by ESS. Persistent ESS favors local lipid build-up, inflammation, oxidative stress, and matrix breakdown, with subsequent plaque progression and further remodeling [109]. Advanced plaques in areas of severe stenosis are submitted to considerable shear stress that promotes plaque destabilization [110].

2.3.2. Fractional Flow Reserve (FFR)

FFR is calculated as the ratio between the maximum blood flow within a diseased coronay artery and the theoretical maximum flow in a normal coronary artery. An FFR of 1.0 is considered normal, while values of less than 0.75–0.80 are acknowledged by most as associated with myocardial ischemia [111]. FFR values >0.8 but <1 are considered indicative of a hemodinamically unsignificant stenosis, while values <0.75 reflect significant stenoses. In earlier works, values between 0.75–0.80 represented a grey area and were interpreted according to the clinical context. Investigators estimated that the cut-off value for FFR could be extended to 0.80, thus improving sensitivity without significantly compromising specificity. The cut-off value of 0.80 was already used in the FAME 1 and FAME 2 trials and proved to be clinically valid [112, 113]. This is now the recommended ischemic reference standard for the invasive assessment of myocardial ischemia [114]. Invasive coronary angiography is the established clinical standard for coronary artery disease assessment, with IVUS providing the advantage of intramural and transmural coronary artery imaging. OCT offers an even more accurate visualization of the coronary arteries [115]. The use of these additional invasive imaging methods can facilitate therapeutical decisions regarding revascularization and help guide percutaneous coronary interven-

http://dx.doi.org/10.5772/61393

tions, leading to better postprocedural results. However, in current clinical practice, the reported rates of use for these techniques in assessing intermediate (40–70%) coronary stenoses are fairly low, 20.3% for IVUS and 6.1% for FFR [116].

In the Percutaneous Coronary Intervention of Functionally Non-significant Stenosis (DEFER) Study [117], investigators evaluated 181 patients with stable ischemic heart disease and FFR > 0.75 across an intermediate stenosis. These patients were randomized to either percutaneous coronary interventions or to deferral of percutaneous coronary interventions with medical treatment. At 5-year follow-up, patients in the deferred group had a significantly decreased (less than half) rate of death or myocardial infarction by comparison with the percutaneous coronary interventions group. In the Fractional Flow Reserve versus Angiography for Multivessel Evaluation (FAME) trial [113], 1,005 patients with multivessel disease were randomized to either FFR- or angiography-guided percutaneous coronary interventions. In patients with FFR-guided interventions, the composite rate of death, MI, or repeated revascularization at 1 year was significantly lower (13.2% vs. 18.3%, $P<0.02$). The Fractional Flow Reserve versus Angiography for Multivessel Evaluation 2 (FAME 2) trial [113] compared the outcomes of FFR-guided percutaneous coronary interventions with optimal medical therapy against optimal medical therapy alone in a group of 888 patients with stable ischemic heart disease. In this trial, unlike in others such as COURAGE, only patients having at least one lesion with FFR <0.80 were enrolled [118].

FFR assessment of lesions with 50% to 70% diameter narrowing revealed that only 35% of the lesions were hemodynamically significant. Interestingly, in severe lesions with 71% to 90% diameter stenoses, 20% were not hemodynamically significant based on FFR and did not require percutaneous coronary interventions. These results endorse the hypothesis that FFR can have essential clinical implications regarding revascularization decisions even in more severe angiographic stenoses and, particularly when noninvasive data is discordant with coronary angiography [119]. In patients with multivessel coronary artery disease, FFR can be performed, allowing an accurate determination of the Functional SYNTAX Score, and subsequently, a better selection of patients that could benefit from percutaneous coronary intervention rather than being submitted to coronary artery by-pass graft [120]. The use of CCTA for non-invasive anatomic assessment has increased considerably and the method is considered an accurate tool for detecting or excluding CAD [6, 5]. FFR-CT is a recently developed method based on computational fluid dynamics to calculate coronary blood flow, pressure, and FFR based on routinely acquired CCTA datasets [121, 122, 123, 124, 125, 126, 127, 128, 129].

3. Clinical implications of napkin-ring sign plaque for prognosis and management

Recent research has shown that the napkin-ring sign is associated with future cardiac events, frequently corresponding to the culprit lesion in ACS [53]. In the study by Otsuka et al., 895 patients were evaluated by CCTA and followed up for 2.3±0.8 years; in this population, the presence of the napkin-ring sign on CCTA was strongly associated with ACS events: 24 patients (2.6%) experienced ACS events, of which 41% developed plaques with napkin-ring sign during the follow-up period [53]. Kashiwagi et al. conducted a CCTA-based study on 273 patients with either ACS or stable angina. In their research, the authors described the napkin-ring sign as the presence of a ring of high attenuation and the CT attenuation of a ring presenting higher than those of the adjacent plaque and no greater than 130 HU. The napkin-ring sign was more frequently encountered in culprit lesions (12.7% vs. 2.8%, $p<0.01$). Moreover, napkin-ring sign plaques were associated with a higher remodeling index and lower CT attenuation (1.15 ± 0.12 vs. 1.02 ± 0.12, $p<0.01$ and 39.9 ± 22.8 HU vs.72.7 ± 26.6 HU, $p<0.01$) [50]. Similar results were obtained in another study in which the napkin-ring sign was more common in patients developing ACS than in those with stable angina [28].

Besides the napkin-ring sign, other imaging characteristics such as large plaque volume, low CT attenuation, positive remodeling, and spotty calcification were proved to be correlated with a higher risk of acute events [130]. Motoyama et al. found that positive remodeling and low attenuation correlated best with the development of ACS, [74] which is consistent with results from other studies [131, 132]. Considering the results of the previously mentioned studies, one can conclude that the identification of CCTA aspects suggesting vulnerable lesions may be useful for several reasons. Firstly, although statins are known to reduce the incidence of acute cardiovascular events [133], proving their effect on a certain individual is challenging. CCTA may help identify coronary artery lesions regression, but, as it is not routinely performed, there is not enough data to support this hypothesis. Risk stratification in asymptomatic individuals has also been taken into account as a possible use for CCTA, but the actual ability of MDCT for detecting small non-stenotic plaques is yet to be established [134].

In conclusion CCTA is used extensively nowadays as a non-invasive imaging method for the evaluation of patients suspected of CAD and the napkin-ring sign described on CCTA has been designated as a valid element for identifying vulnerable plaques, indicating an increased probability of rupture, and was shown to correlate with a higher incidence of cardiovascular events.

Author details

Lucia Agoston-Coldea[1,2], Carmen Cionca[2] and Silvia Lupu[3]

1 Iuliu Hatieganu University of Medicine and Pharmacy, Cluj-Napoca, Romania

2 Hiperdia Diagnostic Imaging Center, Cluj-Napoca, Romania

3 University of Medicine and Pharmacy of Targu Mures, Romania

References

[1] Naghavi M, Libby P, Falk E, Casscells SW, Litovsky S, Rumberger J, Badimon JJ, Stefanadis C, Moreno P, Pasterkamp G, Fayad Z, Stone PH, Waxman S, Raggi P, Madjid M, Zarrabi A, Burke A, Yuan C, Fitzgerald PJ, Siscovick DS, de Korte CL, Aikawa M, Juhani Airaksinen KE, Assmann G, Becker CR, Chesebro JH, Farb A, Galis ZS, Jackson C, Jang IK, Koenig W, Lodder RA, March K, Demirovic J, Navab M, Priori SG, Rekhter MD, Bahr R, Grundy SM, Mehran R, Colombo A, Boerwinkle E, Ballantyne C, Insull W Jr, Schwartz RS, Vogel R, Serruys PW, Hansson GK, Faxon DP, Kaul S, Drexler H, Greenland P, Muller JE, Virmani R, Ridker PM, Zipes DP, Shah PK, Willerson JT. From vulnerable plaque to vulnerable patient: A call for new definitions and risk assessment strategies: Part I. Circulation. 2003;108:1664-1672. DOI: 10.1161/01.CIR.0000087480.94275.97.

[2] Naghavi M, Libby P, Falk E, Casscells SW, Litovsky S, Rumberger J, Badimon JJ, Stefanadis C, Moreno P, Pasterkamp G, Fayad Z, Stone PH, Waxman S, Raggi P, Madjid M, Zarrabi A, Burke A, Yuan C, Fitzgerald PJ, Siscovick DS, de Korte CL, Aikawa M, Airaksinen KE, Assmann G, Becker CR, Chesebro JH, Farb A, Galis ZS, Jackson C, Jang IK, Koenig W, Lodder RA, March K, Demirovic J, Navab M, Priori SG, Rekhter MD, Bahr R, Grundy SM, Mehran R, Colombo A, Boerwinkle E, Ballantyne C, Insull W Jr, Schwartz RS, Vogel R, Serruys PW, Hansson GK, Faxon DP, Kaul S, Drexler H, Greenland P, Muller JE, Virmani R, Ridker PM, Zipes DP, Shah PK, Willerson JT. From vulnerable plaque to vulnerable patient: A call for new definitions and risk assessment strategies: Part II. Circulation. 2003;108:1772-1778. DOI: 10.1161/01.CIR.0000087481.55887.C9.

[3] Taylor AJ, Merz CN, Udelson JE. 34th Bethesda Conference: Executive summary—can atherosclerosis imaging techniques improve the detection of patients at risk for ischemic heart disease? J Am Coll Cardiol. 2003;41:1860-1862. DOI:10.1016/S0735-1097(03)00363-2.

[4] Virmani R, Burke AP, Farb A, Kolodgie FD. Pathology of the vulnerable plaque. J Am Coll Cardiol. 2006;47:C13-18. DOI:10.1016/ j.jacc.2005.10.065.

[5] Budoff MJ, Dowe D, Jollis JG, Gitter M, Sutherland J, Halamert E, Scherer M, Bellinger R, Martin A, Benton R, Delago A, Min JK. Diagnostic performance of 64-multidetector-row coronary computed tomographic angiography for evaluation of coronary artery stenosis in individuals without known coronary artery disease. J Am Coll Cardiol. 2008;52:1724-1732. DOI: 10.1016/j.jacc.2008.07.031.

[6] Meijboom WB, Meijs MF, Schuijf JD, Cramer MJ, Mollet NR, van Mieghem CA, Nieman K, van Werkhoven JM, Pundziute G, Weustink AC, de Vos AM, Pugliese F, Rensing B, Jukema JW, Bax JJ, Prokop M, Doevendans PA, Hunink MG, Krestin GP, de Feyter PJ. Diagnostic accuracy of 64-slice computed tomography coronary angiogra-

phy: A prospective, multicenter, multivendor study. J Am Coll Cardiol. 2008;52:2135-2144. DOI: 10.1016/ j.jacc. 2008.08.058.

[7] Pundziute G, Schuijf JD, Jukema JW, Decramer I, Sarno G, Vanhoenacker PK, Boersma E, Reiber JH, Schalij MJ, Wijns W, Bax JJ. Evaluation of plaque characteristics in acute coronary syndromes: Non-invasive assessment with multi-slice computed tomography and invasive evaluation with intravascular ultrasound radiofrequency data analysis. Eur Heart J. 2008;29:2373-2381. DOI: 10.1093/eurheartj/ehn356.

[8] Achenbach S, Moselewski F, Ropers D, Ferencik M, Hoffmann U, MacNeill B, Pohle K, Baum U, Anders K, Jang IK, Daniel WG, Brady TJ. Detection of calcified and non-calcified coronary atherosclerotic plaque by contrast-enhanced, submillimeter multidetector spiral computed tomography: A segment-based comparison with intravascular ultrasound. Circulation. 2004;109:14-17. DOI: 10.1161/01.CIR. 0000111517.69230.0F.

[9] Petranovic M, Soni A, Bezzera H, Loureiro R, Sarwar A, Raffel C, Pomerantsev E, Jang IK, Brady TJ, Achenbach S, Cury RC. Assessment of nonstenotic coronary lesions by 64-slice multidetector computed tomography in comparison to intravascular ultrasound: Evaluation of nonculprit coronary lesions. J Cardiovasc Comput Tomogr. 2009;3:24-31. DOI: 10.1016/j.jcct.2008.12.005.

[10] Duewell P, Kono H, Rayner KJ, Sirois CM, Vladimer G, Bauernfeind FG, Abela GS, Franchi L, Nuñez G, Schnurr M, Espevik T, Lien E, Fitzgerald KA, Rock KL, Moore KJ, Wright SD, Hornung V, Latz E. NLRP3 inflammasomes are required for atherogenesis and activated by cholesterol crystals. Nature. 2010;464:1357-1361. DOI: 10.1038/nature08938.

[11] Stary HC, Chandler AB, Glagov S, Guyton JR, Insull W Jr, Rosenfeld ME, Schaffer SA, Schwartz CJ, Wagner WD, Wissler RW. A definition of initial, fatty streak, and intermediate lesions of atherosclerosis. A report from the Committee on Vascular Lesions of the Council on Arteriosclerosis, American Heart Association. Circulation. 1994;89:2462-2478. DOI: 10.1161/01.CIR.89.5.2462.

[12] Stary HC, Chandler AB, Dinsmore RE, Fuster V, Glagov S, Insull W Jr, Rosenfeld ME, Schwartz CJ, Wagner WD, Wissler RW. A definition of advanced types of atherosclerotic lesions and a histological classification of atherosclerosis. A report from the Committee on Vascular Lesions of the Council on Arteriosclerosis, American Heart Association. Arterioscler Thromb Vasc Biol. 1995;15:1512-1531. DOI: 10.1161/01.ATV.15.9.1512.

[13] Virmani R, Kolodgie FD, Burke AP, Farb A, Schwartz SM. Lessons from sudden coronary death: A comprehensive morphological classification scheme for atherosclerotic lesions. Arterioscler Thromb Vasc Biol. 2000;20:1262-1275. DOI: 10.1161/01.ATV. 20.5.1262.

[14] Nakashima Y, Wight TN, Sueishi K. Early atherosclerosis in humans: Role of diffuse intimal thickening and extracellular matrix proteoglycans. Cardiovasc Res. 2008;79:14-23. DOI: 10.1093/cvr/cvn099.

[15] Liao X, Sluimer JC, Wang Y, Subramanian M, Brown K, Pattison JS, Robbins J, Martinez J, Tabas I. Macrophage autophagy plays a protective role in advanced atherosclerosis. Cell Metab. 2012;15:545-553. DOI: 10.1016/j.cmet.2012.01.022.

[16] van der Wal AC, Becker AE, van der Loos CM, Das PK. Site of intimal rupture or erosion of thrombosed coronary atherosclerotic plaques is characterized by an inflammatory process irrespective of the dominant plaque morphology. Circulation. 1994;89:36-44. DOI: 10.1161/01.CIR.89.1.36.

[17] Nakashima Y, Fujii H, Sumiyoshi S, Wight TN, Sueishi K. Early human atherosclerosis: Accumulation of lipid and proteoglycans in intimal thickenings followed by macrophage infiltration. Arterioscler Thromb Vasc Biol. 2007;27:1159-1165. DOI: 10.1161/ATVBAHA.106.134080.

[18] Ohayon J, Finet G, Gharib AM, Herzka DA, Tracqui P, Heroux J, Rioufol G, Kotys MS, Elagha A, Pettigrew RI. Necrotic core thickness and positive arterial remodeling index: emergent biomechanical factors for evaluating the risk of plaque rupture. Am J Physiol Heart Circ Physiol. 2008;295:H717-727. DOI: 10.1152/ajpheart.00005.2008.

[19] Dhawan SS, Avati Nanjundappa RP, Branch JR, Taylor WR, Quyyumi AA, Jo H, McDaniel MC, Suo J, Giddens D, Samady H. Shear stress and plaque development. Expert Rev Cardiovasc Ther. 2010;8:545-556. DOI: 10.1586/erc.10.28.

[20] Papaspyridonos M, Smith A, Burnand KG, Taylor P, Padayachee S, Suckling KE, James CH, Greaves DR, Patel L. Novel candidate genes in unstable areas of human atherosclerotic plaques. Arterioscler Thromb Vasc Biol. 2006;26:1837-1844. DOI: 10.1161/ 01.ATV.0000229695.68416.76.

[21] Kolodgie FD, Gold HK, Burke AP, Fowler DR, Kruth HS, Weber DK, Farb A, Guerrero LJ, Hayase M, Kutys R, Narula J, Finn AV, Virmani R. Intraplaque hemorrhage and progression of coronary atheroma. N Engl J Med. 2003;349:2316-2325. DOI: 10.1056/ NEJMoa035655.

[22] Sluimer JC, Kolodgie FD, Bijnens AP, Maxfield K, Pacheco E, Kutys B, Duimel H, Frederik PM, van Hinsbergh VW, Virmani R, Daemen MJ. Thin-walled microvessels in human coronary atherosclerotic plaques show incomplete endothelial junctions relevance of compromised structural integrity for intraplaque microvascular leakage. J Am Coll Cardiol. 2009;53:1517-1527. DOI: 10.1016/j.jacc.2008.12.056.

[23] Mann J, Davies MJ. Mechanisms of progression in native coronary artery disease: Role of healed plaque disruption. Heart. 1999;82:265-268. DOI:10.1136/hrt.82.3.265.

[24] Arbustini E, Dal Bello B, Morbini P, Burke AP, Bocciarelli M, Specchia G, Virmani R. Plaque erosion is a major substrate for coronary thrombosis in acute myocardial infarction. Heart. 1999;82:269-272. DOI:10.1136/ hrt.82.3.269.

[25] Kramer MC, Rittersma SZ, de Winter RJ, Ladich ER, Fowler DR, Liang YH, Kutys R, Carter-Monroe N, Kolodgie FD, van der Wal AC, Virmani R. Relationship of thrombus healing to underlying plaque morphology in sudden coronary death. J Am Coll Cardiol. 2010;55:122-132. DOI: 10.1016/j.jacc.2009.09.007.

[26] Maurovich-Horvat P, Hoffmann U, Vorpahl M, Nakano M, Virmani R, Alkadhi H. The napkin-ring sign: CT signature of high risk coronary plaques? J Am Coll Cardiol Img. 2010;3:440-444. DOI: 10.1016/j.jcmg.2010.02.003.

[27] Tanaka A, Shimada K, Yoshida K, Jissyo S, Tanaka H, Sakamoto M, Matsuba K, Imanishi T, Akasaka T, Yoshikawa J. Non-invasive assessment of plaque rupture by 64-slice multidetector computed tomography—comparison with intravascular ultrasound. Circ J. 2008;72:1276-1281. DOI: 10.1253/circj.72.1276.

[28] Pflederer T, Marwan M, Schepis T, Ropers D, Seltmann M, Muschiol G, Daniel WG, Achenbach S. Characterization of culprit lesions in acute coronary syndromes using coronary dual-source CT angiography. Atherosclerosis. 2010;211:437-444. DOI: 10.1016/j.atherosclerosis.2010.02.001.

[29] Aziz K, Berger K, Claycombe K, Huang R, Patel R, Abela GS. Noninvasive detection and localization of vulnerable plaque and arterial thrombosis with computed tomography angiography/positron emission tomography. Circulation. 2008;117:2061-2070. DOI: 10.1161/CirculationAHA.106.652313.

[30] Youssef G, Budoff M. Role of Computed Tomography Coronary Angiography in the Detection of Vulnerable Plaque, Where Does it Stand Among Others? Angiol. 2013:1:2. DOI: 10.4172/2329-9495.1000111.

[31] Vancraeynest D, Pasquet A, Roelants V, Gerber BL, Vanoverschelde JL. Imaging the vulnerable plaque. J Am Coll Cardiol. 2011;57:1961-1979. DOI: 10.1016/j.jacc. 2011.02.018.

[32] Toutouzas K, Stathogiannis K, Synetos A, Karanasos A, Stefanadis C. Vulnerable atherosclerotic plaque: From the basic research laboratory to the clinic. Cardiology. 2012;123:248-253. DOI: 10.1159/000345291.

[33] Hong MK, Mintz GS, Lee CW, Kim YH, Lee SW, Song JM, Han KH, Kang DH, Song JK, Kim JJ, Park SW, Park SJ. Comparison of coronary plaque rupture between stable angina and acute myocardial infarction: A three-vessel intravascular ultrasound study in 235 patients. Circulation. 2004;110:928-933. DOI: 10.1161/ 01.CIR.0000139858. 69915.2E.

[34] Stone GW, Maehara A, Lansky AJ, de Bruyne B, Cristea E, Mintz GS, Mehran R, McPherson J, Farhat N, Marso SP, Parise H, Templin B, White R, Zhang Z, Serruys

PW; PROSPECT Investigators. A prospective natural-history study of coronary atherosclerosis. N Engl J Med. 2011;364:226-235. DOI: 10.1056/NEJMoa1002358.

[35] Cheng JM, Garcia-Garcia HM, de Boer SP, Kardys I, Heo JH, Akkerhuis KM, Oemrawsingh RM, van Domburg RT, Ligthart J, Witberg KT, Regar E, Serruys PW, van Geuns RJ, Boersma E. In vivo detection of high-risk coronary plaques by radiofrequency intravascular ultrasound and cardiovascular outcome: Results of the ATHEROREMO-IVUS study. Eur Heart J. 2014;35:639-647. DOI:10.1093/eurheartj/eht484.

[36] Tian J, Dauerman H, Toma C, Samady H, Itoh T, Kuramitsu S, Domei T, Jia H, Vergallo R, Soeda T, Hu S, Minami Y, Lee H, Yu B, Jang IK. Prevalence and characteristics of TCFA and degree of coronary artery stenosis: An OCT, IVUS, and angiographic study. J Am Coll Cardiol. 2014;64:672-680. DOI:10.1016/j.jacc.2014.05.052.

[37] Schoenhagen P, Ziada KM, Kapadia SR, Crowe TD, Nissen SE, Tuzcu EM. Extent and direction of arterial remodeling in stable versus unstable coronary syndromes: an intravascular ultrasound study. Circulation. 2000;101:598-603. DOI: 10.1161/01.CIR.101.6.598.

[38] Ehara S, Kobayashi Y, Yoshiyama M, Shimada K, Shimada Y, Fukuda D, Nakamura Y, Yamashita H, Yamagishi H, Takeuchi K, Naruko T, Haze K, Becker AE, Yoshikawa J, Ueda M. Spotty calcification typifies the culprit plaque in patients with acute myocardial infarction: An intravascular ultrasound study. Circulation. 2004;110:3424-3429. DOI: 10.1161/01.CIR.0000148131.41425.E9.

[39] Rodriguez-Granillo GA, García-García HM, Mc Fadden EP, Valgimigli M, Aoki J, de Feyter P, Serruys PW. In vivo intravascular ultrasound-derived thin-cap fibroatheroma detection using ultrasound radiofrequency data analysis. J Am Coll Cardiol. 2005;46:2038-2042. DOI:10.1016/j.jacc.2005.07.064.

[40] Hong MK, Mintz GS, Lee CW, Suh J, Kim JH, Park DW, Lee SW, Kim YH, Cheong SS, Kim JJ, Park SW, Park SJ. Comparison of virtual histology to intravascular ultrasound of culprit coronary lesions in acute coronary syndrome and target coronary lesions instable angina pectoris. Am J Cardiol. 2007;100:953-999. DOI: 10.1016/j.amjcard.2007.04.034.

[41] Hong YJ, Jeong MH, Choi YH, Park SY, Rhew SH, Jeong HC, Cho JY, Jang SY, Lee KH, Park KH, Sim DS, Yoon NS, Yoon HJ, Kim KH, Park HW, Kim JH, Ahn Y, Cho JG, Park JC, Kang JC. Comparison of Coronary Plaque Components between Non-Culprit Lesions in Patients with Acute Coronary Syndrome and Target Lesions in Patients with Stable Angina: Virtual Histology-Intravascular Ultrasound Analysis. Korean Circ J. 2013;43:607-614. DOI: 10.4070/kcj.2013.43.9.607.

[42] Patwari P, Weissman NJ, Boppart SA, Jesser C, Stamper D, Fujimoto JG, Brezinski ME. Assessment of coronary plaque with optical coherence tomography and high-

frequency ultrasound. Am J Cardiol. 2000;85:641-644. DOI: 10.1016/S0002-9149(99)00825-5.

[43] Kume T, Akasaka T, Kawamoto T, Watanabe N, Toyota E, Neishi Y, Sukmawan R, Sadahira Y, Yoshida K. Assessment of coronary intima media thickness by optical coherence tomography: comparison with intravascular ultrasound. Circ J. 2005;69:903-907. DOI:10.1253/circj.69.903.

[44] Motoyama S, Kondo T, Sarai M, Sugiura A, Harigaya H, Sato T, Inoue K, Okumura M, Ishii J, Anno H, Virmani R, Ozaki Y, Hishida H, Narula J. Multislice computed tomographic characteristics of coronary lesions in acute coronary syndromes. J Am Coll Cardiol. 2007;50:319-326. DOI:10.1016/j.jacc.2007.03.044.

[45] Hoffmann U, Moselewski F, Nieman K, Jang IK, Ferencik M, Rahman AM, Cury RC, Abbara S, Joneidi-Jafari H, Achenbach S, Brady TJ. Noninvasive assessment of plaque morphology and composition in culprit and stable lesions in acute coronary syndrome and stable lesions in stable angina by multidetector computed tomography. J Am Coll Cardiol. 2006;47:1655-1662. DOI:10.1016/j.jacc.2006.01.041.

[46] Tearney GJ, Regar E, Akasaka T, Adriaenssens T, Barlis P, Bezerra HG, Bouma B, Bruining N, Cho JM, Chowdhary S, Costa MA, de Silva R, Dijkstra J, Di Mario C, Dudek D, Falk E, Feldman MD, Fitzgerald P, Garcia-Garcia HM, Gonzalo N, Granada JF, Guagliumi G, Holm NR, Honda Y, Ikeno F, Kawasaki M, Kochman J, Koltowski L, Kubo T, Kume T, Kyono H, Lam CC, Lamouche G, Lee DP, Leon MB, Maehara A, Manfrini O, Mintz GS, Mizuno K, Morel MA, Nadkarni S, Okura H, Otake H, Pietrasik A, Prati F, Räber L, Radu MD, Rieber J, Riga M, Rollins A, Rosenberg M, Sirbu V, Serruys PW, Shimada K, Shinke T, Shite J, Siegel E, Sonoda S, Suter M, Takarada S, Tanaka A, Terashima M, Thim T, Uemura S, Ughi GJ, van Beusekom HM, van der Steen AF, van Es GA, van Soest G, Virmani R, Waxman S, Weissman NJ, Weisz G. International Working Group for Intravascular Optical Coherence Tomography (IWG-IVOCT). Consensus standards for acquisition, measurement, and reporting of intravascular optical coherence tomography studies: A report from the International Working Group for Intravascular Optical Coherence Tomography Standardization and Validation. J Am Coll Cardiol. 2012;59:1058-1072. DOI: 10.1016/j.jacc.2011.09.079.

[47] Kashiwagi M, Tanaka A, Kitabata H, Tsujioka H, Kataiwa H, Komukai K, Tanimoto T, Takemoto K, Takarada S, Kubo T, Hirata K, Nakamura N, Mizukoshi M, Imanishi T, Akasaka T. Feasibility of noninvasive assessment of thin-cap fibroatheroma by multidetector computed tomography. J Am Coll Cardiol Img. 2009;2:1412-1419. DOI: 10.1016/j.jcmg.2009.09.012.

[48] Narula J, Garg P, Achenbach S, Motoyama S, Virmani R, Strauss HW. Arithmetic of vulnerable plaques for noninvasive imaging. Nat Clin Pract Cardiovasc Med. 2008;5 Suppl 2:S2-10. DOI: 10.1038/ncpcardio1247.

[49] Maurovich-Horvat P, Schlett CL, Alkadhi H, Nakano M, Otsuka F, Stolzmann P, Scheffel H, Ferencik M, Kriegel MF, Seifarth H, Virmani R, Hoffmann U. The napkin

ring sign indicates advanced atherosclerotic lesions in coronary CT angiography. JACC Cardiovasc Imaging. 2012;5:1243-1252. DOI:10.1016/j.jcmg.2012.03.019.

[50] Kashiwagi M, Tanaka A, Shimada K, Kitabata H, Komukai K, Nishiguchi T, Ozaki Y,Tanimoto T, Kubo T, Hirata K, Mizukoshi M, Akasaka T. Distribution, frequency and clinical implications of napkin-ring sign assessed by multidetector computed tomography. J Cardiol. 2013;61:399-403. DOI: 10.1016/j.jjcc.2013.01.004.

[51] Seifarth H, Schlett CL, Nakano M, Otsuka F, Károlyi M, Liew G, Maurovich-Horvat P, Alkadhi H, Virmani R, Hoffmann U. Histopathological correlates of the napkin-ring sign plaque in coronary CT angiography. Atherosclerosis. 2012;224:90-96. DOI: 10.1016/j.atherosclerosis.2012.06.021.

[52] Hamon M, Morello R, Riddell JW, Hamon M: Coronary arteries. diagnostic performance of 16- versus 64-section spiral CT compared with invasive coronary angiography—meta-analysis. Radiology. 2007;245:720-731. DOI:10.1148/radiol. 2453061899.

[53] Otsuka K, Fukuda S, Tanaka A, Nakanishi K, Taguchi H, Yoshikawa J, Shimada K, Yoshiyama M. Napkin-ring sign on coronary CT angiography for the prediction of acute coronary syndrome. JACC Cardiovasc Imaging. 2013;6:448-457. DOI: 10.1016/ j.jcmg. 2012.09.016.

[54] Fujimoto S, Kondo T, Narula J. Evaluation of plaque morphology by coronary CT angiography. Cardiol Clin. 2012;30:69-75. DOI: 10.1016/j.ccl.2011.10.002.

[55] Narula J, Achenbach S. Napkin-ring necrotic cores: Defining circumferential extent of necrotic cores in unstable plaques. JACC Cardiovasc Imaging. 2009;2:1436-1438. DOI: 10.1016/j.jcmg.2009.10.004.

[56] Raff GL, Gallagher MJ, O'Neill WW, Goldstein JA. Diagnostic accuracy of noninvasive coronary angiography using 64-slice spiral computed tomography. J Am Coll Cardiol. 2005;46:552-557. DOI:10.1016/j.jacc.2005.05.056.

[57] Hadamitzky M, Freissmuth B, Meyer T, Hein F, Kastrati A, Martinoff S, Schömig A, Hausleiter J. Prognostic value of coronary computed tomographic angiography for prediction of cardiac events in patients with suspected coronary artery disease. JACC Cardiovasc Imaging. 2009;2:404-411. DOI: 10.1016/j.jcmg.2008.11.015.

[58] Chow BJ, Wells GA, Chen L, Yam Y, Galiwango P, Abraham A, Sheth T, Dennie C, Beanlands RS, Ruddy TD. Prognostic value of 64- slice cardiac computed tomography severity of coronary artery disease, coronary atherosclerosis, and left ventricular ejection fraction. J Am Coll Cardiol. 2010;55:1017-1028. DOI: 10.1016/j.jacc. 2009.10.039.

[59] Kristensen TS, Kofoed KF, Kühl JT, Nielsen WB, Nielsen MB, Kelbæk H. Prognostic implications of nonobstructive coronary plaques in patients with non-ST-segment elevation myocardial infarction: A multidetector computed tomography study. J Am Coll Cardiol. 2011;58:502-509. DOI: 10.1016/ j.jacc.2011.01.058.

[60] Abdulla J, Asferg C, Kofoed KF. Prognostic value of absence or presence of coronary artery disease determined by 64-slice computed tomography coronary angiography a systematic review and meta-analysis. Int J Cardiovasc Imaging. 2011;27:413-420. DOI: 10.1007/s10554-010-9652-x.

[61] Voros S. What are the potential advantagesand disadvantages of volumetric CT scanning? J Cardiovasc Comput Tomogr. 2009;3:67-70. DOI: 10.1016/j.jcct.2008.12.010.

[62] Kristanto W, van Ooijen PM, Greuter MJ, Groen JM, Vliegenthart R, Oudkerk M. Non-calcified coronary atherosclerotic plaque visualization on CT: Effects of contrast-enhancement and lipid-content fractions. Int J Cardiovasc Imaging. 2013;29:1137-1148. DOI 10.1007/s10554-012-0176-4.

[63] Becker CR, Nikolaou K, Muders M, Babaryka G, Crispin A, Schoepf UJ, Loehrs U, Reiser MF. Ex vivo coronary atherosclerotic plaque characterization with multi-detector-row CT. Eur Radiol. 2003;13:2094-2098. DOI: 10.1007/ s00330-003-1889-5.

[64] Pohle K, Achenbach S, Macneill B, Ropers D, Ferencik M, Moselewski F, Hoffmann U, Brady TJ, Jang IK, Daniel WG. Characterization of non-calcified coronary atherosclerotic plaque by multi-detector row CT: Comparison to IVUS. Atherosclerosis. 2007;190:174-180. DOI: 10.1016/j.atherosclerosis.2006.01.013.

[65] Schroeder S, Kuettner A, Wojak T, Janzen J, Heuschmid M, Athanasiou T, Beck T, Burgstahler C, Herdeg C, Claussen CD, Kopp AF. Non-invasive evaluation of atherosclerosis with contrast enhanced 16 slice spiral computed tomography: Results of ex vivo investigations. Heart. 2004;90:1471-1475. DOI:10.1136/hrt.2004.037861.

[66] Nakazawa G, Tanabe K, Onuma Y, Yachi S, Aoki J, Yamamoto H, Higashikuni Y, Yagishita A, Nakajima H, Hara K. Efficacy of culprit plaque assessment by 64-slice multidetector computed tomography to predict transient no-reflow phenomenon during percutaneous coronary intervention. Am Heart J. 2008;155:1150-1157. DOI: 10.1016/ j.ahj.2008.01.006.

[67] Leber AW, Becker A, Knez A, von Ziegler F, Sirol M, Nikolaou K, Ohnesorge B, Fayad ZA, Becker CR, Reiser M, Steinbeck G, Boekstegers P. Accuracy of 64-slice computed tomography to classify and quantify plaque volumes in the proximal coronary system: A comparative study using intravascular ultrasound. J Am Coll Cardiol. 2006;47:672-677. DOI:10.1016/j.jacc.2005.10.058.

[68] Sun J, Zhang Z, Lu B, Yu W, Yang Y, Zhou Y, Wang Y, Fan Z. Identification and quantification of coronary atherosclerotic plaques: A comparison of 64-MDCT and intravascular ultrasound. Am J Roentgenol. 2008;190:748-754. DOI: 10.2214/AJR. 07.2763.

[69] Schepis T, Marwan M, Pflederer T, Seltmann M, Ropers D, Daniel WG, Achenbach S. Quantification of noncalcified coronary atherosclerotic plaques with Dual Source Computed Tomography: Comparison to intravascular ultrasound. Heart. 2010;96:610-615. DOI: 10.1136/hrt.2009.184226.

[70] Otsuka M, Bruining N, Van Pelt NC, Mollet NR, Ligthart JM, Vourvouri E, Hamers R, De Jaegere P, Wijns W, Van Domburg RT, Stone GW, Veldhof S, Verheye S, Dudek D, Serruys PW, Krestin GP, De Feyter PJ. Quantification of coronary plaque by 64-slice computed tomography: A comparison with quantitative intracoronary ultrasound. Invest Radiol. 2008;43:314-321. DOI: 10.1097/RLI.0b013e31816a88a9.

[71] Springer I, Dewey M. Comparison of multislice computed tomography with intravascular ultrasound for detection and characterization of coronary artery plaques: a systematic review. Eur J Radiol. 2009;71:275-282. DOI: 10.1016/j.ejrad.2008.04.035.

[72] Hoffmann H, Frieler K, Hamm B, Dewey M. Intra- and interobserver variability in detection and assessment of calcified and noncalcified coronary artery plaques using 64-slice computed tomography: Variability in coronary plaque measurement using MSCT. Int J Cardiovasc Imaging. 2008;24:735-742. DOI: 10.1007/s10554-008-9299-z.

[73] Pflederer T, Schmid M, Ropers D, Ropers U, Komatsu S, Daniel WG, Achenbach S. Interobserver variability of 64-slice computed tomography for the quantification of non-calcified coronary atherosclerotic plaque. Rofo. 2007;179:953-957. DOI: 10.1055/s-2007-963113.

[74] Motoyama S, Sarai M, Harigaya H, Anno H, Inoue K, Hara T, Naruse H, Ishii J, Hishida H, Wong ND, Virmani R, Kondo T, Ozaki Y, Narula J. Computed tomographic angiography characteristics of atherosclerotic plaques subsequently resulting in acute coronary syndrome. J Am Coll Cardiol. 2009;54:49-57. DOI: 10.1016/j.jacc.2009.02.068.

[75] Motoyama S, Kondo T, Anno H, Sugiura A, Ito Y, Mori K, Ishii J, Sato T, Inoue K, Sarai M, Hishida H, Narula J. Atherosclerotic plaque characterization by 0.5-mm-slice multislice computed tomographic imaging. Circ J. 2007;71:363-366. DOI: 10.1253/circj.71.363.

[76] Cademartiri F, Mollet NR, Runza G, Bruining N, Hamers R, Somers P, Knaapen M, Verheye S, Midiri M, Krestin GP, de Feyter PJ: Influence of intracoronary attenuation on coronary plaque measurements using multislice computed tomography: observations in an ex vivo model of coronary computed tomography angiography. Eur Radiol. 2005;15:1426-1431. DOI: 10.1007/s00330-005-2697-x.

[77] Cademartiri F, La Grutta L, Runza G, Palumbo A, Maffei E, Mollet NR, Bartolotta TV, Somers P, Knaapen M, Verheye S, Midiri M, Hamers R, Bruining N: Influence of convolution filtering on coronary plaque attenuation values: observations in an ex vivo model of multislice computed tomography coronary angiography. Eur Radiol. 2007;17:1842-1849. DOI: 10.1007/s00330-006-0548-z.

[78] Schroeder S, Flohr T, Kopp AF, Meisner C, Kuettner A, Herdeg C, Baumbach A, Ohnesorge B. Accuracy of density measurements within plaque located in artificial coronary arteries by X-ray multislice CT: Results of a phantom study. J Comput Assist Tomogr. 2001;25:900-906.

[79] Falk E, Nakano M, Bentzon JF, Finn AV, Virmani R. Update on acute coronary syndromes: The pathologists' view. Eur Heart J. 2013;34:719-728. DOI: 10.1093/eurheartj/ehs411.

[80] Aikawa E, Nahrendorf M, Figueiredo JL, Swirski FK, Shtatland T, Kohler RH, Jaffer FA, Aikawa M, Weissleder R. Osteogenesis associates with inflammation in early-stage atherosclerosis evaluated by molecular imaging in vivo. Circulation. 2007;116:2841-2850. DOI: 10.1161/CIRCULATIONAHA.107.732867.

[81] Flammer AJ, Gössl M, Widmer RJ, Reriani M, Lennon R, Loeffler D, Shonyo S, Simari RD, Lerman LO, Khosla S, Lerman A. Osteocalcin positive CD133þ/CD34-/KDRþ progenitor cells as an independent marker for unstable atherosclerosis. Eur Heart J. 2012;33:2963-2969. DOI: 10.1093/eurheartj/ehs234.

[82] Johnson RC, Leopold JA, Loscalzo J. Vascular calcification: Pathobiological mechanisms and clinical implications. Circ Res. 2006;99:1044-1059. DOI: 10.1161/01.RES.0000249379.55535.21.

[83] Watabe H, Sato A, Akiyama D, Kakefuda Y, Adachi T, Ojima E, Hoshi T, Murakoshi N, Ishizu T, Seo Y, Aonuma K. Impact of coronary plaquecomposition on cardiac troponin elevation after percutaneous coronary intervention in stable angina pectoris: a computed tomography analysis. J Am Coll Cardiol. 2012;59:1881-1888. DOI: 10.1016/j.jacc.2012.01.051.

[84] Fujii K, Carlier SG, Mintz GS, Takebayashi H, Yasuda T, Costa RA, Moussa I, Dangas G, Mehran R, Lansky AJ, Kreps EM, Collins M, Stone GW, Moses JW, Leon MB. Intravascular ultrasound study of patterns of calcium in ruptured coronary plaques. Am J Cardiol. 2005;96:352-357. DOI: 10.1016/j.amjcard.2005.03.074.

[85] Kataoka Y, Wolski K, Uno K, Puri R, Tuzcu EM, Nissen SE, Nicholls SJ. Spotty calcification as a marker of accelerated progression of coronary atherosclerosis: Insights from serial intravascular ultrasound. J Am Coll Cardiol. 2012;59:1592-1597. DOI: 10.1016/j.jacc.2012.03.012.

[86] Yumoto K, Anzai T, Aoki H, Inoue A, Funada S, Nishiyama H, Tanaka S, Kowase S, Shirai Y, Kurosaki K, Nogami A, Daida H, Kato K. Calcified plaque rupture and very late stent thrombosis after bare-metal stent implantation. Cardiovasc Interv Ther. 2011;26:252-259. DOI: 10.1007/s12928-011-0070-3.

[87] Nieman K, Cademartiri F, Lemos PA, Raaijmakers R, Pattynama PM, de Feyter PJ. Reliable noninvasive coronary angiography with fast submillimeter multislice spiral computed tomography. Circulation. 2002;106:2051-2054. DOI: 10.1161/01.CIR.0000037222.58317.3D.

[88] Sangiorgi G, Rumberger JA, Severson A, Edwards WD, Gregoire J, Fitzpatrick LA, Schwartz RS. Arterial calcification and not lumen stenosis is highly correlated with atherosclerotic plaque burden in humans: a histologic study of 723 coronary artery

segments using nondecalcifying methodology. J Am Coll Cardiol. 1998;31:126-133. DOI: 10.1016/S0735-1097(97)00443-9.

[89] Brodoefel H, Burgstahler C, Sabir A, Yam CS, Khosa F, Claussen CD, Clouse ME. Coronary plaque quantification by voxel analysis: Dual-source MDCT angiography versus intravascular sonography. AJR Am J Roentgenol. 2009;192:W84-89. DOI: 10.2214/AJR.08.1381.

[90] Boogers MJ, Broersen A, van Velzen JE, de Graaf FR, El-Naggar HM, Kitslaar PH, Dijkstra J, Delgado V, Boersma E, de Roos A, Schuijf JD, Schalij MJ, Reiber JH, Bax JJ, Jukema JW. Automated quantification of coronary plaque with computed tomography: Comparison with intravascular ultrasound using a dedicated registration algorithm for fusion-based quantification. Eur Heart J. 2012;33:1007-1016. DOI: 10.1093/eurheartj/ehr465.

[91] Dey D, Cheng VY, Slomka PJ, Nakazato R, Ramesh A, Gurudevan S, Germano G, Berman DS. Automated 3-dimensional quantification of noncalcified and calcified coronary plaque from coronary CT angiography. J Cardiovasc Comput Tomogr. 2009;3:372-382. DOI: 10.1016/j.jcct.2009.09.004.

[92] Dey D, Schepis T, Marwan M, Slomka PJ, Berman DS, Achenbach S. Automated three dimensional quantification of noncalcified coronary plaque from coronary CT angiography: Comparison with intravascular US. Radiology. 2010;257:516-522. DOI: 10.1148/radiol.10100681.

[93] Schuhbaeck A, Dey D, Otaki Y, Slomka P, Kral BG, Achenbach S, Berman DS, Fishman EK, Lai S, Lai H. Interscan reproducibility of quantitative coronary plaque volume and composition from CT coronary angiography using an automated method. Eur Radiol. 2014;24:2300-8. DOI: 10.1007/s00330-014-3253-3.

[94] Papadopoulou SL, Neefjes LA, Garcia-Garcia HM, Flu WJ, Rossi A, Dharampal AS, Kitslaar PH, Mollet NR, Veldhof S, Nieman K, Stone GW, Serruys PW, Krestin GP, de Feyter PJ. Natural history of coronary atherosclerosis by multislice computed tomography. JACC Cardiovasc Imaging. 2012;5(3 Suppl):S28-37. DOI: 10.1016/j.jcmg.2012.01.009.

[95] Papadopoulou SL, Garcia-Garcia HM, Rossi A, Girasis C, Dharampal AS, Kitslaar PH, Krestin GP, de Feyter PJ. Reproducibility of computed tomography angiography data analysis using semiautomated plaque quantification software: implications for the design of longitudinal studies. Int J Cardiovasc Imaging. 2013;29:1095-104. DOI: 10.1007/s10554-012-0167-5.

[96] Blackmon KN, Streck J, Thilo C, Bastarrika G, Costello P, Schoepf UJ. Reproducibility of automated noncalcified coronary artery plaque burden assessment at coronary CT angiography. J Thorac Imaging. 2009;24:96-102. DOI: 10.1097/RTI.0b013e31819b674b.

[97] Leber AW, Johnson T, Becker A, von Ziegler F, Tittus J, Nikolaou K, Reiser M, Steinbeck G, Becker CR, Knez A. Diagnostic accuracy of dual-source multi-slice CT-coro-

nary angiography in patients with an intermediate pretest likelihood for coronary artery disease. Eur Heart J. 2007;28:2354-2360. DOI: 10.1093/eurheartj/ehm294.

[98] Agatston AS, Janowitz WR, Hildner FJ, Zusmer NR, Viamonte M Jr, Detrano R. Quantification of coronary artery calcium using ultrafast computed tomography. J Am Coll Cardiol. 1990;15:827-832. DOI:10.1016/0735-1097(90)90282-T.

[99] Oudkerk M, Stillman AE, Halliburton SS, Kalender WA, Möhlenkamp S, McCollough CH, Vliegenthart R, Shaw LJ, Stanford W, Taylor AJ, van Ooijen PM, Wexler L, Raggi P. Coronary artery calcium screening: Current status and recommendations from the European Society of Cardiac Radiology and North American Society for Cardiovascular Imaging. Eur Radiol. 2008;18:2785-807. DOI: 10.1007/s00330-008-1095-6.

[100] Greenland P, LaBree L, Azen SP, Doherty TM, Detrano RC. Coronary artery calcium score combined with Framingham score for risk prediction in asymptomatic individuals. JAMA. 2004;291:210-215. DOI: 10.1001/jama.291.2.210.

[101] Vliegenthart R, Oudkerk M, Hofman A Oei HH, van Dijck W, van Rooij FJ, Witteman JC. Coronary calcification improves cardiovascular risk prediction in the elderly. Circulation. 2005;112:572-527. DOI: 10.1161/CIRCULATIONAHA.104.488916.

[102] Achenbach S. Can CT detect the vulnerable coronary plaque? Int J Cardiovasc Imaging. 2008;24:311-312. DOI: 10.1007/s10554-007-9281-1.

[103] Kolodgie FD, Burke AP, Farb A, Gold HK, Yuan J, Narula J, Finn AV, Virmani R. The thin-cap fibroatheroma: A type of vulnerable plaque: The major precursor lesion to acute coronary syndromes. Curr Opin Cardiol. 2011;16:285-292.

[104] Heidenreich PA, Trogdon JG, Khavjou OA, Butler J, Dracup K, Ezekowitz MD, Finkelstein EA, Hong Y, Johnston SC, Khera A, Lloyd-Jones DM, Nelson SA, Nichol G, Orenstein D, Wilson PW, Woo YJ. Forecasting the future of cardiovascular disease in the United States: a policy statement from the American Heart Association. Circulation. 2011;123:933-944. DOI: 10.1161/ CIR.0b013e31820a55f5.

[105] van der Giessen AG, Toepker MH, Donelly PM, Bamberg F, Schlett CL, Raffle C, Irlbeck T, Lee H, van Walsum T, Maurovich-Horvat P, Gijsen FJ, Wentzel JJ, Hoffmann U. Reproducibility, accuracy, and predictors of accuracy for the detection of coronary atherosclerotic plaque composition by computed tomography: An ex vivo comparison to intravascular ultrasound. Invest Radiol. 2010;45:693-701. DOI: 10.1097/RLI.0b013e3181e0a541.

[106] Schulman-Marcus J, Danad I, Truong QA: State-of-the-Art Updates on Cardiac Computed Tomographic Angiography for Assessing Coronary Artery Disease. Curr Treat Options Cardiovasc Med. 2015;17:398. DOI: 10.1007/s11936-015-0398-6.

[107] Wentzel JJ, Janssen E, Vos J, Schuurbiers JC, Krams R, Serruys PW, de Feyter PJ, Slager CJ. Extension of increased atherosclerotic wall thickness into high shear stress re-

gions is associated with loss of compensatory remodeling. Circulation. 2003;108:17-23. DOI: 10.1161/01.CIR.0000078637.21322.D3.

[108] Feldman CL, Ilegbusi OJ, Hu Z, Nesto R, Waxman S, Stone PH. Determination of in vivo velocity and endothelial shear stress patterns with phasic flow in human coronary arteries: A methodology to predict progression of coronary atherosclerosis. Am Heart J 2002; 143:931-939. DOI: 10.1067/mhj.2002.123118.

[109] Chatzizisis YS, Coskun AU, Jonas M, Edelman ER, Feldman CL, Stone PH. Role of endothelial shear stress in the natural history of coronary atherosclerosis and vascular remodeling: Molecular, cellular, and vascular behavior J Am Coll Cardiol. 2007;49:2379-2393. DOI:10.1016/j.jacc.2007.02.059.

[110] Wentzel JJ, Chatzizisis YS, Gijsen FJ, Giannoglou GD, Feldman CL, Stone PH. Endothelial shear stress in the evolution of coronary atherosclerotic plaque and vascular remodelling: Current understanding and remaining questions. Cardiovasc Res. 2012;96:234-243. DOI: 10.1093/cvr/cvs217.

[111] Pijls NH, De Bruyne B, Peels K, Van Der Voort PH, Bonnier HJ, Bartunek J Koolen JJ, Koolen JJ. Measurement of fractional flow reserve to assess the functional severity of coronary-artery stenoses. N Engl J Med. 1996;334:1703-1708. DOI: 10.1056/NEJM199606273342604.

[112] Tonino PA, De Bruyne B, Pijls NH, Siebert U, Ikeno F, van' t Veer M, Klauss V, Manoharan G, Engstrøm T, Oldroyd KG, Ver Lee PN, MacCarthy PA, Fearon WF. Fractional flow reserve versus angiography for guiding percutaneous coronary intervention. N Engl J Med. 2009;360:213-224. DOI: 10.1056/NEJMoa0807611.

[113] De Bruyne B, Pijls NH, Kalesan B, Barbato E, Tonino PA, Piroth Z, Jagic N, Möbius-Winkler S, Rioufol G, Witt N, Kala P, MacCarthy P, Engström T, Oldroyd KG, Mavromatis K, Manoharan G, Verlee P, Frobert O, Curzen N, Johnson JB, Jüni P, Fearon WF. Fractional flow reserve-guided PCI versus medical therapy in stable coronary disease. N Engl J Med. 2012;367:991-1001. DOI: 10.1056/NEJMoa1205361.

[114] Melikian N, De Bondt P, Tonino P, De Winter O, Wyffels Bartunek J, Heyndrickx GR, Fearon WF, Pijils NHJ, Wijns W, De Bruyne B. Fractional flow research and myocardial perfusion imaging in patients with angiographic multivessel coronary artery disease. JACC Cardiovasc Interv. 2010;3:307-314. DOI: 10.1016/j.jcin.2009.12.010.

[115] Christou MA, Siontis GC, Katritsis DG, Ioannidis JP. Metaanalysis of fractional flow reserve versus quantitative coronary angiography and noninvasive imaging for evaluation of myocardial ischemia. Am J Cardiol. 2007;99:450-456. DOI: 10.1016/j.amjcard.2006.09.092.

[116] Dattilo PB, Prasad A, Honeycutt E, Wang TY, Messenger JC. Contemporary patterns of fractional flow reserve and intravascular ultrasound use among patients undergoing percutaneous coronary intervention in the United States: Insights from the Na-

tional Cardiovascular Data Registry. J Am Coll Cardiol. 2012;60:2337-2339. DOI: 10.1016/j.jacc.2012.08.990.

[117] Pijls NH, van Schaardenburgh P, Manoharan G, Boersma E, Bech JW, et al. Percutaneous coronary intervention of functionally nonsignificant stenosis: 5-year follow-up of the DEFER Study. J Am Coll Cardiol. 2007;49:2105-2111. DOI:10.1016/j.jacc.2007.01.087.

[118] Boden WE, O'Rourke RA, Teo KK, Hartigan PM, Maron DJ, Kostuk WJ, Knudtson M, Dada M, Casperson P, Harris CL, Chaitman BR, Shaw L, Gosselin G, Nawaz S, Title LM, Gau G, Blaustein AS, Booth DC, Bates ER, Spertus JA, Berman DS, Mancini GB, Weintraub WS. Optimal medical therapy with or without PCI for stable coronary disease. N Engl J Med. 2007;356:1503-1516. DOI: 10.1056/NEJMoa070829.

[119] Lotfi A, Jeremias A, Fearon WF, Feldman MD, Mehran R, Messenger JC, Grines CL, Dean LS, Kern MJ, Klein LW. Expert Consensus Statement on the Use of Fractional Flow Reserve, Intravascular Ultrasound, and Optical Coherence Tomography: A Consensus Statement of the Society of Cardiovascular Angiography and Interventions. Catheter Cardiovasc Interv. 2014;83:509-518. DOI: 10.1002/ccd.25222.

[120] Nam CW, Mangiacapra F, Entjes R, Chung IS, Sels JW, Tonino PA, De Bruyne B, Pijls NH, Fearon WF; FAME Study Investigators. Functional SYNTAX Score for risk assessment in multivessel coronary artery disease. J Am Coll Cardiol. 2011;58:1211-1218. DOI: 10.1016/j.jacc.2011.06.020.

[121] Koo BK, Erglis A, Doh JH, Daniels DV, Jegere S, Kim HS, Dunning A, DeFrance T, Lansky A, Leipsic J, Min JK. Diagnosis of ischemia-causing coronary stenoses by noninvasive fractional flow reserve computed from coronary computed tomographic angiograms. Results from the prospective multicenter DISCOVER-FLOW (Diagnosis of Ischemia-Causing Stenoses Obtained Via Noninvasive Fractional Flow Reserve) study. J Am Coll Cardiol. 2011;58:1989-1997. DOI: 10.1016/j.jacc. 2011.06.066.

[122] Taylor CA, Fonte TA, Min JK. Computational fluid dynamics applied to cardiac computed tomography for noninvasive quantification of fractional flow reserve: Scientific basis. J Am Coll Cardiol. 2013;61:2233-2241. DOI: 10.1016/j.jacc.2012.11.083.

[123] Min JK, Leipsic J, Pencina MJ, Berman DS, Koo BK, van Mieghem C, Erglis A, Lin FY, Dunning AM, Apruzzese P, Budoff MJ, Cole JH, Jaffer FA, Leon MB, Malpeso J, Mancini GB, Park SJ, Schwartz RS, Shaw LJ, Mauri L. Diagnostic accuracy of fractional flow reserve from anatomic CT angiography. JAMA. 2012;308:1237-1245. DOI: 10.1001/2012.jama.11274.

[124] Nørgaard BL, Leipsic J, Gaur S, Seneviratne S, Ko BS, Ito H, Jensen JM, Mauri L, De Bruyne B, Bezerra H, Osawa K, Marwan M, Naber C, Erglis A, Park SJ, Christiansen EH, Kaltoft A, Lassen JF, Bøtker HE, Achenbach S; NXT Trial Study Group. Diagnostic performance of noninvasive fractional flow reserve derived from coronary computed tomography angiography in suspected coronary artery disease: the NXT trial

(Analysis of Coronary Blood Flow Using CT Angiography: Next Steps). J Am Coll Cardiol. 2014;63:1145-1155. DOI:10.1016/j.jacc.2013.11.043.

[125] Abbara S, Arbab-Zadeh A, Callister TQ, Desai MY, Mamuya W, Thomson L, Weigold WG. SCCT guidelines for performance of coronary computed tomographic angiography: A report of the Society of Cardiovascular Computed Tomography Guidelines Committee. J Cardiovasc Comput Tomogr. 2009;3:190-204. DOI:10.1016/j.jcct.2009.03. 004.

[126] Leipsic J, Yang TH, Thompson A, Koo BK, Mancini GB, Taylor C, Budoff MJ, Park HB, Berman DS, Min JK. Technical factors and patient preparation prior to coronary CT angiography and diagnostic performance of non-invasive fractional flow reserve: Results from the determination of fractional flow reserve by anatomic computed angiography (DeFACTO) study. AJR Am J Roentgenol. 2014;202:989-994. DOI:10.2214/AJR.13.11441.

[127] Patel MR. Detecting obstructive coronary disease with CT angiography and noninvasive fractional flow reserve. JAMA. 2012;308:1269-1270. DOI: 10.1001/2012.jama.11383.

[128] Montalescot G, Sechtem U, Achenbach S, Andreotti F, Arden C, Budaj A, Bugiardini R, Crea F, Cuisset T, Di Mario C, Ferreira JR, Gersh BJ, Gitt AK, Hulot JS, Marx N, Opie LH, Pfisterer M, Prescott E, Ruschitzka F, Sabaté M, Senior R, Taggart DP, van der Wall EE, Vrints CJ; ESC Committee for Practice Guidelines, Zamorano JL, Achenbach S, Baumgartner H, Bax JJ, Bueno H, Dean V, Deaton C, Erol C, Fagard R, Ferrari R, Hasdai D, Hoes AW, Kirchhof P, Knuuti J, Kolh P, Lancellotti P, Linhart A, Nihoyannopoulos P, Piepoli MF, Ponikowski P, Sirnes PA, Tamargo JL, Tendera M, Torbicki A, Wijns W, Windecker S; Document Reviewers, Knuuti J, Valgimigli M, Bueno H, Claeys MJ, Donner-Banzhoff N, Erol C, Frank H, Funck-Brentano C, Gaemperli O, Gonzalez-Juanatey JR, Hamilos M, Hasdai D, Husted S, James SK, Kervinen K, Kolh P, Kristensen SD, Lancellotti P, Maggioni AP, Piepoli MF, Pries AR, Romeo F, Rydén L, Simoons ML, Sirnes PA, Steg PG, Timmis A, Wijns W, Windecker S, Yildirir A, Zamorano JL. 2013 ESC guidelines on the management of stable coronary artery disease: The task force on the management of stable coronary artery disease of the European Society of Cardiology. Eur Heart J. 2013;34:2949-3003. DOI: 10.1093/eurheartj/eht296.

[129] Tonino PA, Fearon WF, De Bruyne B, Oldroyd KG, Leesar MA, Ver Lee PN, Maccarthy PA, Van't Veer M, Pijls NH. Angiographic versus functional severity of coronary artery stenoses in the FAME study fractional flow reserve versus angiography in multivessel evaluation. J Am Coll Cardiol. 2010;55:2816-2821. DOI: 10.1016/ j.jacc.2009.11.096.

[130] Maurovich-Horvat P, Ferencik M, Voros S, Merkely B, Hoffmann U. Comprehensive plaque assessment by coronary CT angiography. Nat Rev Cardiol. 2014;11:390-402. DOI: 10.1038/nrcardio.2014.60.

[131] Nakanishi K, Fukuda S, Shimada K, Ehara S, Inanami H, Matsumoto K, Taguchi H, Muro T, Yoshikawa J, Yoshiyama M. Non-obstructive low attenuation coronary plaque predicts three-year acute coronary syndrome events in patients with hypertension: multidetector computed tomographic study. J Cardiol. 2012;59:167-175. DOI: 10.1016/j.jjcc. 2011.11.010.

[132] Utsunomiya M, Hara H, Moroi M, Sugi K, Nakamura M. Relationship between tissue characterization with 40 MHz intravascular ultrasound imaging and 64-slice computed tomography. J Cardiol 2011;57:297-302. DOI: 10.1016/j.jjcc.2011.01.016.

[133] Ridker PM, Danielson E, Fonseca FA, Genest J, Gotto Jr AM, Kastelein JJ, Koenig W, Libby P, Lorenzatti AJ, MacFadyen JG, Nordestgaard BG, Shepherd J, Willerson JT, Glynn RJ, JUPITER Study Group. Rosuvastatin to prevent vascular events in men and women with elevated C-reactive protein. N Engl J Med. 2008;359:2195-2207. DOI: 10.1056/NEJMoa0807646.

[134] Fayad ZA, Fuster V, Nikolaou K, Becker C. Computed tomography and magnetic resonance imaging for noninvasive coronary angiography and plaque imaging: Current and potential future concepts. Circulation. 2002;106:2026-2034. DOI: 10.1161/01.CIR.0000034392.34211.FC.

Section 2

Surgical Treatment of Coronary Lesions

Chapter 6

Coronary Artery Bypass Surgery

Kaan Kırali and Hakan Saçlı

Additional information is available at the end of the chapter

http://dx.doi.org/10.5772/61404

Abstract

Surgical treatment of coronary artery disease should increase regional coronary flow reserve and not increase any early or late morbidity and mortality more than the other treatment modalities. In the past 50 years, surgical treatment of coronary artery disease has been adapted rapidly worldwide and several techniques have been developed to decrease total surgical risks and to improve early and late results with the highest level of quality of life. In spite of the last guidelines that offer stents for single or multiple vessels disease, the fact is that surgical revascularization has better outcomes in all groups of coronary artery patients. In the past two decades, the main target has been to limit or eliminate side effects of extracorporeal circulation and cardioplegia (off-pump), and general anesthesia (awake coronary bypass). The prime goal of surgical revascularization is to obtain complete revascularization by bypassing all severe stenotic coronary arteries having a diameter larger than 1 mm. Surgical revascularization with cardiopulmonary bypass through a full sternotomy remains the most widely used surgical technique. With the development of stabilization devices, off-pump procedures can be safely performed in most patients with single or multivessel disease. Minimal invasive and/or robotic surgery is an attractive procedure to catch invasive cardiology. The gold standard strategy involves single graft to single target vessel bypass, especially the left internal mammary artery to the left anterior descending artery. The early cumulative mortality rate is below 3%, but lower than 1% in lower-risk patients. There are some variables most predictive of early mortality: older age, female, reoperation, non-elective surgery, left ventricular dysfunction, accelerated atherosclerosis. The survival rate is higher than 65% for 15 years. Late mortality is dependent not only on non-use of internal mammarian artery, closure of grafts, progression of native arterial disease but also on comorbidities. Satisfactory quality of life after surgery depends on the long-term duration of the freedom from angina, heart failure, rehospitalization and reintervention, and improvement of the exercise capacity. Return of angina during the first 6 months depends on incomplete revascularization or graft failure, whereas progression of native-vessel disease and grafts are serious risk factors for the late recurrence of angina. Venous graft occlusion is the most common reason for reintervention, and native vessel disease is the second.

Keywords: Coronary artery bypass, arterial graft, revascularization, off-pump, awake

1. Introduction

Coronary artery disease (CAD) is the most common pathology which prepossesses cardiologists and cardiac surgeons in the past century. It was the most common (38.8%) cause of death in Turkey in 2013 [1]. Ischemic heart disease was also the most common reason of mortality in the world as reported by the World Health Organization in 2012 [2]. Coronary artery disease is caused by an atherosclerotic plaque which narrows the internal lumen of the coronary artery. This lesion decreases coronary arterial blood flow and oxygen supply to the myocardium, and causes several symptoms such as chest pain, dyspnea, syncope, sometimes pulmonary edema. The low blood flow through the coronary artery territory cannot increase and support the increasing daily-life effort capacity, and the increased demand of oxygenated blood supply starts angina pectoris. There are several examinations such as exercise test, myocardial perfusion scintigraphy and computed tomography, but biplane coronary angiography is the gold standard for diagnosis. An improved understanding of the pathophysiology of CAD has forwarded efforts to increase myocardial blood supply. According to the result of angiography, patients should be treated either medically or with invasive treatment modalities. Because myocardial revascularization prolongs survival, relieves angina, and improves quality of life, percutaneous coronary intervention and coronary artery bypass surgery (CABG) can be the only treatment strategies to perform this revascularization. The general condition of patients is the decisive factor to select the best acceptable revascularization strategy. The most adequate surgical technique will be selected according to the degree and number of the affected coronary artery lesions, lesion type, and lesion location. The potential aim of the minimally invasive techniques is to reduce postoperative patient discomfort, to decrease bleeding and wound infection, and to shorten recovery times.

2. History

The first method to establish blood supply to the ischemic myocardium is to place the pedicled pectoralis muscle flap on the pericardium performed by Beck in 1935 [3]. The following 10 years passed with the developments such as chemical pericarditis and revascularization through the coronary sinus. Beck I operation (abrasion of the pericardium and epicardium + application of an inflammatory agent + partial occlusion of the coronary sinus) was described in 1945 and Beck II operation (total or partial ligation of the coronary sinus + brachial artery bypass between the descending aorta and the coronary sinus) was introduced in 1947. Vineberg described the direct implantation of internal mammarian artery (IMA) into the myocardium in 1950 [4]. A modification of the Vineberg procedure (anastomosis of a long saphenous vein between the aorta and the apex of the heart) was performed by Smith in 1955. The first successful coronary endarterectomy was performed by Bailey in 1956 [5]. Goetz performed the first successful planned CABG operation in 1960 [6]. The first patch graft technique to enlarge the obstructed left main coronary artery was performed by Effler in 1962 [7]. The first usage of a saphenous vein as an aorta–coronary artery bypass conduit was described by Sabiston in 1962 [8]. Favalaro placed a saphenous vein between the ascending aorta (side-to-end) and the right coronary artery (RCA) (end-to-end) in 1960s. [9] The official start of CABG surgery happened at the end of 1960s and saphenous vein grafts were used in all major branches with the same technique as we use nowadays [10]. Kolessov performed the first successful left internal mammary artery (LIMA) to the left anterior descending (LAD) coronary artery anastomosis on the beating heart through a left thoracotomy in 1964 [11]. Internal mammary artery grafts have been the first choice and gold standard for LAD revascularization after their superior long-term patency became known [12].

After all of the developments in cardiac surgery, the cornerstone is the development of the cardiopulmonary bypass machine. This staged development has brought CABG surgery as a standard treatment modality after 1960s. The first stage was the discovery of heparin in 1915, which opened the door for open heart surgery. The second stage was the development of a heart–lung machine. The first successful open heart procedures on a human utilizing the heart–lung machine were total left-sided heart bypass procedures, where the patient's own lungs were used to oxygenate the blood. The right-sided heart bypass procedure was performed by Dodrill and colleagues in 1952 [13]. The first successful total cardiopulmonary bypass (CPB) procedure using a heart–lung machine was performed by Gibbon to close an atrial septal defect in 1953 [14]. The third stage was the development of membrane oxygenators in the 1960s. The first successful usage of a membrane oxygenator for extracorporeal circulation was performed by Hill and colleagues in 1972 [15]. The fourth stage was using a potassium-based cardioplegia solution to protect myocardium during open heart surgery. Melrose and colleagues presented the first experimental study with blood cardioplegia in 1955, but toxicity of this solution prevented usage of this cardioplegia for several years [16]. Several types of crystalloid cardioplegia solution with different elements were tried to protect myocardium after a significant protection of myocardium during potassium-induced cardiac arrest was demonstrated in 1973 [17]. Follette and colleagues reintroduced the technique of blood cardioplegia in 1978 [18].

After all of the developments in the conventional CABG surgery, the next step has been to minimize the standard surgical revascularization procedure using different techniques. Coronary bypass surgery is performed without opening a cardiac chamber and it is not necessary to use extracorporeal circulation. Continuing ventilation of the lungs eliminates the use of any oxygenator and keeping a beating heart eliminates any pump. Even though the first CABG procedures were performed with off-pump technique, cardiac arrest during on-pump technique has pressurized beating heart surgery. Ankeney tried to increase the interest of the off-pump revascularization in 1972, but it took only 10 years to be able to perform off-pump CABG routinely [19]. Benetti [20] and Buffolo [21] popularized this strategy in 1980s. The first cases were revascularization of anteriorly located coronary arteries. Three limiting factors have inhibited ideal myocardial revascularization: adequate exposure, blood flow, and motion. The technical advances regarding exposure and stabilization have facilitated complete revascularization. Several new strategies have been developed for off-pump CABG. First strategy was to stabilize the beating heart with different devices [22]. Second strategy was to position the beating heart for the adequate exposure of all epicardial coronary arteries [23]. Third strategy was to minimize surgical intervention with different minimal invasive approaches [24]. Last step was to avoid general anesthesia to minimize respiratory side effects [25], whereas Kırali and colleagues [26] performed off-pump complete arterial revascularization with using bilateral IMAs for in awake patients. Harvesting IMAs was the other issue for off-pump surgery. Endoscopic IMA harvesting was used, but it did not widespread [27]. Today, we are facing fully endoscopic off-pump myocardial revascularization-assisted robotic surgery. Loulmet [28] was the first to report a successfully completed robotic CABG, but conversion was very common in early series. Stepwise progression of robotic technology and development of specific procedures will result in simpler robotic CABG in the near future [29].

3. General information

Coronary artery disease varies enormously from patient to patient; therefore, recommendations to patients on the basis of predictions and comparisons of outcomes between CABG and the other treatment options are of little value. Surgical treatment of CAD should increase the regional coronary flow reserve and not increase any early or late morbidity and mortality more than the other treatment modalities. Patient-specific features, risks, and predictions are required to offer patients the surgical treatment. Because anginal symptoms are very subjective for both patients and surgeons and there is a weak correlation between the severity of symptoms and the involvement of coronary arteries, the gold standard biplane coronary angiography is the only option to decide which surgical revascularization strategy to use. Perfusion imaging and echocardiography examinations can diagnose associated cardiac pathologies, which require surgical intervention at the same time. Computed tomographic angiography is a new option, but not a suitable alternative, and gives more detailed information about distal vascular bed or ostial lesions. Intravascular ultrasound and fractional flow reserve can clarify the severity of intermediate lesions.

Myocardial revascularization represents an effective treatment strategy shown to prolong survival. In the past 50 years, surgical treatment of CAD has been adapted rapidly worldwide because CABG provides excellent short- and mid-term results in the management of ischemic heart disease with the highest level of quality of life. But long-term results of surgical revascularization are affected by failure of conduits, and late patency of conduits is affected by graft-type, coronary runoff, and severity of distal native vessel atherosclerosis. Several techniques have been developed to decrease total surgical risks and to improve early and late outcomes, but CABG surgery with or without CPB through median sternotomy remains the standard surgical intervention despite an increasing risk profile and diffusing coronary artery involvement. The aim of CABG is to increase the blood supply in coronary arteries by obtaining complete revascularization of all severe stenotic epicardial coronary arteries with a diameter larger than 1 mm. However, optimal patency rates can be obtained in saphenous vein grafts with a distal lumen of ≥ 2 mm. Most patients undergoing CABG have extensive three-system disease, often with important stenoses in more than three coronary branches. The standard strategy involves usage of LIMA to the LAD and saphenous veins to the remaining coronary arteries, whereas full arterial revascularization is preferred in young population. "Single graft to single target vessel bypass" is the gold standard for myocardial revascularization, but in some situations sequential bypass or complex configuration of conduits can be used for complete revascularization in the presence of inadequate venous grafts. The condition of the distal coronary vasculature is important for the outcome of bypass conduits, and the rate of CAD progression appears to be three to six times higher in grafted native coronary arteries than that in no grafted native vessels. If coronary arteries are diffusely diseased (> 10 mm) or occluded, several surgical techniques can be chosen to complete surgical revascularization as explained in the next chapter.

Indication for surgical revascularization depends on the need of improvement in the quality and/or duration of life. Despite the increase of CAD, nowadays, the indications for CABG have changed a little, but became more limited. Aggressive percutaneous coronary interventions (PCI) suppress surgery and minimal invasive surgical procedures force surgery. The last guidelines offer stents for single or multiple vessels disease, but the fact that surgical revascularization has better outcomes in all groups of CAD patients and stents is best used if there are no anatomic indications for CABG. The decision to perform myocardial revascularization with stent or CABG depends mainly on coronary anatomy, left ventricular function, and other medical or non-medical comorbidities that may affect the patient's risk. Patients with more extensive and severe coronary atherosclerosis could have more increasing benefit from surgery over stent therapy.

4. Indications

The only base for the indication of surgical myocardial revascularization is the positive benefits of CABG against no treatment, medical treatment, or treatment by PCI. Regardless of symptoms, indication for CABG is determined by the clinical status of the patient and patient-specific predictors. The main purpose is to improve the quality of life and to prolong the life expectancy. The number of the affected vessels, the degree and the localization of lesions are important to make this decision. 2011 ACCF/AHA Guideline for CABG supports surgical revascularization for patients with extensive and severe multivessel CAD, especially associated with left ventricular dysfunction (LVD), renal insufficiency, and/or diabetes mellitus (Table 1) [30]. In the real world, patients with proximal LAD lesion must be sent to surgical revascularization regardless of the number of affected coronary arteries, but cardiologists like to revascularize these patients with stent regardless of the superiority of LIMA-LAD anastomosis (Figure 1). Although patients with LVD would benefit from CABG more, the real data suggest that poor left ventricular function increases early mortality after surgery. Patients with good left ventricular function can have better prognosis than patients with LVD. Risks and benefits of CABG become more uncertain when resting left ventricular ejection fraction (LVEF) is less than 30%, particularly when it is less than 20%. The only exception is myocardial hibernation which causes severe reduction in resting LVEF. Stable angina requires elective myocardial revascularization, but unstable angina or non-ST-segment elevation acute coronary syndrome or non-Q-wave myocardial infarction requires priority CABG to prevent patients from transmural myocardial infarction. In the early period (< 4 h) after acute transmural myocardial infarction, emergency CABG can be a lifesaving procedure, but some patients cannot be salvaged. Myocardial re-revascularization can be necessary when myocardial ischemia returns after CABG, and stent implantation is the first choice for restenosis of grafted coronary arteries or vein grafts.

Revascularization	CABG			DES		
	No-risk	DM	LVD	No-risk	DM	LVD
1-vessel	N	N	N	Y	Y	Y
Proximal LAD	Y	Y	Y	N	N	N
2-vessel without LAD	N	N	N	Y	Y	Y
2-vessel with LAD	Y	Y	Y	Y	Y	Y
2-vessel + proximal LAD	Y	Y	Y	N	N	N
3-vessel	Y	Y	Y	C	C	C
3-vessel + proximal LAD	Y	Y	Y	N	N	N
LMC ± other lesions	Y	Y	Y	N	N	N

CABG = coronary artery bypass grafting; DES = drug eliting stent; DM = diabetes mellitus; LAD = left anterior descending artery; LMC = left main coronary artery disease; LVD = left ventricular dysfunction.
*Y = yes; N = no; C = controversial

Figure 1. The reality of myocardial revascularization strategies in patients with isolated coronary artery disease.

Asymptomatic CAD	
Class I	
	1. LMC stenosis
	2. LMCE disease
	3. Three-vessel disease
Class IIa	
	1. Proximal LAD (one- or two-vessel)
Class IIb	
	1. One- or two-vessel disease not involving proximal LAD
	(if a large territory at risk on noninvasive studies or LVEF < 50%, IIa and IIb become class I indications)
Stable Angina	
Class I	
	1. LMC stenosis

	2. LMCE disease
	3. Three-vessel disease
	4. Two-vessel disease with proximal LAD stenosis and LVEF < 50% or demonstrable ischemia
	5. One- or two-vessel disease without proximal LAD stenosis but with a large territory at risk and high-risk criteria on noninvasive testing
	6. Disabling angina refractory to medical therapy
Class IIa	
	1. Proximal LAD stenosis with one-vessel disease
	2. One- or two-vessel disease without proximal Lad stenosis, but with a moderate territory at risk and demonstrable ischemia
Unstable Angina / Non-ST-Segment Elevation MI (NSTEMI)	
Class I	
	1. LMC stenosis
	2. LMCE disease
	3. Ongoing ischemia not responsive to maximal nonsurgical therapy
Class IIa	
	1. Proximal LAD stenosis with one- or two-vessel disease
Class IIb	
	1. One- or two-vessel disease without proximal LAD stenosis when PCI not possible (becomes class I if high-risk criteria on noninvasive testing)
ST-Segment Elevation (Q wave) MI	
Class I	
	1. Failed PCI with persistent pain or shock and anatomically feasible
	2. Persistent or recurrent ischemia refractory to medical treatment with acceptable anatomy who have a significant territory at risk and not a candidate for PCI
	3. Requires surgical repair of post-infarct VSD or MR
	4. Cardiogenic shock in patients < 75 years of age who have ST elevation, LBBB, or a posterior MI within 18 hours onset
	5. Life-threatening ventricular arrhythmias in the presence of ≥ 50% LMC stenosis or three-vessel disease
Class IIa	
	1. Primary reperfusion in patients who have failed fibrinolytics or PCI and are in the early stages (6-12 h) of an evolving STEMI
	2. Mortality with CABG is elevated the first 3-7 days after STEMI/NSTEMI. After 7 days, criteria for CABG in previous section apply.
Poor LV Function	

Class I	
	1. LMC
	2. LMCE
	3. Proximal LAD stenosis and two- to three-vessel disease
Class IIa	
	1. Significant viable territory and noncontractile myocardium
Life-Threatening ventricular Arrhythmias	
Class I	
	1. LMC
	2. Three-vessel disease
Class IIa	
	1. Bypassable one- or two-vessel disease
	2. Proximal LAD disease and one- or two-vessel disease
	These become class I indications if arrhythmia is resuscitated cardiac death or sustained ventricular tachycardia
Failed PCI	
Class I	
	1. Ongoing ischemia with significant territory at risk
	2. Shock
Class IIa	
	1. Foreign body in critical position
	2. Shock with coagulopathy and no previous sternotomy
Class IIb	
	1. Shock with coagulopathy and previous sternotomy
Previous CABG	
Class I	
	1. Disabling angina refractory to medical therapy
	2. Nonpatent previous bypass grafts, but with class I indications for native CAD
Class IIa	
	1. Large territory at risk
	2. Vein grafts supplying LAD or large territory are "/> 50% stenosed

Class I: Conditions for which there is evidence and/or general agreement that a given procedure or treatment is useful and effective

http://dx.doi.org/10.5772/61404

Class II: Conditions for which there is conflicting evidence and/or a divergence of opinion about the usefulness or efficacy of a procedure
Class IIa: Weight of evidence/opinion is in favor of usefulness/efficacy
Class IIb: Usefulness/efficacy is less well established by evidence/opinion
Class III: Conditions for which there is evidence and/or general agreement that the procedure/treatment is not useful/ effective and in some cases may be harmful

ACC = American College of Cardiology; AHA = American Heart Association; CABG = coronary artery bypass grafting; CAD = coronary artery disease; LAD = left anterior descending artery; LBBB = left bundle branch block, LMC = left main coronary artery; LMCE = left main coronary equivalent; LVEF = left ventricular ejection fraction; MI = myocardial infarction; MR = mitral regurgitation; NSTEMI = non-ST elevation myocardial infarction; PCI = percutaneous transluminal coronary angioplasty; STEMI = ST elevation myocardial infarction; VSD = ventricular septal defect

Table 1. AHA/ACC guidlines for CABG

Myocardial revascularization in special circumstances is another important issue (Table 2). The common denominator of these distressed conditions is the accelerated risk of surgery. Intraoperative mortality and morbidity increase after CABG due to the multi-organ dysfunction. Prolonged intubation, requiring ultrafiltration or hemodialysis, mechanical hemodynamic support, and/or infection risk can be very harmful despite full multisystem treatment. Nowadays, an aggressive strategy is favored to early myocardial revascularization in acute coronary syndrome, and surgical indication can be extended for these patients, but stent implantation is the first choice in the majority of this population. Surgical treatment has the advantage to bypass all occluded and/or stenotic coronary arteries at the same time, which suppresses early adverse outcomes. Left main or left main equivalent disease should be treated surgically, and this pathology is not a contraindication to use arterial grafts in any situation, especially for LIMA to LAD anastomosis. Severe LVD is not considered as an indication for surgery, but patients with hibernating or stunned myocardium can benefit from CABG. The only surgical indication for patients with severe LVD is the possibility of full revascularization during CABG. Otherwise, stent implantation should be the preferred approach. Total occlusion is not a contraindication for stent; but if it cannot be applied, surgery will be the alternative treatment. The important point is the diffuse involvement of atherosclerosis, which needs endarterectomy or long-segment anastomosis, and the choice of the acceptable revascularization procedure, which will be particularly influenced by the presence of comorbidities, especially in the elderly patients; but they cannot prevent usual surgery. In general, women have a higher risk for perioperative complications, but this adverse outcome can be explained by the presentation of female population at older ages with more extensive CAD, associated risk factors, LVD, and smaller body size. Diabetes is characterized by an inflammatory, proliferative, and prothrombotic state with more diffuse atherosclerosis, which may have a role in the increased risk of restenosis and occlusion. The first option is the complete revascularization, which is more often performed surgically than percutaneously. Coronary artery disease is a common reason of mortality among patients with end-stage renal failure and CABG is the option for myocardial revascularization. The main problem is the excessive atherosclerosis with severe calcification on the aortic wall and in the coronary arteries, which make surgery difficult. Recurrent ischemia after CABG or stent implantation is an indication of re-

revascularization. Severe stenosis must be treated with stent after previous CABG, but CABG is the first option for re-revascularization after previous PCIs.

1. Acute coronary syndrome
2. Left main or left main equivalent (proximal LAD and Cx) disease
3. Severe left ventricular dysfunction
4. Total occlusions
5. The elderly population
6. The female population
7. Diabetes mellitus
8. End-stage renal disease
9. Previous myocardial revascularization (CABG or stent)

Table 2. Special circumstances for myocardial revascularization

5. Bypass conduits

Conduits for CABG are the base of surgical myocardial revascularization, because they are critical to the success of the procedure. Easy harvesting, simple implantation, long-term patency, and possible side effects must be taken into consideration during the preference of usable conduits for each patient to avoid an uneventful postoperative outcome and to achieve better long-term survival. Arterial grafts are favorable because of their long-term patency and resistance against atherosclerosis, which is related to the differences in biological characteristics between veins and arteries. Early vein graft failure (stenosis or occlusion) is the most important drawback of venous conduits; nevertheless, using venous grafts is still an integral part of coronary surgery. There are some differences between venous and arterial conduits, which may affect the long-term patency rate (Table 3).

1. Veins are more susceptible to vasoactive substances than arteries.
2. The venous wall is supplied by the vaso vasorum whereas the arterial wall may be supplied through the lumen in addition to the vaso vasorum.
3. The arterial endothelium may secrete more endothelium-derived relaxing factor and nitric oxide.
4. The structure of veins is more suited to low pressure whereas the artery to high pressure.

Table 3. Differences between venous and arterial grafts

5.1. Arterial grafts

Arterial grafts are not similar in anatomy or function, and there are differences regarding to contractility and endothelial function. Commonly harvested arterial conduits relate to different groups of arteries in the body (Table 4). The most important variation is the structural histology of arteries, whereas some arteries (Type II and III) contain more smooth muscle cells in their wall, thus are less elastic, or some arteries (Type I) contain more elastic laminae, thus are more elastic. Arterial grafts can develop spasm during surgical harvesting and handling, but the IMA shows the lowest vasospasm rate. Internal mammary artery releases more nitric oxide and endothelium-derived relaxing factor than the other arterial conduits. The reactivity of the arterial conduits changes along the length of arteries and the main mid-portion of them is less reactive than distal or proximal portions. This is the reason why the small and highly vasospastic distal part of the arterial grafts is trimmed before anastomosis. This part of conduits contains relatively smoother muscle cells and has a smaller diameter. The incidence of atherosclerotic changes in arterial conduits is rare and lower than in coronary arteries. Based on the superior long-term patency of the IMA, orientation to the other arteries has been popularized. The radial artery (RA) and the gastroepiploic artery (GEA) have been used for complete revascularization. Their usage has decreased in the past decade due to their lower patency rate, where the early occlusion of both grafts depends on higher response to vasoconstructive situations like the inotropic support, the low cardiac output syndrome (LCOS), and usage of different spasmogens.

A. Type I (somatic arteries; less spastic)
1. Internal mammary artery
2. Inferior epigastric artery
3. Subscapular artery
B. Type II (splanchnic = visceral arteries; spastic)
1. Gastroepiploic artery
2. Splenic artery
3. Inferior mesenteric artery
C. Type III (limb arteries; spastic)
1. Radial artery
2. Ulnar artery
3. Lateral femoral circumflex artery

Table 4. Arterial grafts

5.1.1. Internal mammary artery

The IMAs lie vertically and slightly laterally at a short distance from both margins of the sternum. The length of in situ left IMA is slightly longer than the right and ranges from 15 to 25 cm (mean 20 ± 2 cm). The IMA bifurcates into its terminal branches (musculophrenic and superior epigastric arteries) at the level of the sixth rib, and the in situ IMA should be cut before this distal bifurcation to get the acceptable intraluminal diameter for IMA–coronary artery anastomosis. Excessive traction, stretching, clamping, or misplaced metal clips during harvesting should be avoided to get a nontraumatized IMA without any injury (hematoma, dissection, rupture). We prefer to harvest the IMA using semi-skeletonized technique, which allows an increasing luminal diameter, providing a longer graft, allowing more distal anastomosis and sequential grafting. The full length of this IMA prevents any tension on the conduit, but some associated maneuvers can be needed to avoid stress on the IMA [31]. Making a window on the pericardium at the left side of the pulmonary artery, where the LIMA is lied down into the pericardium, prevents also the stretch of the LIMA [32]. The full length of the right IMA (RIMA) allows anterior (on the front of the heart) or lateral (through the transverse sinus) wall revascularization with optimal long-term patency, but the RCA revascularization is more difficult due to the distance of the distal segments [33].

5.1.2. Radial artery

The radial artery with higher patency rate according to saphenous vein can be a second alternative bypass conduit instead of vein grafts. The RA can have more atherosclerotic changes at the time of harvest than the IMA. The RA is very vasoreactive, and therefore is very sensitive to competitive flow. In the past two decades, using the RA as a pedicled arterial graft has been the preferred conduit as the second bypass graft, but the mid- and long-term patency rates are controversial. The failure of the RA grafts depends on three general ways: complete occlusion, string sign, or focal stenosis. The graft failure rate is the highest at the right system and equal to the saphenous vein graft [34]. The mid-term patency on the left coronary system is higher if the proximal anastomosis is performed on the ascending aorta [35]. Because the IMAs have higher long-term patency rates than the RA and the acceptable approach is using both IMAs for the left coronary system, usage of the RA has not increased and the saphenous vein is a more practicable conduit with a comparable patency rate than the RA for the right system [36]. The patient's nondominant arm is chosen for harvest, but the extremity must have adequate ulnar collateral circulation and the recurrent radial branch should be left intact [37]. The harvest of the left RA can be performed easily and simultaneously with the LIMA. Transient paresthesia, numbness, and thumb weakness could be seen, but the symptoms resolve with time [38].

5.1.3. Gastroepiploic artery

The gastroepiploic artery has been used as an alternative conduit or as part of an all-arterial revascularization strategy. The widespread use of the GEA has not been adopted due to the increased harvesting time, the potential abdominal complications, and inadequate early- and long-term patency rates. Opening the abdomen is a serious intervention and the GEA may be used only in patients who require any abdominal aortic surgery [39]. This arterial conduit has been used usually for the RCA revascularization because the in situ right GEA can reach only to the distal branches of the RCA.

5.1.4. Other arteries

Bilateral IMAs and the RA are often adequate to get full arterial complete myocardial revascularization. These grafts can be used in situ or in combined fashion, and distal anastomoses can be made single or sequential. Revascularization with the other arterial conduits has been left as an anecdotal use in the literature. Maybe, they can be used during redo or tredo CABG operations if there is no another conduits left. The studies on these arterial grafts have been left as academic researches [40].

5.2. Venous grafts

5.2.1. Greater saphenous vein

The saphenous vein is one of the most commonly used conduits in CABG. The early- and long-term patency of vein grafts is worse than that of arterial grafts, and one third of the vein grafts shows an important reduction in flow compared with the early postoperative period. Second disadvantage is easy kinking or torsion after anastomosis, which can cause fatal myocardial ischemia. However, its easiness to harvest, availability, usability, resistance to spasm, and acceptable long-term patency rate make vein grafts the second choice for revascularization conduits. There are no detrimental effects of harvest technique on vein morphology, endothelial structure or function, or graft patency. Saphenous vein can be harvested with an open (conventional = standard) or endoscopic technique. Endoscopic or minimal invasive harvest techniques could be more harmless. Open harvesting can be achieved with a complete or bridged approach. In reality, no-touch technique during open-vein harvest, in which the vein is removed with a pedicle of surrounding tissue, prevents vein injury and prolongs long-term durability. Specifically, vein grafts must not be grasped with forceps, stretched, or overdistended to avoid any endothelial damage. All venous tributaries should be ligated or clipped away from the vein itself and the lumen of the graft should not be injured, narrowed, or left with a blind sac on the side branches.

5.2.2. Other veins

Alternative venous grafts such as the lesser saphenous and cephalic veins are seldom secondary choice for vein graft. The lesser saphenous vein could be harvested with the same technique performed during standard vein harvest. Arm veins have significantly lower patency rate than saphenous veins, and for that reason, they are not used as a venous conduit.

6. Surgical procedures

Coronary bypass surgery can be performed with different techniques. The most common approach for CABG is on-pump revascularization via median sternotomy and under general anesthesia. Patients' characteristics and risk factors forward surgeons to prefer the appropriate approach for each individual case. Different techniques, variant approaches, new technologies, surgeon experience, and associated cardiovascular or organ pathologies restrict or direct cardiac surgeons to specific CABG procedures (Table 5). The benefits of off-pump techniques can be more evident for patients with high risk, especially for complications associated with cardiopulmonary bypass (CPB) and aortic manipulation. Myocardial protection prevents perioperative infarction and/or postischemic ventricular dysfunction (Table 6). Although considerable progress has been made in this field, the ideal technique has not yet to be discovered due to complex nature of ischemia–reperfusion cascade during surgical revascularization.

A. Arrested heart surgery with CPB
B. Fibrillating heart surgery with CPB
C. Beating heart surgery with circulatory support (central or peripheral)
1. Veno-arterial support (CPB, ECMO)
2. Atrio-arterial support (LHB devices)
3. Veno-venous support (RHB devices)
4. IABP support
D. Beating heart surgery without CPB
1. Standard off-pump through the median sternotomy (OPCAB)
2. Minimal invasive off-pump (MIDCAB)
3. Endoscobic off-pump (OP-TECAB)
4. Robotically assisted off pump (BHTECAB)
5. Awake off-pump (ACAB)

Table 5. Surgical revascularization techniques

A. Arrested heart (cardioplegic) surgery
1. Crystalloid cardioplegia (hypothermic)
2. Blood cardioplegia (cold – warm – tepid)
a) Antegrade (intermittent, continuous)
b) Retrograde (continuous)
c) Combined
i. Antegrade (arrest) – retrograde (continuous)
ii. antegrade (arrest and intermittent) – conduits (intermittent)
iii. antegrade (arrest) – retrograde (continuous) – conduits (intermittent)
B. Beating heart surgery
1. off-pump CABG
2. on-pump CABG
C. Fibrillating heart surgery
1. Intermittent aortic cross-clamping with fibrillation
2. Systemic hypothermia and elective fibrillatory arrest

Table 6. Myocardial protection

http://dx.doi.org/10.5772/61404

6.1. On-Pump CABG

On-pump CABG surgery is the standard conventional technique for myocardial revascularization which is performed via CPB. Despite the fact that off-pump CABG was the first performed technique, on-pump CABG has been used widespread around the world and became the first choice for surgery. An empty, nonbeating heart, a bloodless surgical field, and an easy exposure are essential reasons to prefer on-pump CABG for success of the revascularization procedure. Cardiopulmonary bypass technique includes several stages: cannulation, extracorporeal circulation, myocardial protection, distal with/without proximal anastomoses, and weaning from CPB.

Arterial cannulation for inflow and venous cannulation for outflow are necessary to establish extracorporeal circulation. Arterial cannulation is performed mostly on the ascending aorta, but in case of a contraindication, alternative arteries (femoral or axillary artery) can be preferred. The right atrium is the first choice for venous cannulation; but if there is a contraindication, femoral vein can be used. After inserting the cannulas and finishing harvest of grafts, cardiopulmonary bypass machine starts to work. Blood comes out from the right atrium to the venous blood reservoir, then passes through the oxygenator and is sent to the aorta with a pump. A roller or centrifugal pump is used to continue body perfusion with an acceptable arterial pressure.

Extracorporeal circulation for support during cardiac surgery is uniform, because blood contacting to foreign, nonendothelial surfaces is collected in the reservoir and continuously recirculated throughout the body after oxygenated in the oxygenator. The heart and lung machine has some side effects on the body, which increases early and late morbidity and mortality. There are several adverse effects which cause organ dysfunctions (Table 7). The inflammatory reaction to CPB starts a powerful thrombotic stimulus and the production, release, and circulation of vasoactive and cytotoxic substances that influence the whole body. The inflammatory response produces the cytotoxic compounds and activates neutrophils and monocytes that will destroy organ and tissue cells. On the other hand, the body is able to resist and repair the most part of the cellular damage, although some abnormalities may appear later. The body temperature is lowered according to surgical procedures, but usually mild hypothermic (32–34°C) body perfusion is preferred for isolated CABG procedures to avoid cold or warm body temperature.

A systemic inflammatory response
Releasing cytokines
Metabolic changes
Ischemia-reperfusion injury
Activation of the clotting cascade
Micro-embolization

Table 7. Adverse effects of cardiopulmonary bypass

After cross-clamping the ascending aorta, cardiac arrest is achieved with a cardioplegic solution. Cardioplegic solutions containing a variety of chemical agents are used to arrest the heart rapidly in diastole, create a bloodless anastomotic field, and prevent myocardium against ischemia-reperfusion injury. Blood cardioplegia is chosen for myocardial protection of the arrested heart. Both cold (4–10°C) and warm (37°C) blood cardioplegic solutions have temperature-related advantages and disadvantages. But, tepid (29–32°C) blood cardioplegic solution is the other effective alternative to reduce anaerobic lactic acid released during the arrest period. The best and easiest way to prepare blood cardioplegic solution is to get isothermic (= body perfusion temperature; 32–34°C) blood directly from the pump. The most common cause of postoperative LCOS is inadequate myocardial preservation. There are many different ways of administering the cardioplegic solution: intermittent antegrade ± antegrade via grafts, continuous retrograde, or combined. Continuous retrograde cardioplegia is preferred for severe LMC lesions or diffuse multivessel disease; intermittent antegrade cardioplegia can preserve the myocardium in the other cases effectively. Noncardioplegic surgery is used very seldom, and elective fibrillatory arrest with systemic hypothermia is particularly applicable in case of severely calcified "porcelain aorta", where clamping the ascending aorta may be associated with increased risk of stroke and aortic dissection.

On-pump coronary artery bypass gives an advantage to the surgeon to make the distal anastomoses safely and confidently. Arteriotomy sites should be chosen as accurate as possible to reach the largest-sized coronary target, but distal enough to keep away from obstruction or significant atherosclerotic stenosis. If any target coronary artery has an intramyocardial course, this coronary artery must be opened at the epicardial indentation (for the LAD) or the myocardium on the reflection of the coronary artery can be divided with tight sharp dissection until the coronary artery is reached (for the Cx). The coronary arteriotomy must be performed at least 1.5 times the luminal diameter of the distal coronary artery to get acceptable blood flow, and the distal end of the conduit should be cut vertically at least the luminal diameter of the coronary artery to avoid any anastomotic kinking. Longer incision is not necessary and cannot increase blood supply; but if the graft has a wide diameter, the coronary arteriotomy should be kept open as long as to perform a successful anastomosis. The aim of the anastomosis is to connect the graft and the target coronary artery with fully endothelial approximation affording minimal resistance to flow. Sequential grafting permits efficient use of grafts and the distal anastomosis must be performed on the largest target vessel. The most important drawback of sequential grafting is the source of two or more distal targets on a single graft, where the flow could not be enough for this large myocardial area. For that reason, sequential anastomoses must be performed only on the branches of the same coronary artery. The LAD artery should be revascularized alone or sequential on itself. With the same reason, the IMA should be anastomosed on the LAD alone. Any composite grafting on the IMA (T- or Y-grafting) can increase the risk of inadequate perfusion of the LAD. Coronary arteriotomy and anastomotic technique in diffuse diseased coronary arteries are discussed in the next chapter. Proximal anastomoses are performed after the distal anastomoses under the same cross-clamp or after releasing the cross-clamp under the side-clamp during the rewarming. If the ascending aorta is severely calcific, proximal anastomoses can be performed on the in situ IMAs or

http://dx.doi.org/10.5772/61404

brachiocephalic artery, or on the prosthetic tubular graft after the replacement of the ascending aorta.

On completion of all distal with/without proximal anastomoses, the aortic cross-clamp is removed and the heart begins to beat. The patient is prepared for conversion from mechanic circulation to native circulation, and during this period the bypass grafts are checked for kinks, twists, or tension and for presence of hemostasis. Persistency or regional wall motion abnormalities may require bypass graft revision or replacement of additional bypass graft.

6.2. Off-Pump CABG

The conventional on-pump CABG can be harmful for patients because of the side effects of the heart–lung machine causing fatal complications like stroke, renal, or respiratory failure. Although off-pump revascularization procedures have gained popularity because of the avoidance of the heart–lung machine during surgery in the past two decades, off-pump CABG appears to have reached a plateau, and currently approximately 20% of all CABG procedures are performed on the beating heart without CPB. The main refuse is to success uncomplicated distal anastomoses on the beating heart, which needs bloodless and immobile anastomotic area. Coronary collateral circulation is not necessary until 15 min; but if the anastomotic duration will be longer, an intracoronary shunt may be used to prevent intraoperative ischemia [41].

6.3. OPCAB

Ideal candidates for off-pump coronary artery bypass (OPCAB) include those undergoing primary CABG with good target anatomy and preserved ventricular function. The benefit may be small in low-risk patients, but it is also not so much in high-risk patients. High-risk patients with diffuse multivessel disease and/or LVD cannot tolerate longer ischemia during distal anastomosis, cardiac manipulation, and/or displacement, which cause ventricular arrhythmia or hemodynamic deterioration. Standard OPCAB is performed through the median sternotomy, and cardiac positioners and stabilizers increase the ability of the manipulation of heart with minimal hemodynamic compromise during lateral and/or inferior wall revascularization. A suction-based positioner is placed at the apex to pull the heart in the appropriate direction. The heart is not compressed, anatomo-functional geometry is keeped, and cardiac positioning is usually well tolerated. Then, a stabilizer is established with minimal tension on the epicardium to get a motionless anastomotic area. Some maneuvers may be used to get better exposure such as Trendelenburg position, turning the table toward any side, deep traction stitches; but usually they are not necessary. Medical support can be necessary to stabilize the arterial blood pressure and pulse rate. Anesthesia management is important not to make a per-operative myocardial infarction and life-threatening arrhythmia during distal anastomoses. Heparinization dose is lower than that in the standard on-pump CABG surgery. A soft silastic retractor tape is placed around the proximal segment of the lesion for transient occlusion of coronary blood flow, whereas a second tape could be placed around the distal segment in the presence of strong coronary backflow. The field is kept free of blood with a humidified CO_2 or O_2 blower.

Careful attention must be paid to the sequence of grafting because regional myocardial perfusion is temporarily interrupted in the beating heart (Table 8). As a general rule, the collateralized vessel is grafted first and the collateralizing vessel grafted last. Additional option is a "proximal first" approach. But in our experience, the priority for grafting belongs to the in situ LIMA conduit and LIMA-LAD anastomosis is performed first. There is no doubt to manipulate the heart after this anastomosis, which is the main safety valve of the off-pump revascularization.

First, to revascularize the LAD with in situ LIMA to get fully LAD perfusion immediately after finishing the anastomosis.
Second, to anastomose the other in situ conduits to the target vessels (first IMA-LAD, then IMA-Cx, then RGEA-RCPD)
Third, to perform distal anastomoses of completely occluded or collateralized coronary arteries first, and then to perform proximal anastomoses.
to perform proximal anastomoses first, and then to perform distal anastomoses.
Fourth, to use an intracoronary shunt when beware of a large, dominant RCA with moderated proximal stenosis.
Fifth, to pass small or intramyocardial vessels on the lateral wall with an appropriate lesion for stent.
Sixth, to avoid any sequential grafting and to apply one-to-one bypass grafting.
Seventh, to keep away from endarterectomy if not total occluded coronary artery is present.
Eight, to convert on-pump beating heart surgery if moderate MR is present in patients with Cx and/or distal RCA lesions.

Table 8. Sequence of grafting in OPCAB

6.4. MIDCAB

Minimally invasive direct coronary artery bypass (MIDCAB) procedures have evolved to minimize surgical trauma caused by CPB and aortic manipulation, to avoid wound complications developed by full median sternotomy and open harvesting techniques for bypass conduits, and to prevent respiratory troubles caused by prolonged mechanical ventilation. Only contraindication is emergent revascularization, and severe chronic obstructive pulmonary disease may also not be ideally suited to minithoracotomies. This surgical strategy is a very attractive procedure for coronary patients due to excellent cosmetic and an early and quick recovery. This approach has begun with the single LAD revascularization, but then it has been generalized to multivessel CABG. Another situation for MIDCAB is hybrid procedures, where all coronary arteries that required revascularization (except the LAD) are stented. There are several procedures to perform MIDCAB for single or multiple coronary artery revascularization (Table 9). The main difference of some MIDCAB techniques is the selective right lung ventilation and fast-track approach for extubation.

http://dx.doi.org/10.5772/61404

A. Incisional (avoid from sternotomy)
1. Mini-thoracotomy (MIDCAB)
2. Mini-sternotomy
a) Reversed-J-inferior partial sternotomy
b) T-sternotomy
3. Rib cage lifting technique
4. Subxiphoidal approach
B. Instrumental
1. Conventional
2. Endoscopic
3. Robotic assisted fully endoscopic (TECAB)
C. Respiratuar (avoid from extended mechanical ventilation)
1. Limited mechanic ventilation (fast track anesthesia = intraoperative extubation)
2. Spontaneous ventilation with high thoracic epidural anesthesia (ACAB)
D. Circulatuar (avoid from cardiopulmonary bypass)
1. Off-pump
2. Partial support
a) ECMO
b) IABP
E. Myocardial (avoid from cardioplegia)
1. Off-pump
2. On-pump on the beating heart
3. Ventricular fibrillation
F. Proximal anastomotic (avoid from aortic manipulation)
1. Special devices for proximal anastomoses on the ascending aorta
2. Proximal anastomoses on the LIMA (T- or Y-graft)
3. All in situ arterial grafts

Table 9. Minimal invasive surgical techniques

6.4.1. Minithoracotomy

Standard MIDCAB is usually performed through a left anterior minithoracotomy. The skin incision is made 5–6 cm long in the fourth intercostal space, but removal of a rib is not necessary in any case. This approach is used for single vessel bypass (LIMA-LAD), and the anastomosis is performed with/without any stabilizator. Rib dislocation or fracture is very seldom. After the completion of the anastomosis, the rest of the operation is standard and the patient can be extubated in the operating room or in a couple of hours in the intensive care unit. The patient can be discharged on the 3rd or 4th postoperative day. Because this approach is a highly demanding technical procedure and must be performed by experienced surgeons, this single-vessel CABG procedure will remain an alternative revascularization strategy to stent for patients with complex proximal LAD lesion, chronic occlusions, and in-stent restenosis.

6.4.2. *Ministernotomy*

This approach is preferred mostly by unexperienced surgeons because of similar technical manipulations of the full median sternotomy procedure. The sternotomy is performed partially and divided from xiphoid to the second intercostal space in a down to up direction. Then, the sternum is transected obliquely to the left side (reverse-J-inferior ministernotomy) for single-vessel CABG or the sternum is cut bilaterally (T-sternotomy) for multivessel CABG. These both partial lower median sternotomy techniques leave the manubrium intact to preserve the continuity and stability of the superior thoracal aperture for early and late postoperative recovery. Furthermore, conversion to full sternotomy is more practical than the other small thoracotomy techniques. Only reverse-J-inferior ministernotomy can obstruct proximal anastomosis on the ascending aorta if any free graft is used for bypass surgery [42]. The rest of the surgical revascularization is similar to the conventional CABG procedures. Reverse-J-inferior sternotomy approach preserves respiratory function postoperatively and accelerates the early postoperative recovery, especially in ACAB [43]. T-ministernotomy causes less chest tube drainage, and shorter recovery with early discharge [44].

6.5. TECAB

Robotically assisted totally endoscopic coronary bypass surgery (TECAB) is the most advanced form of less invasive surgical coronary revascularization, which can be an elegant surgical component to hybrid revascularization. However, procedural complexity and a steep learning curve have limited its penetrance in the surgical community. The procedure can be applied on on-pump or off-pump. There are several instruments for anastomoses, but on-pump is more acceptable. Peripheral cannulation is the main disadvantage in some patients, who are not candidates for TECAB.

6.6. ACAB

Awake coronary artery bypass (ACAB) surgery has been offered as a new and unique technique to decrease the adverse effects of general anesthesia. This new modality of CABG combines the minimal invasive nature of MIDCAB with the avoidance of endotracheal intubation and mechanical ventilation. Due to its nature, ACAB offers several advantages over general anesthesia, including better analgesia, decreased myocardial ischemia, improved pulmonary function, reduced stress response, and discharge in couple days of surgery. Cardiac sympatholysis achieves bradycardia, coronary and arterial grafts' vasodilatation and prevents arrhythmia. The aim of this technique is to provide somatosensory and motor block at the T1 and T8 levels and motor block of the intercostal muscles while preserving diaphragmatic respiration. Thoracic sympatholysis allows complete arterial revascularization with bilateral

http://dx.doi.org/10.5772/61404

IMAs with/without RA [45]. A perfect understanding and cooperation between patient and anesthesiologist is necessary for ACAB, while an excellent collaboration between cardiac surgeon and anesthesiologist provides a flawless procedure. Combining advanced anesthetic and high-level surgical merit, this alternative CABG procedure makes surgical treatment feasible and suitable for patients who are not candidates for conventional general anesthesia with endotracheal intubation.

7. Special circumstances

Coronary artery surgery is not unique because of other tissue and/or organ pathologies (Table 10). Coronary revascularization can be performed isolated in patients with single- or multi-vessel disease or combined with other coronary artery interventions and/or cardiac procedures. Associated non-coronary arterial pathologies can make CABG procedures more complex. Surgical strategies for diffuse CAD are discussed in the next chapter.

A. Associated cardiac pathologies
1. Ascending aorta diseases
2. Left ventricular dysfunction
3. Ischemic mitral insufficiency
4. Valvular lesions
5. Congenital pathologies
6. Coronary anomalies
B. Acute coronary syndrome
C. Associated acute mechanical complications of myocardial infarction
1. Mitral regurgitation
2. Ventricular septal defect
3. Free wall rupture
4. Congestive heart failure
D. Associated non-coronary arterial pathologies
1. Carotid artery disease
2. Abdominal aorta pathologies
3. Peripheral arterial diseases
4. Venous diseases
E. Combined diseases
1. Renal disease
2. Diabetes mellitus
3. Malignancy
4. Chronic obstructive pulmonary disease

Table 10. Special situations

Ascending Aorta Pathologies

Ascending aortic pathologies can be treated with different methods. Ascending aortic atherosclerosis can be a very important risk factor for distal embolization, especially for stroke. Epiaortic ultrasound is the only method to identify the extent of atherosclerosis of the ascending aorta. Severe atherosclerosis of the ascending aorta forwards surgeons to the right axillary or femoral artery cannulation. Coronary bypass is performed with "no-touch technique" using only pedicled arterial conduits or composite grafts (T- or Y-graft). If aortic valve replacement is required, the ascending aorta replacement will be performed. Ascending aortic aneurysm and/or dissection required a composite graft replacement during CABG; proximal anastomoses can be performed easily on the tubular graft or composite conduits can be used.

Left Ventricular Dysfunction

Nowadays, most patients with multivessel disease are candidates for surgical revascularization, but the depressed left ventricular function could be a serious contraindication for surgery or risk factor for early adverse outcomes. Resting regional perfusion defects and LV systolic function are improved after CABG in at least 65% of patients with LVD. However, preoperatively depressed resting global left ventricular systolic function cannot change less than 2 weeks after surgery. If this improvement fails to occur, incomplete revascularization or early graft failure is usually found. When preoperative global LVD is severe (LVEF < 30%), myocardial scarring is usually greater and limits recovery of left ventricular function. Complete revascularization is more effective than CABG strategy for myocardial recovery, and there is no reason to prefer OPCAB with incomplete revascularization [46].

Ischemic Mitral Regurgitation

Ischemic LVD represents the first leading cause for mitral regurgitation (MR), which can alter the spatial relationship between the papillary muscles and chordae tendineae and thereby results in functional MR. Some degree of functional MR is found approximately 30% of patients undergoing CABG. In most cases, MR develops from tethering of the posterior leaflet because of regional LVD. The incidence and severity of MR vary inversely with the LVEF and directly with the left ventricular end-diastolic pressure. Correction of reversible ischemia changes the left ventricular geometry and functional MR can decrease or it can be corrected intraoperatively using a ring. The new designed 3D mitral rings are useful, but MR can worsen with time if the left ventricular remodeling continues.

Valvular Pathologies

Nonischemic mitral valve diseases are not common with CAD, but they are not contraindications for coronary surgery. Mitral stenosis is rare, but mitral valve resection with subvalvular apparatus does not decrease left ventricular function. Degenerative mitral valve regurgitation can be associated with LVD; in this situation, subvalvular apparatus should be preserved to prevent the limited left ventricular function. Tricuspid regurgitation is a rare pathology and seen mostly secondary to the left-side valvular diseases, and can be a sign of pulmonary hypertension.

http://dx.doi.org/10.5772/61404

Degenerative aortic stenosis is the most common associated cardiac pathology because of advanced age of CAD patients. Aortic stenosis can be moderate or severe, but asymptomatic. The decision for aortic stenosis may be mixed. If CABG is the decisive indication, the indication for moderate aortic stenosis is more flexible and aortic valve replacement should be performed to prevent patients from reoperation. Aortic valve stenosis with moderate signs (mean gradient > 30 mmHg; aortic valve area 1–1.5 cm^2), pathologic bicuspid aortic valve, or severe annulo-valvular calcification can indicate for associated aortic valve replacement. Stentless biological valves must be the first choice if the aorticoventricular continuity is not disturbed [47].

Acute Coronary Syndrome

Acute coronary syndromes cover a wide spectrum of CAD, while non-ST-segment elevation is the best and risk-free indication for early CABG, if stent implantation is ineffective. Isolated and limited elevation of troponin is not a contraindication for early surgical treatment. Surgical revascularization can be postponed in patients with transmural myocardial infarction without life-threatening complications. But, acute hemodynamic deterioration is a serious and often fatal complication of ongoing myocardial infarction, and delay of CABG can be disadvantageous.

Carotid Artery Disease

Carotid artery disease is an important risk factor of stroke after CABG, especially in the older age group, and the prevalence is higher than 30%. Routine carotid sonographic evaluation is the most widely used preoperative screening test to detect important asymptomatic carotid artery stenosis. If the preoperative carotid Doppler study demonstrates significant stenosis (>80%), it must be verified by arteriography. Combined surgical revascularization has been used in most centers with two different approaches: concomitant or staged. In both approaches, carotid endarterectomy is performed primarily to prevent stroke. When a concomitant procedure is performed, carotid endarterectomy can be performed during hypothermic CPB before CABG, which provides additional brain protection [48]. Neither strategy has not been proved to be superior to another, and an individualized approach is most appropriate. Preoperative stenting is a more suitable alternative approach to combine carotid endarterectomy and CABG.

Abdominal Aortic Disease

When an abdominal aortic pathology is elective, it should be postponed after CABG. The combination of an abdominal aortic aneurysm and CAD can be seen more common in elderly patients. A combined procedure can be necessary in patients with unstable CAD and abdominal aortic aneurysm. Combined surgical treatment using CBP is a safe and effective strategy. Because conventional surgery can increase complications postoperatively, any minimal invasive combined approach can improve early postoperative outcomes.

Peripheral Vascular Disease

Patients with CAD and peripheral atherosclerosis are older and have more widespread vascular disease with/without end-organ damage. Coronary atherosclerosis is usually diffuse and requires more complicated surgical revascularization. Left subclavian artery stenosis is a major contraindication for harvesting LIMA, but left subclavian artery bypass or stent implantation can increase LIMA flow. In this situation, RIMA can be used as a pedicled graft to LAD, or LIMA can be used as a free graft. Iliac artery stenosis with LIMA collateral circulation is another contraindication for LIMA-LAD anastomosis, but peripheral artery revascularization can solve this problem. Except severe peripheral stenosis, staged surgical approach should be preferred (CABG first).

Chronic Renal Failure

One of the main reasons of death in 40 to 50% of patients on hemodialysis is coronary atherosclerosis. It is well known that cardiac pathologies have more serious outcomes if the established renal failure is concomitant, especially the progression of the CAD is more accelerated in hemodialysis patients. Calcification of the coronary territory is a serious complication of long-term hemodialysis and complicates surgical revascularization. Cerebral and/or visceral vascular complications related to accelerated atherosclerosis and particle embolization after CABG are seen more often in patients with end-stage renal failure than in other patients. Hemodialysis-dependent patients are at high risk of CPB-related complications such as bleeding, volume overload, and cerebrovascular events during conventional CABG, whereas OPCAB surgery can be the optimum revascularization strategy to prevent these complications [49].

Malignancy

Recently, cardiac disease and malignancy are seen together more frequently in patients undergoing surgical revascularization. Cancer therapy should be applied as soon as possible after diagnosis; however, patients with high risk of a major cardiac event should take cardiac surgery as a priority. Conventional open cardiac surgery causes a transient immunosuppression due to increasing immunoregulatory factors. Although these biochemical changes are short term and not likely to induce carcinogenesis, they may lead to cancer surveillance with the spread and growth potential of coexisting cancer cells. Overall mortality increases after open heart surgery, and a shorter time interval (especially < 2 years) between the cancer diagnosis and subsequent cardiac surgical intervention can aggravate cancer-specific deaths. Results of a multicenter research show that on-pump CABG surgery with CPB increases significantly the relative risk of skin melanoma, cancer of the lung and bronchus, and overall cancer incidence when compared with those patients who underwent OPCAB [50]. Off-pump myocardial revascularization must be preferred over the use of CPB in combined surgery to prevent the adverse effects of the extracorporeal circulation, especially during lung surgery [51]. Further researches may obtain optimal strategies for management of cancer patients with cardiovascular comorbidities.

Chronic Obstructive Pulmonary Disease

Chronic obstructive pulmonary disease (COPD) is often considered as a risk factor for postoperative outcomes after CABG, but the presence and worsening of COPD do not show any increase in mortality following surgical revascularization in patients with COPD compared with normal patients. However, severe COPD patients have more frequent pulmonary infections, atrial fibrillation, and a longer hospital stay when they are compared with mild to

http://dx.doi.org/10.5772/61404

moderate COPD patients and patients with normal spirometry. Cardiopulmonary bypass has adverse effects on the alveolar stability by activation of the complement cascade, sequestration of the neutrophil in the pulmonary vascular territory, release of the oxygen-derived free radicals, and change of the composition of alveolar surfactant. Atelectasis is the most observed complication after CPB and mechanical ventilation, especially in the first two days after the operation. Because patients with COPD are affected negatively from adverse effects of both CPB and full median sternotomy in the mean of postoperative pulmonary complications, it seems more advantageous that this patient group will be operated on using OPCAB, especially with minimal invasive techniques [52].

8. Outcomes

Because CABG is probably the most performed procedure in cardiac surgery, an enormous amount of information is available about morbidity and mortality, and also long-term survival. Comparison with stent can never give us the real world results, because every patient has his/her specific risk analysis. The early mortality and morbidity rates for isolated CABG are stabilized (Table 11) [53].

Preoperative Characteristics	
Age (years)	65 (58 – 73)
Male	74.8%
Body Mass Index	29 (26 – 33)
Hypertension	88.3%
Dyslipidemia	87.5%
Diabetes Mellitus	46%
Peripheral vascular disease	14.4%
Stroke	7.3%
Dialysis	4.8%
Cardiac Characteristics	
Previous myocardial infarction	47%
Previous stent	25.3%
Previous CABG	1.32%
Presentation of NSTEMI	23.7%
Three-vessel disease	79.4%
Left main disease	33.8%
Proximal LAD disease	56.9%

Operative Characteristics	
Elective	42.2%
OPCAB	16.6%
Full median sternotomy	98.5%
IMA harvesting technique (standard direct vision)	98.9%
IMA use	100%
LIMA	94%
BIMA	5.1%
Operation durations (minutes)	
Cardiopulmonary bypass	91 (71 – 115)
Skin-to-skin	225 (183 – 275)
Operating room	301 (253 – 359)
Any blood products used	31.4%
RBC	2 units
Early Outcomes	
Operative mortality	1.5%
Mortality or morbidity	11.8%
Permanent stroke	1.2%
Re-exploration	2.2%
Renal failure required dialysis	1.8%
Prolonged ventilation	8.2%
Mediastinitis	0.3%
Surgical site infection	1.2%
Sepsis	0.7%

Table 11. STS-database for isolated CABG (July 2011 – March 2013; N = 197.672)

Operative Mortality

The risk profile of patients with isolated CAD has changed in the past decade and they have more complicated comorbidities: older age, LVD, accelerated coronary atherosclerosis, a higher burden of non-coronary atherosclerotic disease, re-operation, emergency operation, multi-stent application, multi-organ pathologies. However, early outcomes after CABG continue to improve and the early cumulative mortality rate is below 2%, lower than 1% in lower-risk patients. The most common reasons for death are heart failure (65%), neurologic events (7.5%), hemorrhage (7%), respiratory failure (5.5%), and dysrhythmia (5.5%).

Long-Term Survival

http://dx.doi.org/10.5772/61404

The survival rate after isolated CABG is higher than 98% for the first month and 97% for first year, 92% for 5 years, 80% for 10 years, 65% for 15 years, and 51% for 20 years. Late mortality depends on non-use of ITA, closure of grafts, progression of native coronary atherosclerosis, and also comorbidities. Procedure-related factors that influence long-term survival include complete revascularization, selection of bypass grafts, and intraoperative myocardial protection. Mortality rate is the highest in the first month, but it is parallel to that of general population after the first postoperative year. Time-related prevalence of sudden death is low after CABG (at least, 95% for the first 10 years) and the most significant risk factor for sudden death is LVD.

Quality of Life

Satisfactory quality of life after CABG is the most important and favorable outcome for all patients who quantify that according to freedom from angina, heart failure, re-hospitalization or re-intervention, and to improvement of a reasonable exercise capacity. Maximal exercise capacity is generally improved at least for 3 to 10 years after CABG, whereas degree of recovery and ultimate exercise capacity reached depend on preoperative LV function, completeness of revascularization, and long-term graft patency. When preoperative global LV dysfunction is severe (EF < 30%), myocardial scarring usually affects a wide area and limits improvement of LV function. But, incomplete revascularization of viable myocardium is the primary cause of the failure of postoperative recovery. Global LV function during exercise begins to increase noticeably 2 weeks after CABG in most patients; however, when it still does not improve in 3 months after CABG, one or more bypass grafts are usually occluded or stenosed.

Recurring Myocardial Ischemia

Return of angina is the most common post-CABG ischemic event. Freedom from angina is approximately 95% at 1 year, 80% at 5 years, 60% at 10 years, 40% at 15 years, and 20% at 20 years. Return of angina during the first 6 months depends on incomplete revascularization or graft failure, whereas progression of native-vessel disease and grafts are serious risk factors for the late recurrence of angina. Including perioperative myocardial infarction, the overall freedom from new myocardial infarction after first surgical complete revascularization is 95% at least 5 years, 85% at 10 years, 75% at 15 years, 55% at 20 years. The overall freedom from any re-intervention (stent or re-CABG) is about 97% at 5 years, 90% at 10 years, 70% at 15 years, and 50% at 20 years. Venous graft occlusion (incidence: 15% at the first year, and 60% at 10 years) is the most common reason for re-intervention, and progression of atherosclerosis in the native coronary arteries (incidence: 50% at 10 years) is the second. Using IMA(s) reduces the frequency of reoperation, but not the frequency of stent implantation. Requirement of reoperation begins to rise noticeably after 5 years and it is usually preferred when the left main or LAD disease is life threatening. Because the operative risk is double in the second CABG than those in the primary, stent implantation with the assistance of embolic protection devices for stenotic vein grafts or native vessels is used more often in symptomatic patients with patent IMA-LAD anastomosis.

Early Postoperative Complications

1. Perioperative myocardial infarction is defined by appearance of new Q waves or significant elevation of myocardial biomarkers. It relates with early or late death and also with

postoperative ischemic cardiomyopathy. It depends on inadequate myocardial preservation, incomplete revascularization or graft failure. Prevalence of perioperative myocardial infarction is between 2.5 and 5%. Early renewing or completing revascularization of the target vessels can be lifesaving.

2. Low cardiac output syndrome varies between 4 and 9% and develops during or after the operation and increases operative mortality 10- to 15-fold. Inotropic supports with/without intra-aortic balloon pump support or mechanical circulation support must be used to maintain a systolic blood pressure > 90 mmHg or a cardiac index > 2.2 L/min/m^2.

3. Adverse neurologic events after surgery can be major or minor. Type 1 deficits (stupor, coma) are more fatal, but the incidence is lower than 1.5%. Severe atherosclerosis of the ascending aorta and/or severe stenosis with/without any calcification in the carotid arteries are the most common risk factors for the type 1 neurologic events. Type 2 deficits are characterized by deterioration of intellectual function and memory, but it is more difficult to characterize. The risk factors are CPB, aortic manipulation, or air embolization. Off-pump is not superior to on-pump, but avoidance of proximal anastomoses on the ascending aorta can prevent type 2 neurologic deficits.

4. Renal failure can develop after cardiac surgery and the incidence of renal dysfunction not requiring dialysis rises to 6.5%, but requiring hemodialysis is below 1.5%. Operative mortality rate is directly related to patients' renal functions: proximately 1% with good renal function, 20% with renal dysfunction, 60% with renal dysfunction and dialysis. Older age (< 70 years), LVD, diabetes mellitus with silent renal dysfunction, preoperative renal dysfunction (creatinine > 2 mg/dL), and LCOS are the major risk factors for postoperative renal failure. Off-pump CABG can be a more appropriate alternative for complete revascularization in patients with chronic renal failure or patients with estimated postoperative renal dysfunction.

5. Deep sternal wound infection carries a mortality rate of 25%. Obesity and diabetes are strong independent risk factors for mediastinitis, whereas reoperation, re-exploration for bleeding, and blood transfusions are other variables. The use of bilateral IMAs does not increase mediastinitis risk, especially with skeletonization technique. However, bilateral IMA harvest must be avoided in obese diabetic women or patients with severe COPD. In spite of all the recent advances in open cardiac surgery, mediastinitis still is an important risk factor for early mortality, but it does not affect the graft patency [54].

Author details

Kaan Kırali* and Hakan Saçlı

*Address all correspondence to: kaankirali@sakarya.edu.tr

Department of Cardiovascular Surgery, Faculty of Medicine, Sakarya University, Turkey

References

[1] Turkey Statistical Agency 2013 Statistical Analysis, 1 April 2014 issue: 16162.

[2] World Health Organization (WHO) Data 2012.

[3] Beck CS. Coronary artery disease: physiologic concepts; surgical operation. Ann Surg 1957;145(4):439–60.

[4] Vineberg A, Miller G. Internal mammary coronary anastomosis in the surgical treatment of coronary artery insufficiency. Can Med Assoc J 1951;64(3):204–10.

[5] May AM, Bailey CP. Coronary endarterectomy. J Int Coll Surg 1958;29(2 Part I):160–3.

[6] Goetz RH, Rohman M, Haller JD, Dee R, Rosenak SS. Internal mammary-coronary artery anastomosis. A nonsuture method employing tantalum rings. J Thorac Cardiovasc Surg 1961;41:378–86.

[7] Effler DB, Sones FM Jr, Favaloro R, Groves LK. Coronary endarterotomy with patch-graft reconstruction: clinical experience with 34 cases. Ann Surg 1965;162(4):590–601.

[8] Sabiston DC, Jr. Surgery of the coronary circulation. J R Coll Surg Edinb 1963;8:105–21.

[9] Favalaro RG. Saphenous vein autograft replacement of severe segmental coronary artery occlusion. Operative technique. Ann Thorac Surg 1968;5(4):334–9.

[10] Johnson WD, Flemma RJ, Lepley D Jr, Ellison EH. Extended treatment of severe coronary artery disease: total surgical approach. Ann Surg 1969;170(3):460–70.

[11] Kolessov VI. Mammary artery-coronary artery anastomosis as method of treatment for angina pectoris. J Thorac Cardiovasc Surg 1967;54(4):535–44.

[12] Loop FD, Lytle BW, Cosgrove DM, et al. Influence of the internal mammary artery graft on 10-year survival and other cardiac events. New Engl J Med 1986;314(1):1–6.

[13] Dodrill FD, Hill E, Gerish RA, Johnson A. Pulmonary valvuloplasty under direct vision using the mechanical heart for a complete bypass of the right heart in a patient with congenital pulmonary stenosis. J Thorac Surg 1953;26(6):584–94.

[14] Gibbon JH Jr. Application of a mechanical heart and lung apparatus to cardiac surgery. Minn Med 1954;37(3):171–85.

[15] Hill JD, O'Brien TG, Murray JJ, et al. Prolonged extracorporeal oxygenation for acute posttraumatic respiratory failure (shock-lung syndrome): use of the Bramston membrane lung. New Engl J Med 1972;286(12):629–34.

[16] Melrose DG, Dreyer B, Bentall MB, Baker JBE. Elective cardiac arrest. Lancet 1955;269:21–2.

[17] Gay WA Jr, Ebert PA. Functional, metabolic, and morphologic effects of potassium-induced cardioplegia. Surgery 1973;74(2):284–90.

[18] Follette DM, Mulder DG, Maloney JV, Buckberg GD. Advantages of blood cardioplegia over continuous coronary perfusion or intermittent ischemia. Experimental and clinical study. J Thorac Cardiovasc Surg 1978;76(5):604–19.

[19] Ankeney JL. To use or not use the pump oxygenator in coronary bypass operations [editorial]. Ann Thorac Surg 1975;19(1):108–9.

[20] Benetti FJ. Direct coronary surgery with saphenous vein bypass without either cardiopulmonary bypass or cardiac arrest. J Cardiovasc Surg (Torino) 1985;26(3):217–22.

[21] Buffolo E, Andrade JCS, Succi JE, et al. Direct revascularization of the myocardium without extracorporeal circulation. Description of the technic and preliminary results. Arq Bras Cardiol 1982;38(5):365–73.

[22] Ömeroğlu SN, Kırali K, Güler M, et al. Midterm angiographic assessment of coronary artery bypass grafting without cardiopulmonary bypass. Ann Thorac Surg 2000;70(3):844–9.

[23] Eleveli G, Mataracı İ, Büyükbayrak F, Erkin A, Şişmanoğlu M, Kırali K. Complete revascularization with or without cardiopulmonary bypass using arterial grafts: the six-month angiographic results. Turkish J Thorac Cardiovasc Surg 2011;19(1):1–6.

[24] Işık Ö, Dağlar B, Kırali K, et al. Coronary bypass surgery via minithoracotomy on the beating heart. Ann Thorac Surg 1997;63(Suppl1):S57–60.

[25] Karagöz H, Sönmez B, Bakkaloğlu B, et al. Coronary artery bypass grafting in the conscious patient without endotracheal general anesthesia. Ann Thorac Surg 2000;70(1):91–6.

[26] Kırali K, Koçak T, Güzelmeriç F, et al. Off-pump awake coronary revascularization using bilateral internal thoracic arteries. Ann Thorac Surg 2004;78(5):1598–603.

[27] Kırali K, Güler M, Dağlar B, et al. Videothoracoscopic internal mammary artery harvest for coronary artery bypass. Asian Cardiovasc Thorac Ann 1999;7(4):259–62.

[28] Loulmet D, Carpentier A, d'Attellis N, et al. Endoscopic coronary artery bypass grafting with the aid of robotic assisted instruments. J Thorac Cardiovasc Surg 1999;118(1):4–10.

[29] Lehr EJ, Chitwood W Jr, Bonatti J. Technique of totally endoscopic robot-assisted off-pump coronary artery bypass grafting. In: Raja SG and Amrani M. (Eds.) Off-Pump Coronary Artery Bypass Grafting. New York, NY: Nova Science Publishers, Inc. 2012, pp.123–143.

[30] 2011 ACCF/AHA Guideline for coronary artery bypass surgery: executive summary. Circulation 2011;124(23):2610–42.

[31] Mansuroğlu D, Şişmanoğlu M, Ömeroğlu SN, Kırali K, İpek G, Yakut C. A simple method to prevent internal thoracic artery tension: Single pericardio-thoracic suture technique. J Card Surg 2004;19(3):264–6.

[32] Kırali K. Technique of awake off-pump coronary artery bypass surgery. In: Raja SG and Amrani M. Off-pump Coronary Artery Bypass Grafting. New York, NY: Nova Science Publisher, Inc. 2012, p. 205.

[33] Toker ME, Ömeroğlu SN, Kırali K, Balkanay M, Yakut C. Using the bilateral internal mammary artery in the left or right coronary artery system: 5-year comparison of operation techniques and angiographic results. Heart Surg Forum 2005;8(6):345–50.

[34] Mansuroğlu D, Göksedef D, Ömeroğlu SN, et al. Use of radial artery in coronary artery bypass surgery: midterm angiographic results. Turkish J Thorac Cardiovasc Surg 2003;11(2):96–100.

[35] Akıncı E, Uzun K, Erentuğ V, et al. The comparison of the early and midterm results of the proximal anastomosis techniques in sequential radial artery grafting. Turkish J Thorac Cardiovasc Surg 2004;12(4):235–40.

[36] Kaya E, Mansuroğlu D, Göksedef D, et al. Long-term angiographic results of coronary artery bypass surgery with the use of arterial graft combinations. Turkish J Thorac Cardiovasc Surg 2005;13(4):309–13.

[37] Mansuroğlu D, Ömeroğlu SN, Göksedef D, et al. Does radial artery harvesting cause any changes in the forehand circulation during the postoperative period? An angiographic study. Anadolu Kardiyol Derg 2004;4(2):149–52.

[38] Kırali K, Yakut N, Güler M, et al. Radial artery in coronary bypass surgery: anatomical landmarks and harvesting technique. Turkish J Thorac Cardiovasc Surg 1999;7(5): 358–61.

[39] Gürbüz A, Kırali K, Tuncer A, Şişmanoğlu M, Yakut C. Combined transdiaphragmatic MIDCAB with right gastroepiploic artery and abdominal aortic aneurysm repair. Cardiovasc Surg 2000;8(6):503–6.

[40] Bozbuğa NU, Yaymacı B, Kırali K, et al. The morphometric features of the lateral circumflex branch of femoral artery as a potential arterial conduit. Turkish J Thorac Cardiovasc Surg 2001;9(3):145–8.

[41] Kırali K, Mansuroğlu D, Kayalar N, Güzelmeriç F, Alp M, Yakut C. Markers of myocardial ischemia in the evaluation of the effect of left anterior descending coronary artery lesion and collateral circulation on myocardial injury in 1-vessel off-pump coronary bypass surgery. Heart Surg Forum 2003;6(3):143–8.

[42] Kırali K, Kayalar N, Koçak T, Yakut C. Reversed-J inferior sternotomy for awake coronary bypass. Eur J Cardiothorac Surg 2005;27(5):923–4.

[43] Kırali K, Kayalar N, Özen Y, Sareyyüpoğlu B, Güzelmeriç F, Koçak T, Yakut C. Reversed-J inferior versus full median sternotomy: which is better for awake coronary bypass surgery. J Card Surg 2005;20(5):463–8.

[44] Kırali K. (Abstract) Mini-T sternotomy for awake coronary revascularization with bilateral internal thoracic artery. Interactive Cardiovasc Thorac Surg 2004;3(Suppl 1):S64–5.

[45] Kırali K. Composite bilateral internal thoracic artery grafts via standard sternotomy for lateral wall revascularization in conscious patients. Heart Surg Forum 2005;8(6): 340–4.

[46] Kırali K, Rabus MB, Yakut N, et al. Early- and long-term comparison of the on- and off-pump bypass surgery in patients with left ventricular dysfunction. Heart Surg Forum 2002;5(2):177–81.

[47] Kırali K. Stentless bioprostheses for aortic valve replacement. In: Aikawa E (Ed.). Calcific Aortic Valve Disease. In Tech, Croatia, 2013: pp. 411–449 (ISBN 978-953-51-1150-4).

[48] Ozen Y, Aksoy E, Sarikaya S, Aydin E, Altas O, Rabus MB, Kirali K. Effect of hypothermia in patients undergoing simultaneous carotid endarterectomy and coronary artery bypass graft surgery. Cardiovasc J Afr 2015;26(1):17–20.

[49] Erentuğ V, Akıncı E, Kırali K, et al. Complete off-pump coronary revascularization in patients with dialysis-dependent renal disease. Tex Heart Inst J 2004;31(2):153–6.

[50] Pinto CA, Marcella S, August DA, Holland B, Kostis JB, Demissie K. Cardiopulmonary bypass has a modest association with cancer progression: a retrospective cohort study. http://www.ncbi.nlm.nih.gov/pubmed/24180710 BMC Cancer (web) 2013;13:519.

[51] Ömeroğlu SN, Erdoğan HB, Kırali K, et al. Combined coronary artery bypass grafting and lung surgery. Asian Cardiovasc Thorac Ann 2004;12(3):260–2.

[52] Güler M, Kırali K, Toker ME, et al. Different CABG methods in patients with chronic obstructive pulmonary disease. Ann Thorac Surg 2001;71(1):152–7.

[53] Harskamp RE, Brennan JM, Xian Y, et al. Practice patterns and clinical outcomes after hybrid coronary revascularization in the United States. An analysis from the STS adult cardiac database. Circulation 2014;130(11):872–9.

[54] Mansuroğlu D, Ömeroğlu SN, Kaya E, Kırali K, et al. Does mediastinitis affect the graft patency? J Card Surg 2005;20(3):208–11.

Chapter 7

Surgical Treatment in Diffuse Coronary Artery Disease

Kaan Kırali and Yücel Özen

Additional information is available at the end of the chapter

http://dx.doi.org/10.5772/61514

Abstract

Diffuse coronary artery atherosclerosis can be defined as "consecutive or longitudinal" and "complete or partial" obstruction in coronary vessels. Most of the patients with diabetes, hyperlipidemia, chronic renal insufficiency, connective tissue disease, and multi-stented coronary arteries have diffuse atherosclerotic lesions in the coronary territory. Viable large myocardium without necrosis is the only coronary bypass indication in these patients, because it is very difficult to find any healthy area for anastomosis. This type of coronary occlusion frequently stimulates the formation of collateral vessels that protect against extensive myocardial ischemia. The choice of a surgical method also depends on the nature of the coronary artery, and multisegment plaques and healthy-area intervals simplify complete revascularization. On the other hand, a more aggressive treatment modality should be preferred when no soft site can be identified for arteriotomy or there is an extensively diseased area that is not amenable to grafting. The less invasive techniques are "don't touch the plaque" techniques (jumping multi-bypass, sequential bypass, hybrid interventions). Sometimes an aggressive diffuse plaque formation needs to be treated with "touch the plaque" techniques (long-segment anastomosis, patch-plasty, endarterectomy ± patch-plasty). In simple forms, a limited long-segment anastomosis of conduits eliminates the occlusion of the limited atherosclerotic plaque where the whole lesion is opened and cross-covered by the graft. In the accelerated form of coronary arteriosclerosis, the atherosclerotic plaque appears widespread and the full-length lumen of the coronary artery can get very narrow or occluded totally. The long-segment lesion is usually calcified and it inhibits any kind of stitching; however, the plaque can be separated easily from the arterial wall in order to create an appropriate lumen in the total occluded coronary artery. Because the aggressive endarterectomy increases the operation risk, the arteriotomy should be extended until the normal lumen with normal intima in the distal segment of the coronary artery. In general, severity and distribution of coronary arteriosclerosis tend to increase with time but the rate of increase is highly variable and difficult to predict. Although diffuse atherosclerosis is severe enough, it is uncommon to render any patient unsuitable for surgery.

Keywords: Diffuse atherosclerosis, endarterectomy, patch-plasty, sequential bypass, jumping bypass

1. Introduction

Coronary artery disease usually involves the proximal portion of the larger epicardial coronary arteries, but generally not their intramural branches. In most patients, atherosclerotic lesions in coronary territory are segmental and eccentric, and they affect particularly bifurcations and sharp curvatures, whereas the rest of long segments of coronary arteries are plaque-free. Diffuse coronary artery disease can be defined as the presence of multiple atherosclerotic stenoses or long-segment occlusions in coronary territory. Atheromatous materials spread toward distal and retain a long segment of coronary arteries which can obstruct coronary lumen "consecutive or longitudinal" and "complete or partial".

In general, severity and distribution of coronary arteriosclerosis tend to increase with time but the rate of increase is highly variable and difficult to predict. Diffuse atherosclerosis severe enough to render the patient unsuitable for surgery is uncommon. On the other hand, progression of atherosclerosis in the native coronary arteries after coronary bypass surgery is not rare and accelerated atherosclerosis usually is the main contraindication for reoperation. The early and late results of endarterectomy are inferior to those of routine coronary bypass, but it offers a viable alternative not to leaving a territory ungrafted. Rate of aggressive progression of atherosclerosis cannot as yet be examined directly in multivariable risk factor analyses, but this progression can be slowed by intensive lipid-lowering therapy.

The nature of atherosclerotic coronary artery disease is a chronic inflammation and fibroproliferation of large- and medium-sized epicardial arteries consisting of the progressive deposition or degenerative accumulation of lipid-containing plaques on the innermost layer of the arterial wall. The basic mechanism of atherosclerosis is endothelial dysfunction which is characterized by the reduction of the endothelium-derived vasodilators, especially nitric oxide, and an increase in endothelium-derived contracting factors. The immune-inflammatory response involving macrophages, T-lymphocytes and intimal smooth muscle cells tries healing and repairing injured endothelium, stabilizing plaques, protecting rupture, and avoiding thrombosis. If the atherosclerotic stimuli persist over long time, the reparative response may accelerate and target to the progressive occlusion of the arterial lumen. Progressive diffuse coronary artery stenosis involves the following processes: local atheroma, lipid accumulation, biologic stimuli of vessel wall, chronic inflammation, cellular necrosis, plaque formation and complications, and calcification. Arterial wall injury is most often related to age, diabetes, smoking, dyslipidemia, hypertension, hyperuremia, and immunosuppressive therapy, which trigger and accelerate the inflammatory response aimed at restoring arterial wall integrity. During the progression of atherosclerosis, endothelial and smooth muscle cells die by apoptosis, and an atheromatous plaque covers the defects of the endothelium. A vulnerable plaque is a nonobstructive, silent coronary lesion, which suddenly becomes obstructive and symptomatic. Plaque rupture with/without thrombotic complications is the main reason for this acute coronary syndrome with/without complications. The lesions responsible for acute episodes are generally less calcified than plaques responsible for chronic stable angina, because calcification is the last part of the healing response to atherosclerosis and it appears to have no direct link to thrombosis. Because diffuse type of coronary disease is time-consuming, slowly developing occlusions frequently stimulate the formation of collateral vessels that protect myocardium against extensive ischemia. Viable large myocardium without necrosis is the only indication for coronary revascularization in these patients (without mechanical complications of myocardial infarction), because it is very difficult to find any healthy area for anastomosis. Consequently, the relative severity and associated risk balance between focal stenosis and diffuse disease cannot be easily compared when making revascularization decisions [1]. The physiological anatomy of coronary arteries must be detailed for myocardial revascularization, but quantifying the anatomic severity of diffuse lesions is difficult. Lower coronary flow reserve associated with severe diffuse disease may neutralize or override any potential benefit from eliminating stenosis by stents. On the other hand, more diffusely expanded coronary atherosclerosis can cause higher mortality rate during coronary bypass artery grafting (CABG) than focal lesions because of association of more complicated vessels, which are not appropriate for suturing or distal perfusion after anastomosis. Patients with diffuse coronary artery disease can also face a twofold increased risk of in-hospital mortality or major morbidities, which is independent of reoperation [2].

2. Etiology

Most of the patients with diabetes, hyperlipidemia, chronic renal insufficiency, connective tissue disease, heart transplantation, and multi-stented coronary arteries have diffuse atherosclerotic lesions in the coronary territory. All of these diseases affect and accelerate coronary arteriosclerosis differently [3]. Restenosis after first CABG can also be a reason for the diffuse coronary atherosclerosis, but usually these patients have ungraftable diffuse diseased coronary vasculature and none of the specific revascularization methods can be used.

2.1. Diabetes mellitus

Compared with nondiabetic patients, diabetes mellitus increases the incidence of coronary artery disease two to four times as much and accelerates the nature of the atherosclerosis. The nature of coronary artery disease in diabetic patients is clinically challenging because it causes an extensive and diffuse multivessel involvement. Hyperglycemia is directly related to the atherosclerotic development, progression, and instability due to induced endothelial dysfunction (abnormal nitric oxide biology, increased endothelin and angiotensin II, reduced prostacyclin activity), abnormalities in lipid metabolism (high triglyceride and LDL-cholesterol, low HDL-cholesterol), systemic inflammation (increased oxidative stress, accumulation of advanced glycation and products), and disorders in the proteo-fibrinolytic system and platelet biology (thrombosis). Hyperglycemia can deplete the cellular NADPH pool and induce with high levels of fatty acids to oxidative stress on phospholipids and proteins. Insulin resistance is the main actor to the endothelial dysfunction in type II diabetes, and endothelial dysfunction is closely complicated with microangiopathy and atherosclerosis in diabetic patients. Endothelial dysfunction decreases the capacity of nitric oxide synthase enzyme and depleted nitric oxide, which effects endothelial cell-dependent vasodilatation. Overexpression of growth factors causes endothelial cells and vascular smooth muscle proliferation. All of these negative changes accelerate atherosclerosis in all arterial territories, and the involvement of coronary arteries can be very extensive and diffuse with either serious jumping stenoses or long-segment narrowing with/without occlusion. The optimal strategy of coronary revascularization is controversial, but CABG has better long-term survival and freedom from re-interventions [4]. Diabetic patients have a higher restenosis rate after stent implantation and also progression of diffuse disease after stent implantation forms new lesions in diabetic patients than non-diabetic patients more often. Clinical outcomes in CABG patients are similar for diabetic and non-diabetic patients, while outcomes after stent could be worse for diabetic patients [5]. In diabetic patients with multivessel coronary artery disease, rates of death and myocardial infarction in 5 years are significantly lower in patients treated with CABG due to more complete revascularization, which bypasses several lesions and prevents coronary territory against progressive proximal coronary stenosis [6]. On the other hand, the operative risk in patients with diabetes might be a consequence of a preoperatively endothelial dysfunction and an inflammatory response to extracorporeal circulation characterized by an impaired release of interleukin-6 and increased turnover of E-selectin [7]. Simple distal anastomosis for each coronary artery cannot be enough to supply blood along the coronary territory, and most of the diabetic patients with diffuse multivessel coronary artery disease require specific surgical revascularization modalities, which can increase perioperative myocardial damage and operative mortality.

2.2. Hypercholesterolemia

Cholesterol is one of the most important risk factors for the development of premature coronary artery disease, which is characterized without any serious intravascular stenosis. Cholesterol levels and coronary artery disease show a strong and linear relationship, whereas cholesterol levels even in the normal range may inhibit endothelium-dependent vasodilatation in all arterial beds. The pathogenesis of atherosclerosis in the obese population can be related to metabolic syndrome associated with insulin intolerance and dyslipidemia, which cause endothelial dysfunction with decreasing nitric oxide production. Lowering of LDL-cholesterol rather than moderate weight loss is more effective to improve endothelial function, because the coronary vasculature is affected by the atherosclerosis process, and the most atherosclerotic lesions are associated with remarkable neovascularization of the vasa vasorum, which can cause intra-plaque rupture and bleeding. Hypercholesterolemia is one of the most important factors to stimulate this process and its role begins in the early atherosclerotic remodeling before plaque formation [8]. Hyperlipidemia-related coronary lesions are very predisposed to spread lengthways coronary territory and cause diffuse stenosis or occlusion, and calcification is usually associated with this type of atherosclerosis.

2.3. End-stage renal disease

A strong relationship subsists between chronic renal failure and coronary artery disease, and atherosclerosis can be accelerated in patients with end-stage renal disease due to multifactorial reasons [9]. Increased oxidative stress, hyperhomocysteinemia, hyperlipidemia, hyperglycemia and others are also important comorbidities. The main pathology is the impairment of endothelium-dependent vasodilatation. Dialysis-dependent renal failure patients undergoing CABG can have a greater degree of distal and/or diffuse coronary artery disease burden compared with matched patients with silent renal failure. The diffuseness of coronary atherosclerosis in patients with end-stage renal disease can be severe and the intraluminal lesions are usually calcified. Extensive calcification of all arterial structures in the body can inhibit conventional CABG strategies, which increase surgical outcomes. Impaired distal run-off of the coronary arteries is another strong independent predictor of operative mortality. All kinds of complex anastomotic techniques can be used in these patients, and endarterectomy can be very easy to perform to get adequate distal run-off. Restenosis after CABG is not uncommon in this group of patients, especially if saphenous vein is used.

2.4. Connective tissue disease

Several connective tissue diseases (systemic lupus erythematosus, rheumatoid arthritis, systemic sclerosis, Takayasu disease) are characterized by vascular dysfunction and excessive fibrosis. The presence of coronary microvascular dysfunction is the common pathologic change in various chronic inflammatory diseases [10]. Cardiac manifestation of these chronic diseases can be estimated lower, because most of them are asymptomatic. Diffuse form of these pathologies has a distressed clinical course with severe organ involvement. First, an endothelial injury occurs early in the disease process leading to endothelial dysfunction. Myofibroblasts drawn into the arterial wall by cellular growth factors contribute to the thickening of the intimal layer, compromising regional blood flow by narrowing the arterial lumen. In the absence of epicardial coronary stenosis, the abnormal coronary flow is dependent on the structural remodeling of the small coronary arteries and arterioles. Aggressive surgical interventions are usually ineffective, but multi-anastomoses can be applicable. Because diffuse atherosclerosis shows strict adhesions between arterial wall layers, endarterectomy can never satisfy to load out the intra-arterial lumen for appropriate anastomosis.

2.5. Heart transplantation

The occurrence of coronary artery disease is common in posttransplant patients, and atherosclerotic process is different from normally occurring coronary artery disease. This type of atherosclerosis is specific for heart transplanted patients, and it affects the entire length of the coronary arteries, and diffuse intimal proliferation develops without damage to the internal elastic lamina in contrast to classic atherosclerosis. The intimal proliferation developed by smooth muscle cells and macrophages contains cholesterol crystals and lipid components, but calcification is rare. This lesion affects large epicardial coronary arteries as well as the penetrating intramyocardial branches, and occlusion of these small branches is the first reason for acute coronary syndrome. Coronary endothelial vasodilator dysfunction is a common and early indicator for graft atherosclerosis, which is caused by both immunological and classic risk factors. The immunological response is the first stimulus causing endothelial damage and this injury alters endothelial permeability, with consequent myointimal hyperplasia and extracellular matrix synthesis. Alloimmune injury starts when donor antigens expressed from the donor endothelial cells interact with recipient dendritic cells, and the activated macrophages secrete several factors, which stimulate the proliferation of smooth muscle cells and vascular remodeling [11]. Before microvasculature occlusions, stent or standard CABG can be preferred for the treatment of newly developed epicardial lesions, but endarterectomy may not be usually applicable in most diffuse cases, and retransplantation is the only option under these circumstances.

2.6. Multistented coronary arteries

The problem of restenosis after stenting represents a special case of arterial hyperplastic disease and the in-stent restenosis is made from myxomatous tissue, whereas accelerated intimal hyperplasia occludes the distal segment of the same coronary vessel after stenting. Availability of access to healthy coronary wall for revascularization is usually feasible in patients receiving a single stent implantation in one or each coronary artery. However, the distal vascular bed of multi-stented coronary artery is often influenced by the accelerated atherosclerosis and diffusely diseased where it is impossible to find any healthy area for distal anastomosis. Sometimes, open endarterectomy with removal of stent(s) can remain the last option for surgical revascularization.

3. Surgical treatment techniques

Diffuse atherosclerosis has been highly widespread among patients with coronary artery disease in the last two decades, because simple lesions are usually treated with stent interventions in the early phase of the coronary pathology. Diffuse coronary lesion and reduced coronary flow reserve can be silent due to several collaterals, but it might result in severe functional limitation, chronic low-level ischemia, and myocardial remodeling. Low-level ischemia can be a potential driver of both first coronary vasomotor and myocardial dysfunction, and then remodeling in heart failure with preserved ejection fraction. Diffuse atherosclerosis and microvascular dysfunction-associated coronary artery disease comorbid conditions may guide new, more effective, aggressive, and therapeutic interventions for global cardiovascular risk reduction due to complete revascularization. There is no difference in event-free survival between CABG or stent implantation in patients with high coronary flow reserve; however, CABG is significantly more effective than stent in patients with low coronary flow reserve [12]. Diffuseness of coronary artery disease is a serious risk factor for early and late adverse events after coronary revascularization, but the acceptable strategy should be complete revascularization. Standard bypass method (finding an appropriate lumen and performing anastomosis) is usually not possible in the diffusely diseased coronary arteries, and such a region, which may be found at most distal, cannot be expected to bring any benefit. For this reason, in such cases, it is required to apply a complex method other than standard bypass method. When the atherosclerotic stenosis is local, it is technically possible and easy to revascularize the distal segment directly, but in diffuse coronary artery disease or in the presence of diffuse stenotic regions, different techniques should be implemented for complete revascularization.

http://dx.doi.org/10.5772/61514

The treatment of the diffused-type coronary artery disease has always been an issue; however, this scenario is challenging for cardiac surgeons because diffuse atheromatous lesions frequently render epicardial coronary vessels unsuitable for conventional distal grafting. However, there are some strategies to perform a complete revascularization with increasing complexity and mortality risk sequentially in these patients. Second, to attenuate or prevent perioperative infarction and/or postischemic ventricular dysfunction caused by inadequate myocardial protection, there are many different administrative ways for cardioplegic solutions, but the optimal delivery method of cardioplegia also remains controversial. Off-pump bypass can be another option when coronary artery is totally occluded and retrograde flow supplies the myocardium.

The aggressive involvement type of atherosclerosis is the corner stone for coronary revascularization, and the first choice of the aggressive surgical techniques also depends on this nature (Table 1). A coronary artery with multisegment plaques and healthy-area intervals simplifies complete revascularization, and multiple revascularization of this coronary artery with different methods seems applicable by every cardiac team. On the other hand, a more aggressive treatment modality should be preferred when no soft site can be identified for arteriotomy or there is an extensively diseased area not amenable to grafting or no other methods except transplantation. The routine application for arteriotomy in patients with local stenosis is to perform the anastomotic incision proximal enough to get the larger-sized coronary target but distal enough from atherosclerotic lesion. Arteriotomy should be more complicated or extended to get appropriate coronary lumen and anastomotic area in patients with diffuse coronary lesions. The main goal of CABG is to finish complete revascularization using different surgical approaches during open-heart surgery. Using a single graft or multi-grafts or a hybrid procedure (stent + bypass) is a reliable option to revascularize all segments of each coronary artery: **don't touch the plaque techniques**. Sometimes an aggressive plaque formation needs to be touched using extended arteriotomy with/without endarterectomy and patch-plasty: **touch the plaque techniques**.

Don't Touch the Plaque Techniques

1. Jumping bypass technique

This technique is used for revascularization of the same coronary artery with more than one anastomosis (Figure 1). Most patients with diffuse coronary artery disease have multiple severe stenoses along coronary arteries or diseased coronary artery may have critically important side branches before the last stenosis that could not be bypassed. Jumping bypass is performed via single or multiple conduits on the same coronary artery and is the only solution to supply blood throughout the diseased coronary artery, especially for the left anterior descending (LAD) artery and the right coronary artery (RCA). The circumflex artery (Cx) may have multiple major branches and each one does not need to be revascularized consecutively with this technique; on the contrary, these branches should be revascularized separately with sequential grafting. The jumping bypass technique has several advantages to avoid unexpected adverse complications intraoperatively (Table 2). It is the simpler technique to perform complete revascularization in diffuse coronary disease patients. This technique can be applied via different approaches.

A. No-touch the plaque techniques
1. Jumping bypass (the same coronary artery)
a. with multiple grafts
b. with a single graft
c. with a composite graft
d. with a bifurcated graft
2. Sequential bypass (multiple coronary arteries)
a. with a single graft
b. with a composite graft
c. with a bifurcated graft
3. Hybrid revascularization (different coronary arteries)
B. Touch the plaque techniques
1. long-segment anastomosis
2. patch-plasty
3. endarterectomy ± patch-plasty
a. closed
b. open

Table 1. Aggressive bypass strategies for diffusely diseased coronary territory

1. To achieve complete revascularization of the same major coronary artery
2. To supply blood to the myocardium via grafting major side branches of the same coronary artery
3. To avoid more aggressive surgical procedures ("touch the plaque" techniques)
4. To shorten ischemic and cardiopulmonary bypass times
5. To salvage myocardium from perioperative myocardial infarction caused by graft failure

Table 2. Advantages of the jumping bypass technique

a. Jumping grafting with multiple conduits

This approach is the easiest approach, and it is usually used for the LAD revascularization, whereas the RCA is seldom preferred. This jumping bypass approach using more than one conduit is usually preferred in emergency situations to salvage myocardium perioperatively, but it can also be used in elective cases. Two arteriotomies are performed on the same coronary

http://dx.doi.org/10.5772/61514

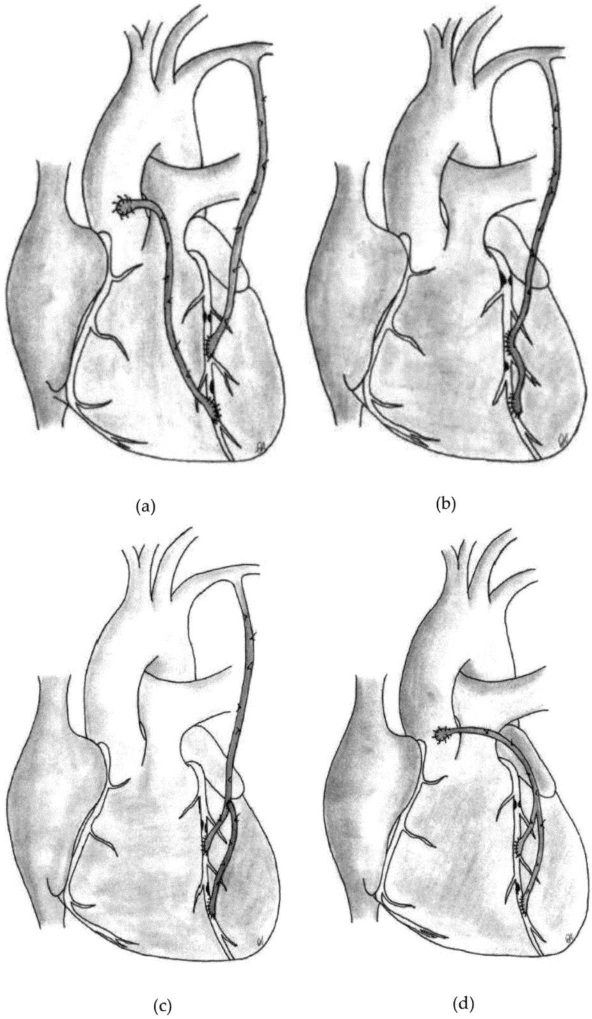

Figure 1. Jumping grafting is an alternative to multi-revascularization of the same coronary artery with multi-segment stenoses. **a)** Jumping grafting with multiple conduits. **b)** Jumping grafting with a single conduit. **c)** Jumping grafting with a composite conduit. **d)** Jumping grafting with a bifurcated conduit.

artery and both are grafted by different conduits (Figure 1a). Two conduits are anastomosed in an end-to-side fashion, and this approach achieves double suppliers with double sources. This approach is usually preferred for the LAD, and the left internal mammarian artery (LIMA) is often anastomosed between the proximal and distal lesions, because the length of LIMA is usually not enough to reach to the distal segment. The distal segment of the coronary artery is revascularized using a second conduit, especially with a vein graft. In elective and planned surgery, the second graft could be an arterial conduit: the right internal thoracic artery (RIMA) or radial artery (RA). In the emergency salvage re-exploration after perioperative myocardial infarction, the saphenous vein graft (SVG) should be chosen for its precipitous harvesting. This approach can be preventative against early graft failure, whereas the second independent conduit can continue to supply blood. This approach is also lifesaving when perioperative myocardial infarction is developed because of the graft failure, and the second graft is anastomosed at the distal part of the affected coronary artery. This alternative procedure is mostly used to salvage myocardium when the LIMA or the other conduit does not work due to any reason perioperatively.

b. Jumping grafting with a single conduit

This approach can be used for the LAD or RCA elective and planned revascularization, but it is not feasible for emergency surgery. This approach is similar to sequential bypass technique, but the only difference is to be a single target vessel requiring multiple anastomoses. If harvesting of a second conduit is not possible due to any reason and the target coronary artery has multiple stenosis, the harvested single graft can be anastomosed on the same coronary artery consecutively (Figure 1b). In situ or free conduits can be used for jumping grafting. The double arteriotomies are made in the direction of the long axis at the mid and distal soft segments of the target coronary artery, and a single proximal arteriotomy is made at the conduit. The two proximal incisions are aligned parallel and the proximal anastomosis is performed in a side-to-side fashion and created kissing anastomosis, which is the critical part of this approach, but "aligned perpendicular and created a diamond-shaped anastomosis" is never used for this anastomosis like the routine sequential bypass technique. The distal end of the graft is anastomosed to the distal arteriotomy on the target coronary artery as the standard end-to-side fashion. Using a larger graft for consecutive anastomoses on the same coronary artery can be performed with a lower technical risk than the LIMA because of its borderline diameter, and the best conduits for this approach are the RA and SVG. This approach is often complication free and consecutive grafting of the same target coronary artery permits efficient use of limited conduits, but it is preferred rarely.

c. Jumping grafting with a composite conduit

This approach can be used for the LAD revascularization. This approach is more time-consuming than the other approaches and needs more attention. A composite conduit can be built as T- or Y-graft with the in situ LIMA. This second graft is usually prepared from a free arterial graft (a short segment of the RA or RIMA), and both free ends of the second arterial conduit are anastomosed on the same coronary artery, whereas the LIMA is anastomosed at the middle part of the second conduit conduit (T-graft) or the LIMA is anastomosed on the LAD, whereas both free ends of the second arterial conduit are anastomosed on the distal segment of the LAD and at the middle part of the LIMA (Y-graft) (Figure 1c). This application arranges uniform distal anastomoses using the same conduit with the same diameter and prevents stealing coronary blood by any larger conduit. In the absence of the second arterial graft, a short SVG can be also used as the composed part.

d. Jumping grafting with a bifurcated conduit

This approach can be used for the LAD or RCA revascularization. This approach is easy to apply, but it is very uncommon to find a bifurcated conduit in the body. The two branches of

http://dx.doi.org/10.5772/61514

the LIMA have a smaller diameter and are very vasospastic, which are not suitable for grafting. The only option is to harvest the SVG with its first major bifurcated branches (Figure 1d). The advantages are avoiding the second proximal anastomosis on the ascending aorta or on the other conduit, any handicap caused by anastomosis between both grafts, and technical difficulties and risks of kissing anastomosis.

2. Sequential bypass technique

This technique is used for revascularization of more than one target coronary arteries or major branches of the same coronary artery with the same conduit. The number of the sequential bypassed vessels depends on the availability of multi-conduits, which allow one or more sequential bypass at the same time. If harvesting adequate conduits is feasible, the true way is bypassing all diseased coronary artery separately as the "one graft-to-one target coronary artery" rule. The main purpose of this technique is the efficient usage of limited conduits to achieve complete revascularization (Table 3). The most distal anastomosis should be to the furthest target coronary artery with an acceptable diameter, and the conduit is anastomosed at several coronary arteries before its proximal anastomosis. The most possible drawback is more than one distal anastomoses with a single proximal source that can cause an aggravated risk of inadequate myocardial perfusion. It cannot be hazardous, if the equal coronary territory is bypassed with the same conduit sequentially. On the other hand, if the distal coronary artery has a small diameter, it would be hazardous, and this smaller distal anastomosis lies under the risk of total occlusion because of preferential graft flow to the larger proximal coronary arteries. All available conduits can be used for sequential grafting, especially the SVG. The RA is usually used for sequential anastomosis during full arterial revascularization [13]. The LIMA should not be used for sequential bypass grafting, if it supplies the LAD flow, but it can be used as a donor for composite T- or Y-grafting of other arterial conduits, especially with the RIMA, in order to achieve complete arterial revascularization. The distal anastomosis is performed with the standard end-to-side technique and all proximal anastomoses with the side-to-side technique. Both the target coronary artery and the conduit are incised longitudinally and aligned perpendicular to each other, and all proximal sequential anastomoses must be constructed in a diamond-shaped fashion to prevent any stenosis, kinking, distortion or tension on the anastomoses and conduit. Both the arteriotomy and the incision on the conduit should not exceed the diameter of the conduit. The distal anastomosis is completed first and the other anastomoses are performed towards the proximal consecutively.

1. To achieve complete revascularization of the different coronary arteries
2. To perform complete revascularization if conduits are inappropriate
3. To supply blood to the myocardium via grafting major side branches of the same or different coronary arteries
4 To avoid more aggressive surgical procedures ("touch the plaque" techniques)
5. To shorten ischemic and cardiopulmonary bypass times
6. To salvage myocardial revascularization intraoperatively when the conduits are shorter for proximal anastomosis on the ascending aorta.

Table 3. Advantages of the sequential bypass technique

a. **Sequential grafting with a single conduit**

This approach can be used for all coronary arteries and is the most used approach for complete revascularization. If harvesting of sufficient conduits is not possible due to any reason and there are a large number of target coronary arteries, the harvested single graft can be anastomosed on the different coronary arteries (RCA-Cx-Diagonal-LAD) or on the several branches of a single coronary artery (Cx 1-3) sequentially (Figure 2a). All free grafts are suitable for this sequential bypass approach. The best conduit for this approach is the SVG or RA. Proximal anastomosis is always performed on the ascending aorta without any concern on the long-term patency [14]. In situ arterial grafts should be used alone to the target coronary artery, especially both IMAs. First, the distal end of the graft is anastomosed to the distal target coronary artery in an end-to-side fashion. The other proximal coronary arteries are bypassed consecutively through the anterior surface of the heart. The small arteriotomies are made in the direction of the long axis of the target coronary artery and small incisions are made at the conduit. The two incisions are aligned perpendicularly creating a diamond-shaped anastomosis and the sequential anastomosis is performed in a side-to-side fashion, which is the critical part of this approach; however, "aligned parallel and created a kissing anastomosis" is never used for this anastomoses. This approach is often complication free, and sequential grafting of the different target coronary arteries permits efficient use of limited conduits.

b. **Sequential grafting with a composite conduit**

This approach can be performed in two different methods. The first method is usually used if the distal SVGs remain shorter for proximal anastomosis on the ascending aorta intraoperatively, especially for revascularization of the Cx-branches. A composite conduit can be built as Y-graft and the second short graft is usually anastomosed on the main conduit, and the most preferred conduits are the SVG and RA (Figure 2b-1). The main graft is anastomosed to the largest target coronary artery first, and the proximal anastomosis of the other shorter graft(s) is performed on this main graft before or after releasing the aortic cross-clamp. The second method is used for complete arterial revascularization of all coronary arteries, but this method is more time-consuming and needs more competency (Figure 2b-2). This composite conduit is prepared for T- or Y-graft and it can reach all surfaces of the heart. The most preferred conduits are the LIMA as a pedicle graft source and the RIMA as a composed part for grafting all target coronary arteries.

c. **Sequential grafting with a bifurcated conduit**

This approach can be used for revascularization of the distal RCA- or Cx-branches (Figure 2c). This approach is easy to apply, but it is very uncommon to find a bifurcated conduit in the body. The advantages are avoiding the second proximal anastomosis on the ascending aorta, any handicap caused by anastomosis between both grafts, and technical difficulties and risks of kissing anastomosis.

3. **Hybrid revascularization**

The standard hybrid coronary revascularization combines the benefits of the LIMA-to-LAD grafting and stent implantation to the other coronary territory. The hybrid revascularization

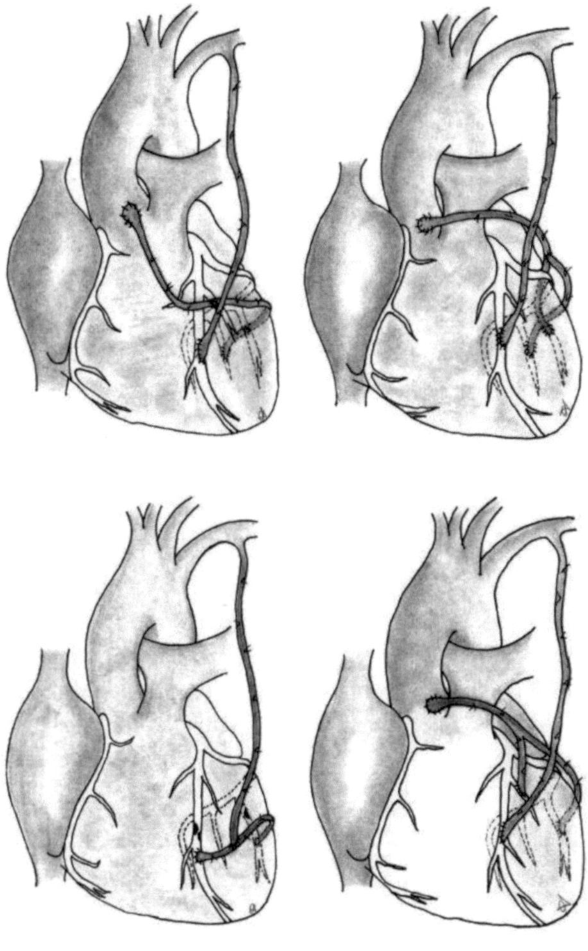

Figure 2. Sequential grafting is the best alternative for the multivessel revascularization in the absence of adequate conduits. **a)** Sequential grafting with a single conduit. **b)** Sequential grafting with a composite conduit: **1-** classic approach with inadequate saphenous vein grafts; **2-** T- or Y- graft for total arterial revascularization. **c)** Sequential grafting with a bifurcated conduit.

technique can be chosen with several indications in patients with diffuse coronary artery disease (Table 4). Patients with severe comorbidities or patients with multiple stenoses may be the best candidates for this procedure. If complete multivessel surgical revascularization increases operative adverse outcomes in high-risk patients, stent implantation in one or more coronary arteries, except the LAD, can be a preventative alternative to complete myocardial revascularization (Table 4). Hybrid revascularization can be performed concomitant or staged. Concomitant hybrid revascularization needs a specific operating room, whereas staged hybrid revascularization can be performed in every clinic. Percutaneous coronary intervention is applied before or after CABG. The decision depends on the severity of proximal lesions which may not be revascularized, and the aim is the avoidance of any perioperative myocardial infarction. Especially proximal or ostial left main or LAD serious stenosis should be treated by stent, if single LIMA-to-LAD grafting cannot achieve complete blood supply to the LAD territory. Ungraftable RCA or Cx vessels with severe stenosis should be treated by percutaneous intervention to achieve complete revascularization.

1. Invisible coronary artery during surgery threatening a huge myocardium
2. Multiple stenosis with a very proximal lesion threatening proximal larger branches
3. To shorten cardiopulmonary and ischemic times
4. Absence of sufficient conduits for complete revascularization
5. Impaired or diseased conduits

Table 4. Indication for hybrid revascularization

Touch the Plaque Techniques

1. Long-segment (1-3 cm) anastomosis

This technique is chosen when the plaque with limited length obstructs the coronary blood flow. This simplest form includes a limited long-segment anastomosis of a conduit to eliminate the occlusion of the limited atherosclerotic plaque (Figure 3). This technique is a prolonged version of the standard anastomosis technique to revascularize proximal and distal segments of the coronary artery and makes jumping grafting with/without a second graft unnecessary. The whole diseased coronary artery segment is opened at full length of the atherosclerotic lesion and the arteriotomy is extended bidirectionally until the healthy coronary artery lumen comes out. The aim of this maneuver is to forward graft blood flow directly into the healthy coronary artery lumen bidirectionally. The distal end of the graft is opened longer than coronary arteriotomy to prevent any tension, tightening, stenosis or inadequately anastomotic length of the conduit, and then the graft is anastomosed on the coronary arteriotomy longitudinally. All attention should be directed to avoid any distal embolization of atherosclerotic debris or to prevent the continuity of the coronary artery.

2. Patch-plasty (> 3 cm) anastomosis

A diffusely diseased coronary artery cannot be grafted by conventional grafting technique and side branches and/or distal segment would not be revascularized. This technique is preferred mostly for the LAD, but the RCA or the Cx artery can be also bypassed with this technique. The patch-plasty technique is necessary if any kind of endarterectomy cannot be applied and the long-segment lesions should be opened in full length. The main principle is to avoid touching the atherosclerotic plaques during the patch reconstruction. The in situ or free conduit can be used alone (Figure 4a) or it can be anastomosed onto the second graft, which is sewn on the long-segment arteriotomy as a hood (Figure 4b). The arteriotomy can be made as long as the length of the attainable epicardial coronary artery, and then a conduit is used to close this arteriotomy without the occlusion of side branches. The graft should also be opened as long as the arteriotomy and anastomosed with a running single suture. In the standard approach, the bites can be taken at the free ends of the arteriotomy to get the largest lumen

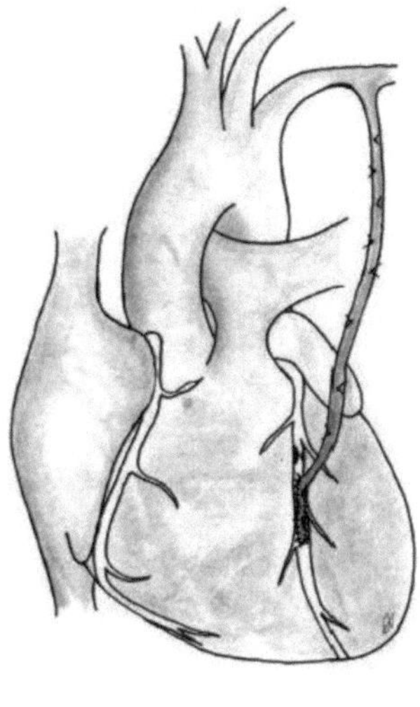

Figure 3. Long-segment anastomosis (1-3 cm) is the simplest alternative to eliminate the distal eccentric lesion.

(Figure 5a). If the lateral walls of the coronary arteriotomy are much calcified, the bites can also be taken very closely to the septal branches, however, this approach needs grafting epicardial side branches separately (Figure 5b). This technique is more useful for the diffusely occluded LAD to perfuse septal branches as far as possible or for the distal major branches of the RCA with septal branches. The Cx artery can be grafted with this technique to make the anastomosis safe.

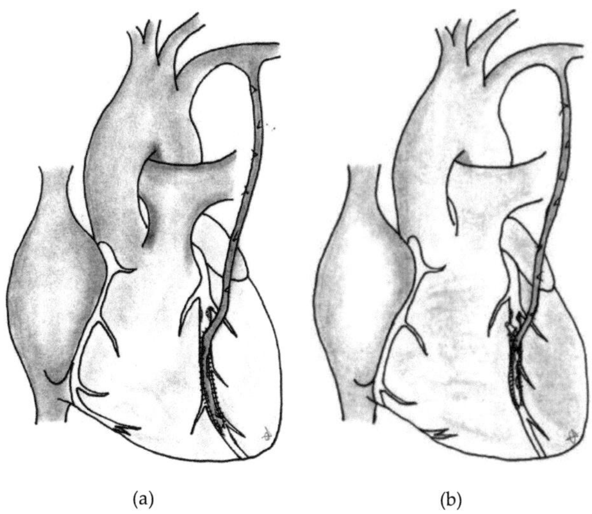

(a) (b)

Figure 4. Patch-plasty is the best alternative to avoid endarterectomy in the extended long-segment (> 3 cm) diffuse coronary artery disease. **a)** The in situ or free conduit is anastomosed onto the long-segment coronary artery as a patch. **b)** The limited second conduit is anastomosed as a hood and the main conduit is anastomosed onto this conduit.

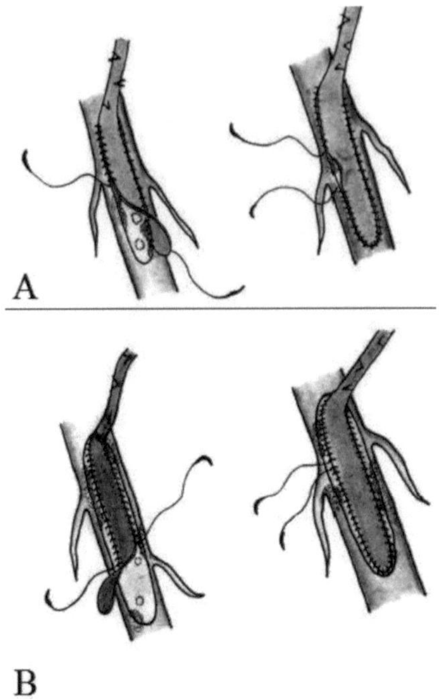

Figure 5. The stitching maneuvers of the patch-plasty technique. **a)** Bites on the free margins of the coronary arteriotomy. **b)** Bites close to the septal branches.

3. Endarterectomy with/without patch-plasty

In the accelerated form of coronary arteriosclerosis, the atherosclerotic plaque appears widespread and the full-length lumen of the coronary artery can be narrowed strictly or occluded totally. Coronary endarterectomy can be applied via off- or on-pump techniques, but the Cx endarterectomy with off-pump technique is used very seldom because it is more difficult and needs more competence [15]. This technique can be often used for every coronary artery, but it is usually preferred for the LAD and RCA [16]. The long-segment lesion is usually calcified and it inhibits any kind of stitching; however, the plaque can be separated easily from the arterial wall. Endarterectomy and graft anastomosis is preferred only to create an appropriate lumen in the total occluded coronary artery due to the removal of the atheromatous material. Long-standing atherosclerosis permits a successful endarterectomy to get adequate distal run-off. All debris and layer until the adventitia should be removed, and then the vessel wall is reconstructed with a conduit. The early occlusion of the endarterected coronary artery is caused by thrombosis or intimal flap formation, but the reason for late occlusion is intimal hyperplasia. The endarterectomy and patch plasty approach has a very satisfactory graft patency compared with the other approaches for the coronary territory [17,18].

a. Closed Endarterectomy

The closed approach is preferred for the LAD or RCA (Figure 6a). Approximately 2 cm arteriotomy is performed and an endarterectomy plane between the medial layer and the adventitia is developed with the coronary scissors. The circumferential plane is performed and the core is pulled out from the distal arterial wall. Distal plaque removal causes usually a better coronary distal bed, but proximal plaque removal via a limited arteriotomy can cause poor outcomes as the native vessel laceration resulting native coronary artery dissection or a native passage of high blood flow from the aorta to the distal coronary resulting competition, and early thrombosis. To optimize the technique, avoiding proximal endarterectomy by the pull-out method and cutting the proximal part without any traction would come along with better results [19]. The core usually is separated cleanly from the distal vessel, but all debris must be cleaned from the septal ostia. If the core branches can be reached, major side branches are endarterectomized separately. The main aim is to get the distal core without any rupture; otherwise the arteriotomy should be extended until the ruptured distal end to continue the closed endarterectomy.

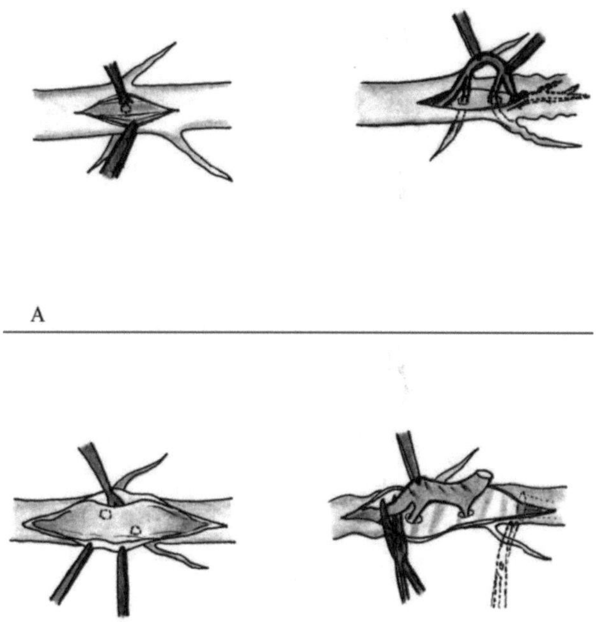

A

B

Figure 6. Endarterectomy is the most aggressive method for coronary bypass surgery. **a)** Closed endarterectomy. **b)** Open endarterectomy.

b. Open Endarterectomy + Patch-plasty

The open approach is a useful procedure for the total occluded LAD (Figure 6b). The open approach prevents any obstruction of septal branches and inadequate endarterectomy of diagonal branches. The arteriotomy is started at the middle segment of the LAD and extended bidirectionally as proximal and distal as possible. If septal branches are easy to be revascularized with long-segment grafting, anastomosis can be finished without endarterectomy. If the direct anastomosis is impossible because of severe calcified vessel wall or no lumen, a long-segment endarterectomy should be performed to separate the core from the adventitia. The core is removed gently and both ends of the core at the ends of the arteriotomy should be cut without any traction. Because aggressive endarterectomy increases the operation risk, the arteriotomy should be extended until the normal lumen with normal intima in the distal and proximal segments of the coronary artery. All coronary arteries have very small lumen and thin wall at the distal, and the arteriotomy should be stopped 2-3 cm before the last bifurcation. The arteriotomy is reconstructed with a long segment of the conduit or a graft patch into which the in situ conduit is anastomosed.

Author details

Kaan Kırali* and Yücel Özen

*Address all correspondence to: imkbkirali@yahoo.com

Department of Cardiovascular Surgery, Koşuyolu Herat and Research Hospital, Istanbul, Turkey

References

[1] Gould KL, Johnson NP. Physiologic severity of diffuse coronary artery disease: Hidden high risk. (Editorial) Circulation 2015;131(1):4-6.

[2] McNeil M, Buth K, Brydie A, MacLaren A, Baskett R. The impact of diffuseness of coronary artery disease on the outcomes of patients undergoing primary and reoperative coronary artery bypass grafting. Eur J Cardiothorac Surg 2007;31(5):827-833.

[3] Hadi HA, Carr CS, Suwaidi JA. Endothelial dysfunction: Cardiovascular risk factors, therapy, and outcome. Vasc Health Risk Manag 2005;1(3):183-198.

[4] Kurlansky P, Herbert M, Prince S, Mack MJ. Improved long-term survival for diabetic patients with surgical versus interventional revascularization. Ann Thorac Surg 2015;99(4):1298–1305.

[5] Kappetein AP, Head SJ, Morice MC, et al. Treatment of complex coronary artery disease in patients with diabetes: 5-year results comparing outcomes of bypass surgery and percutaneous coronary intervention in the SYNTAX trial. Eur J Cardiothorac Surg 2013;43(5):1006-1013.

[6] Fanari Z, Weiss SA, Zhang W, Sonnad SS, Weintraub WS. Meta-analysis of three randomized controlled trials comparing coronary artery bypass grafting with percu-

taneous coronary intervention using drug-eluting stenting in patients with diabetes. Interactive Cardiovasc Thorac Surg 2014;19(6):1002-1007.

[7] Lehle K, Preuner JG, Vogt A, et al. Endothelial cell dysfunction after coronary bypass grafting with extracorporeal circulation in patients with type 2 diabetes mellitus. Eur J Cardiothorac Surg 2007;32(4):611-616.

[8] Galili O, Sattler KJ, Herrmann J, et al. Experimental hypercholesterolemia differentially affects adventitial vasa vasorum and vessel structure of the left internal thoracic and coronary arteries. J Thorac Cardiovasc Surg 2005;129(4):767-772.

[9] Wong D, Thompson G, Buth K, Sullivan J, Ali I. Angiographic coronary diffuseness and outcomes in dialysis patients undergoing coronary artery bypass grafting surgery. Eur J Cardiothorac Surg 2003;24(3):388-392.

[10] Faccini A, Agricola E, Oppizzi M, et al. Coronary microvascular dysfunction in asymptomatic patients affected by systemic sclerosis. Circ J 2015;79(4):825-829.

[11] Vecchiati A, Tellatin S, Angelini A, Iliceto S, Tona F. Coronary microvasculopathy in heart transplantation: Consequences and therapeutic implications. World J Transplant 2014;4(2):93-101.

[12] Taqueti VR, Hachamovitch R, Murthy VL, et al. Global coronary flow reserve is associated with adverse cardiovascular events independently of luminal angiographic severity and modifies the effect of early revascularization. Circulation 2015;131(1): 19-27.

[13] Kaya E, Mansuroglu D, Göksedef D, et al. Long-term angiographic results of coronary artery bypass surgery with the use of arterial graft combinations. Turkish J Thorac Cardiovasc 2005;13(4):309-313.

[14] Akıncı E, Uzun K, Erentuğ V, et al. The comparison of the early and midterm results of the proximal anastomosis techniques in sequential radial artery grafting. Turkish J Thorac Cardiovasc 2004;12(3):235-240.

[15] Kırali K, Sareyyüpoğlu B, Yıldırım Ö, et al [abstract]. Coronary artery endarterectomy: Off-pump or on-pump? 56th International Congress of the European Society for Cardiovascular Surgery, May 17-20, 2007; Venice, Italy. Interact Cardiovasc Thorac Surg 2007;6(Suppl 1):S52.

[16] Kırali K, Yıldırım Ö, Sareyyüpoğlu B, et al [abstract]. Coronary artery endarterectomy: Impact on morbidity and mortality. 56th International Congress of the European Society for Cardiovascular Surgery, May 17-20, 2007; Venice, Italy. Interact Cardiovasc Thorac Surg 2007;6(Suppl 1):S75.

[17] Kırali K, Sareyyüpoğlu B, Yıldırım Ö, et al [abstract]. Left anterior descending coronary artery endarterectomy: 15-year results. 56th International Congress of the European Society for Cardiovascular Surgery, May 17-20, 2007; Venice, Italy. Interact Cardiovasc Thorac Surg 2007;6(Suppl 1):S103.

[18] Kırali K, Yıldırım Ö, Sareyyüpoğlu B, et al [abstract]. Coronary endarterectomy for diffuse right coronary artery disease: 11 years results. 15th Annual Meeting of Asian Society of Cardiovascular Surgery, May 17-20, 2007; Beijing, China.

[19] Sareyyüpoğlu B, Yıldırım Ö, Kırali K. Different results of proximal coronary endarterectomy via conventional pull-out method. Kosuyolu Heart J 2012;15(2):90-91.

Chapter 8

Role and Rationale for Hybrid Coronary Artery Revascularization

Kendal M. Endicott and Gregory D. Trachiotis

Additional information is available at the end of the chapter

http://dx.doi.org/10.5772/61095

Abstract

The optimal revascularization strategy for patients with multi-vessel coronary artery disease remains controversial. The advent of percutaneous coronary intervention (PCI) has challenged the superiority of coronary artery bypass graft (CABG) surgery for multi-vessel disease. In the late 1990s, an integrated approach, now referred to as "hybrid coronary revascularization" (HCR), was pioneered combining CABG and PCI to offer appropriate patients a less invasive option for revascularization while still capitalizing on the superior patency rates of the left internal mammary artery (LIMA) to the left anterior descending (LAD) artery bypass . The operative techniques continue to evolve as well as the timing strategies for intervention and use of anti-platelet therapy. While more research is needed, current data supports hybrid coronary revascularization as a promising technique to optimize outcomes in patients with multi-vessel coronary artery disease.

Keywords: Hybrid Coronary Revascularization, Coronary Artery Disease, Coronary Artery Bypass Grafting, Percutaneous Coronary Intervention, Robotics

1. Introduction

The optimal revascularization strategy for patients with multi-vessel coronary artery disease remains controversial. The advent of percutaneous coronary intervention (PCI) has challenged the superiority of coronary artery bypass graft (CABG) surgery for multi-vessel disease as PCI offers a less invasive option with faster recovery time and lower risk. Despite a survival benefit in high-risk groups and superior long-term freedom from revascularization, trends continue to move toward increasing percutaneous approaches. In the late 1990s, an integrated approach, now referred to as "hybrid coronary revascularization" (HCR), was pioneered combining CABG and PCI to offer appropriate patients a less invasive option for revascularization while still capitalizing on the superior patency rates of the left internal mammary artery (LIMA) to left anterior descending (LAD) artery bypass. The technology has evolved tremendously since the introduction of HCR with some LIMA-LAD grafts now performed completely robotically. As HCR evolves, questions regarding indications, optimal surgical technique, timing, and outcomes as well as cost-benefit analysis continue to permeate current practice and will define the future of HCR in the algorithm of coronary revascularization.

2. Rationale

CABG has long been the established standard of care to treat left main or three vessel coronary artery disease [1]. The therapeutic benefit of this approach lies in the LIMA-LAD revascularization. Patency rates of this anastomosis lie between 95%–98% at 10 years [2]. Radial arterial conduits have been explored as another option for total arterial revascularization; however, results do not compare with the long-term patency of LIMA utilization [3]. Saphenous vein grafts (SVG) also do not provide the same longevity of the LIMA-LAD revascularization. Failure of SVG is multifactorial including technical failure within 30 days, neo-intimal hyperplasia at 1–24 months, and atherosclerotic degeneration beyond 2 years. Patient risk factors such as hyperlipidemia and ongoing tobacco are also associated with accelerated graft failure. Failure rates are estimated as high as 10%–15% at 1 year after CABG with almost 50% total graft occlusion at 10 years [4]. Despite this high failure rate, SVG remain the most commonly used conduit for CABG surgery.

PCI has challenged the superiority of CABG surgery for multi-vessel disease. The use of drug-eluting stents (DES) in particular has provided a less invasive option for revascularization with faster return to normal activities and lower risk of complications. Restenosis rates and stent thrombosis of DES in non-LAD lesions are markedly lower than non-LAD SVG with rates less than 10% and 1%, respectively [5]. In addition, stenting of SVG after thrombosis introduces technical changes with higher peri-procedural rates of complications and in-hospital mortality than stenting of native arteries [4, 6]. Despite data that suggests improved outcomes with many patients including diabetics and those with left main and complex multi-vessel coronary artery disease (CAD) [2], trends continue toward increased PCI over CABG.

The strategy of HCR attempts to capitalize on the superior LIMA-LAD patency rates as well as the minimally invasive PCI approach thus eliminating the need for additional venous or arterial conduits. Patients with multi-vessel disease with significant proximal LAD disease with other lesions suitable for PCI in the left main, left circumflex, or right coronary artery territories are appropriate candidates for HCR [7]. In addition, patients with lack of suitable conduits, prior sternotomy, severe ascending aortic disease, or coronary arteries not amenable for bypass may be suitable HCR candidates. Patients generally not deemed HCR candidates

http://dx.doi.org/10.5772/61095

and thus deferred to conventional CABG include those with chronic total occlusions, highly calcified segments, and diffusely diseased and bifurcation coronary lesions [7]. Table 1 summarizes the clinical and angiographic findings that should be taken into consideration when discussing the option for HCR. Discussions regarding treatment options are best facilitated by a multi-disciplinary approach including both an interventional cardiologist and cardiac surgeon.

	PCI	CABG	HCR
Angiographic Characteristics			
Unprotected Left Main Disease	no	yes	yes
Intra-myocardial LAD	yes	no	no
Complex LAD lesion	no	yes	yes
Complex non-LAD lesions	no	yes	no
Comorbidities			
Advanced Age	yes	no	yes
LVEF <30%	no	yes	yes
Diabetes mellitus	no	yes	yes
Renal insufficiency	no	yes	yes
Severe chronic lung disease	yes	no	no
Prior left thoracotomy	yes	yes	no
Prior sternotomy	yes	no	yes
Limited vascular access	no	yes	no
Lack of available conduits	yes	no	yes
Severe aortic calcification	yes	no	yes
Contraindication for dual anti-platelet therapy	no	yes	no

Table 1. Recommendations for Candidates for Hybrid Coronary Revascularization Versus Conventional Coronary Revascularization [2, 21]

3. Strategies and surgical approach

3.1. Surgical approaches

Minimally invasive cardiac surgery seeks to eliminate two invasive components of conventional CABG: cardiopulmonary bypass (CBP) and sternotomy. The development of stabilizer technology in the early 1990s made available off-pump CABG with the potential advantages of less blood loss, lower incidence of neurologic complications, and less pulmonary complications [8]. In conjunction with sternal sparing incisions as well as robotic techniques, a minimally invasive off-pump option for LIMA-LAD revascularization offers the key to optimizing the HCR option. The techniques described below and in Table 2 discuss the current options for minimally invasive surgical approaches to LIMA-LAD revascularization highlighting key features of the various techniques.

	Thoracic Access	LIMA Harvest	Anastomosis	Single Lung ventilation	CPB	Advantages/Disadvantages
OPCAB (Off-pump CABG)	Midline Sternotomy	Direct Vision	Direct vision with stabilizers	Not Required	No	Avoids risks associated with CBP
MIDCAB (Minimally invasive direct coronary artery bypass grafting)	Left-sided thoracotomy or lower partial sternotomy	Direct Vision	Direct Vision	Improves exposure but not required	Not required but can be performed by femoral cannulation	Avoids aortic cross-clamping and manipulation
Endo-ACAB (Endoscopic atraumatic coronary artery bypass graft surgery)	Limited rib sparing left-sided thoracotomy	Robotic or Thoracoscopic	Hand-Sutured	Required when robot is used	Not required	Decreased morbidity from thoracotomy incision yet allows for hand-sewn anastomosis
TECAB (Totally endoscopic coronary artery bypass graft surgery)	Thoracoscopic	Robotic	Robotic intracorporeal anastomosis	Required	Not required	Minimally invasive, however very technically challenging

Table 2. Surgical Techniques Used for LAD Revascularization During Hybrid Coronary Revascularization

MIDCAB: Minimally invasive direct coronary artery bypass(MIDCAB) grafting refers to an off-pump minimally invasive LIMA-LAD revascularization performed through a small left-sided thoracotomy in the fourth or fifth interspace. Costal cartilage removal or rib disarticulation is sometimes necessary for visualizing. Cardiac stabilization and LAD harvest is performed directly through the wound and does not require endoscopic or robotic skills to master the LAD harvest. Surgeon comfort with off-pump techniques is critical as well as experience with sternal sparing incisions. Single-lung ventilation is optimal for exposure; however chest cavity insufflation is not necessary. A slightly larger thoracotomy incision can allow exposure for harvest of bilateral internal mammary arteries.

Large series published since 1994 have validated short-term LAD-LIMA patency rates of this technique at 95%–97% [8]. The advantage of this technique lies in the avoidance of CBP and aortic manipulation as an off-pump strategy; however, no data exists to suggest differences in

http://dx.doi.org/10.5772/61095

post-operative pain or pulmonary complications from conventional CABG [8]. MIDCAB may have decreased bleeding and infection rates compared to traditional sternotomy, however the need for a thoracotomy incision for the technique has prompted further exploration into various thoracoscopic and robotic techniques to capitalize on the advantages of minimally invasive strategies as discussed in the following.

Endo-ACAB: Endoscopic atraumatic coronary artery bypass (Endo-ACAB) refers to the thoracosocpic or robotic identification of the LAD with LIMA mobilization without violating the integrity of the chest wall (Figure 1). A directed, non-rib spreading or limited rib spreading thoracotomy is then employed for a hand-sewn LIMA-LAD anastomosis on the beating heart. Robotic LIMA mobilization requires single-lung ventilation and insufflation to create space in the anterior mediastinum to facilitate LIMA harvest. After the LIMA is taken down, a pericardial incision is made for identification of the LAD. A small (4–5cm) anterior thoracotomy without disarticulation of costal cartilage is then made to introduce an endoscopic stabilizer via an arm port, which allows for LAD stabilization and hand-sewn anastomosis.

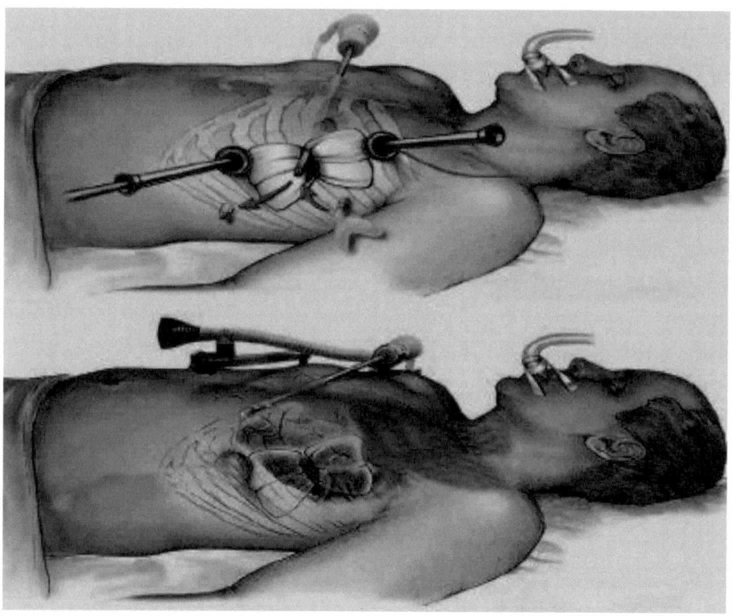

Figure 1. EndoCab technique as described above.

Multiple case series have reported excellent LIMA-LAD patency rates with thoracoscopic Endo-ACAB approaches. In new smaller series with robotic Endo-ACAB approaches, routine post-operative angiography has demonstrated no decline in LIMA-LAD patency rates. In Kiaii's series of 58 patients who underwent one-stage robotic Endo-ACAB HCR, the average length of stay in the ICU and hospital were 1 and 4 days, respectively, leading the authors to suggest benefit to patients in terms of post-operative surgical morbidity and recovery time using more minimally invasive technology [9].

TECAB: Totally endoscopic coronary artery bypass grafting (TECAB) utilizes a robotically sewn, intracorporeal anastomosis, which negates the need for even a small thoracotomy. This technique was first explored on an arrested heart during CBP; however, the associated complications of CPB have led most robotic surgeons to employ an off-pump TECAB. The operation itself is technically challenging without widespread adoption of this technique owning to the need for robotic technology and surgeon expertise.

One of the largest series published in 2012 reported on 226 patients with 5-year outcomes [10]. Perioperative results were consistent with the standards of open CABG. The authors report a dramatically decreased time to recovery owning to the lack of need for sternal precautions. In the 10 cases requiring conversion to thoracotomy, these patients averaged 2- day longer hospital stays with increased ventilator time and return to normal activities [10]. Overall results in other case series support the safety and feasibility of this technique; however, Harskamp reports that only approximately one-third of HCRs from 2011–2013 reported in the Society of Thoracic Adult Cardiac Database utilize robotic technology [11]. Expansion of the TECAB approach is currently limited by the cost and learning curve associated with the implementation of robotic technology.

Graft Assessment: Off-pump (OP) and minimally invasive techniques for LAD-LIMA grafting have appropriately been scrutinized with regard to patency rate outcomes compared to the classical on-pump CABG via a midline sternotomy. The recent Randomized On/Off Bypass (ROOBY) trial as well as other smaller trails have demonstrated that the patency rates of LIMA-LAD grafts between off-pump coronary artery bypass (OPCAB) and conventional CABG were similar (95.3 and 96.2, respectively) [12]. As the HCR approach relies upon the durability and integrity of this anastomosis, the ability of the surgeon to assess the LIMA-LAD graft intra-operatively becomes increasingly important. In fact, the European Society of Cardiology (ESC) and the European Association for Cardio-Thoracic Surgery (EACTS) recommends graft evaluation before leaving the operating room [13].

Graft assessment includes the traditional methods such as inspection, palpation, electrocardiography (ECG), and echocardiography (ECHO). Other methods include conventional coronary angiography, which is the gold standard, transit-time flow measurement (TTFM), and intra-operative fluorescence imaging (IFI). As the causes of early graft failure are often technical, this technology seeks to eliminate these errors by objectively evaluating graft function. Certainly, a clear advantage of single stage HCR with CABG followed by PCI lies in the opportunity for angiographic graft assessment with readily available operative access for reintervention; however, when angiographic assessment is not available, the most commonly utilized technique among cardiovascular surgeons over the last decade has become TTFM. Retrospective studies have demonstrated the ability of TTFM to detect grafts with impaired flow thus predicting graft failure within 6 months after CABG [14]; however, little is known about how TTFM relates to long-term graft patency and patient survival.

TTFM relies on the principles of transit-time ultrasound technology. The surgeon can obtain both quantitative data of average blood flow volume and several calculated derivatives of the flow of blood in the graft displayed in waveform. TTFM cannot, however, differentiate physiologic conditions accounting for low blood flow versus technical quality of a surgical anastomosis. While clear cut-off values for graft revision have not been set, a mean flow <15ml min $^{-1}$ for grafts to the left coronary system and less than 20ml min $^{-1}$ for grafts to the right coronary system were predictive of failure. A pulsatility index (PI) greater than 0.5 is predictive of graft failure. Another important value is the diastolic flow percentage (DF%) or diastolic flow divided by total flow through the graft. This value should be greater than 50% for all grafts and territories and ideally greater than 65%. When the PI and DF% both demonstrate adequate measurements, the graft can be objectively presumed adequate [15]. Figure 2 demonstrates the intra-operative TTFM tracings utilizing the MediStim ASA technology, which is one of the more commonly utilized flowmeters.

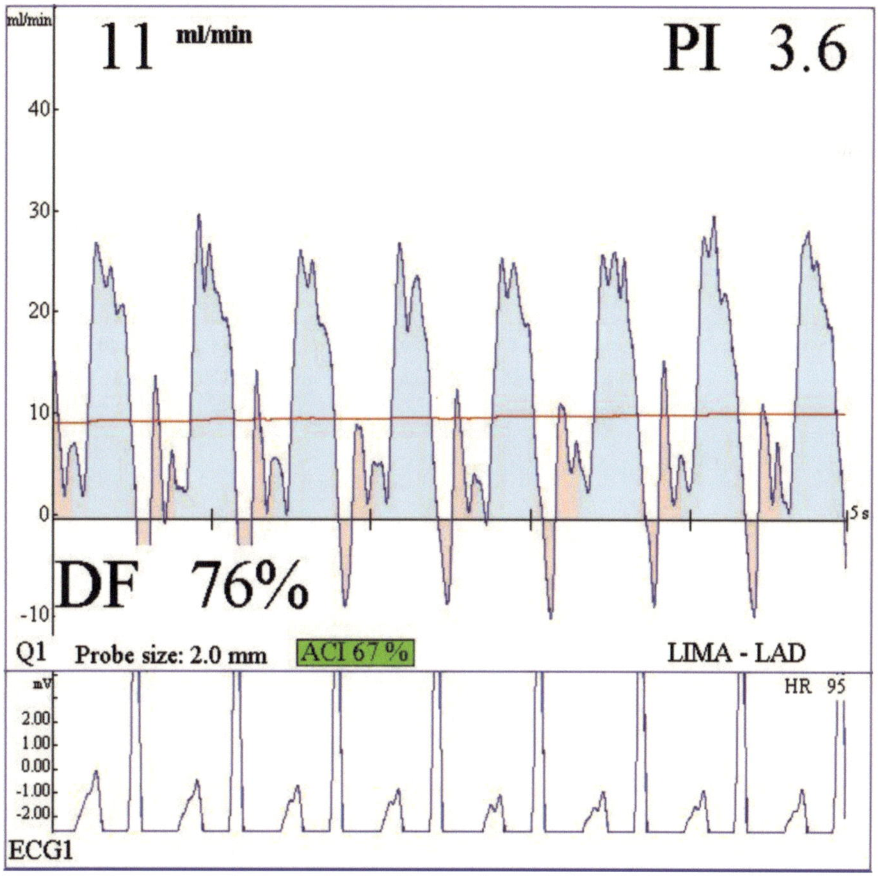

Figure 2. Transit Time Flow Assessment.

3.2. Timing strategies

HCR began in the 1990s as a staged procedure with LIMA-LAD revascularization performed first followed by PCI. The use of DESs and anti-platelet therapy as well as the use of hybrid operating room suites has introduced questions as to the most optimal timing for open and

PCI revascularization. Currently, three options for timing strategies exist: PCI followed by CABG, CABG followed by PCI, and one-stage hybrid HCR. Each option introduces different benefits and challenges, and at this time no clear consensus exists on the optimal strategy for timing of revascularization (Table 3). Patient characteristics, operator skill, and availability of facilities should be considered when choosing the most appropriate approach.

One-Stage HCR	**Two-Stage HCR**	
Simultaneous CABG and PCI	**CABG then PCI**	**PCI then CABG**
Advantages:	**Advantages:**	**Advantages:**
Ability to study LIMA-LAD graft	Ability to study LIMA-LAD graft	Pre-operative angiographic imaging of LIMA size
Protected LAD to allow PCI to high-risk non-LAD lesions	Protected LAD to allow PCI to high-risk non-LAD lesions	Lower risk of ischemia during CABG given non-LAD territory revascularization
Single anesthetic exposure	Reduced risk of post-surgical bleedingas no need for anti-platelet therapy post CABG	Useful in acute coronary syndromeswith non-LAD culprits
Can convert to conventional CABG if PCI fails	After LIMA-LAD revascularization, asymptomatic patients may require no further intervention	If stents unsuccessful, conventional CABG has to be subsequently performed
Single procedure reduces cost and hospital length of stay		
Disadvantages:	**Disadvantages:**	**Disadvantages:**
Requires hybrid suite	Risk of ischemia during CABG in non-LAD lesions	No ability to angiographically evaluate LIMA-LAD anastomosis
Increased risk of post-operative bleeding due to need for anti-platelet after surgery	Unsuccessful PCI may lead to need for surgical reintervention	Increased peri-operative bleeding due to need for anti-platelet therapy
Risk of stent thrombosis due to post-operative inflammatory state		Potential for LAD territory ischemia between stages
CKD patients exposed to dual nephrotoxic insults with surgery and PCI contrast use		Higher risk of stent thrombosis due to inflammatory response of CABG and potential need to hold anti-platelet therapy
High degrees of coordination needed between teams		

Table 3. Advantages and Disadvantages of One and Two-Staged HCR Procedures

One-Stage HCR: Simultaneous CABG and PCI: The advent of hybrid operating room suites has introduced the option for simultaneous CABG and PCI. This approach allows for complete revascularization before leaving the operating room. Routine imaging of the LIMA-LAD anastomosis is also available before chest closure. More aggressive percutaneous approaches can be taken to otherwise challenging lesions given the safety net of open revascularization options. The patient benefits from a single anesthetic exposure and decreased hospitalization time. One ongoing concern however is the post-operative risk of bleeding given the need for dual anti-platelet therapy after DES placement in conjunction with incomplete heparin reversal. Concerns also exist regarding the relationship of the inflammatory response in the post-operative setting and risk for acute stent thrombosis.

Two-Stage: PCI Followed by CABG: This option confers several advantages. In revascularizing the non-LAD lesion first and thus providing collateralization, the potential risks of ischemia during LAD occlusion are minimized. PCI firstly also provides the interventional cardiologist a safety net should revascularization be unsuccessful percutaneously. The most important benefit of this approach occurs in the setting of acute coronary syndrome with a non-LAD culprit. The acutely affected lesion may be stented followed by LAD revascularization at a later time. This strategy does however introduce the difficulty of the need for anti-platelet therapy with DES. Even brief discontinuation of anti-platelet therapy can risk stent thrombosis; however this must be weighed with intra-operative bleeding risk. Investigation is underway regarding the use of newer anti-platelet agents and potential decreased bleeding risk. It again should be noted that the pro-inflammatory trauma from surgery could also put new stents at risk for thrombosis.

Two-Stage: CABG Followed by PCI: This strategy has become the most widely adopted one for HCR. With PCI post-CABG, the concern for surgical bleeding while on anti-platelet therapy is negated. Like hybrid HCR, LIMA-LAD graft patency can be confirmed during PCI angiography. Pre-PCI protection of the LAD also provides the interventional cardiologist the option to approach lesions that would perhaps have otherwise been at higher risk. This includes both left main lesions and diagonal bifurcation lesions [8]. For the minimally invasive surgeon, the unrevascularized collateral lesions could manifest as intra-operative ischemia. Careful attention must be paid to hemodynamics during insufflation, and the use of peripheral CPB should be considered if needed. In the scenario of a PCI complication or failure, this approach could necessitate a return to the operating room with emergent CABG. The optimal time frame for PCI following CABG remains unclear. Some teams opt for PCI during the index hospitalization and thus avoid patient discharge with an incomplete revascularization, however other teams propose a more extended period of waiting from 1 to several weeks. Economic factors also become an increasing concern given questions of reimbursement.

Overall, no clear optimal timing strategy has been clearly defined. While some studies demonstrate increased post-operative bleeding risks on dual-anti-platelet therapy, others suggest that the minimally invasive surgical approaches negate this risk traditionally associated with sternotomy. Harskamp's analysis of recent STS data suggests that the need for post-operative transfusion was actually lower in the one-stage procedure group with comparable reoperation for bleeding [11]. This analysis also reports that patients undergoing one-stage procedures were more likely to have peripheral vascular disease and stroke history compared to other groups [11]. Further studies are needed to outline the specific clinical scenarios and patient characteristics, which should dictate the timing of CABG and PCI. Certainly, cost analysis and patient preferences will also factor into future decision-making regarding timing strategies.

Anti-platelet management: As discussed, the use of anti-platelet therapy is a complicated balance of post-surgical bleeding versus risk of acute stent thrombosis. Currently, no guidelines exist to define the optimal strategy. This question of anti-platelet therapy poses two questions regarding the order of staging as well as timing of initiation of therapy. Different authors have reported their experience with varying strategies and outcomes. In cases of two staged procedures with CABG first, most authors performed CABG on aspirin alone followed by a second anti-platelet agent greater than 4 h post-operatively after ensuring that there were no bleeding complications [16]. In the two stage procedures, which performed PCI first, anti-platelet therapy was begun before PCI and continued uninterrupted during CABG. In one-stage procedures, the most common strategies administered anti-platelet therapy after undergoing the LIMA-LAD graft, just before its completion, or immediately after PCI. Others administered anti-platelet therapy at the induction of anesthesia or in the pre-operative area owning to the fact that maximal platelet inhibition occurs 4–24 h after administration [16]. None of these strategies differed in reported rate of acute stent thrombosis [5]. In some studies, the rate of blood transfusion was actually lower in the HCR group as was the need for reoperation for bleeding [11]. Newer anti-platelet agents that are more potent and have a faster onset of action and reversal have also been employed; however, there is currently no data to support the use of these new agents in HCR.

4. Outcomes

Multiple case series from single institution experiences have been published on HCR since the first report in 1996. This includes a population of over 3,000 patients [16]. Data from these series suggest that in experienced hands, the safety profile of HCR is excellent. Multiple studies comparing outcomes after HCR versus CABG and multi-vessel disease have also been published (Table 4). Among cohort studies, the single-stage HCR was most commonly employed. Across these studies, age averaged around 60 years with a male predominance. Left ventricular ejection fraction (LVEF) was preserved or mildly reduced in the majority of patients. With the exception of data from Leacche et al., overall in-hospital mortality, stroke and reoperation for bleeding rates were comparable and low [0% to 2.6%). The outlier reported by Leacche et al. was among the high SYNTAX-HCR group with a reported in-hospital mortality of 23% leading the authors to suggest that HCR should be approached with caution in patients with high (≥33] SYNTAX scores [17]. These reports collectively suggest that HCR may be a comparable option to CABG in patients with non-LAD lesions accessible by PCI.

Author, Year Type of Study	N	Surgical Technique	Timing of PCI	Age, years	Male, %	LVEF %	SYNTAX Score	In-Hospital Mortality	Follow-Up Period	Survival
Shen et al., 2013 Retrospective, matched cohort study (propensity matched) Recruitment: 2007-2010 (23)	141 HCR 141 CABG 141 PCI	Lower partial mini-sternotomy CABG (on and off pump)	One Stage	62±9.9 62.4±7.8 61.7±10.3	88.7 90.1 87.2	62.7±7.1 62.6±8.0 62.1± 9.3	27.6±7.9 28.2±9.4 26.0±8.2	N/A	30 days	99.3% 97.2% 96.5%
Leacche et al., 2013 Retrospective cohort study (group stratification) Recruitment: 2005-2009 (17)	80 HCR SYNTAX≤32 (67) SYNTAX>32 (13) 301 CABG SYNTAX≤32 (226) SYNTAX>32 (75)	OP 22% OP 31% OP 15% OP 16%	One Stage	62 (32-85) 74 (32-84) 63 (32-89) 62 (32-83)	79 62 75 83	50 (20-70) 50 (20-65) 55 (10-80) 50 (10-70)	N/A	****	30 days	N/A
Bachinsky et al., 2012 Prospective cohort study, no matching Recruitment: 2009-2011 (24)	25 HCR 27 CABG	OP MIDCab (Robotic) 100% OP CABG (thoracotomy)	One Stage	63.2±10.5 66.78±10.7	80 59	55.3±10.4 51.48±12.0	33.52±8 34.89±8.2	0% 4%	30 days	100% 96%
Halkos et al., 2011 Retrospective matched cohort study (propensity matching) Recruitment: 2003-2010 (25)	147 HCR 588 CABG	OP EndoACAB OP CABG	Surgery and PCI within 2-3 day (137); One stage (10)	64.3±12.8 64.3±12.5	38.1 28.6	54.7±8.7 54.6±8.7	N/A	0.7% 0.9%	3.2 years	5-year survival: 86.8% 84.3%
Vassiliades et al., 2009 Retrospective cohort study (no matching, propensity score adjustment) Recruitment: 2003-2007 (26)	91 HCR 4175 CABG	OP EndoACAB OP CABG	85 CABG first 6 PCI first	64.7±13.7 62.8±11.7	40.7 37.3	51.5±9.4 50.9±12.7	N/A	0% 1.8%	3 years	94.0% 89.2%
Zhao et al., 2009 Retrospective cohort study (no matching) Recruitment: 2005-2007 (27)	112 HCR 20 CABG	Reversed-J inferior sternotomy OP CABG	One Stage	63 (32-85) 63 (32-89)	71 76	50 (15-70) 54 (10-72)	N/A	2.6% 1.5%	N/A	N/A
Reicher et al., 2008 Prospective, matched cohort study (propensity matching) 2005-2006 (28)	12 HCR 26 CABG	OP MidCab OP CABG (sternotomy)	CABG first	62±10 64±10	80 83	31 (EF <40%) 27 (EF <40%)	N/A	0% 0%	30 days	100% 100%
Kon et al., 2008 Matched prospective cohort study, unclear matching method Recruitment: 2005-2006 (29)	15 HCR 30 CABG	OP MidCab OP CABG (sternotomy)	One Stage	61±10 65±10	73 63	47±14 45±14	N/A	0% 0%	12 mo.	100% 100%

**** see text

Table 4. Studies Comparing Outcomes After HCR Versus CABG or PCI in the Drug Eluting Stent Era [5, 22]

Harskamp et al. published a meta-analysis in 2014 reporting clinical outcomes after HCR in 1,190 patients in single-center registries [18]. This study incorporated six observational studies (one case control and five propensity adjusted) that included adjustments for differences in baseline characteristics. Comparisons of individual components showed no differences in all-cause mortality, MI, or stroke at one year follow-up (odds ratio: 0.49; 95% confidence interval: 0.2 -1.24; p=0.13), however the HCR group demonstrated a higher repeat revascularization rate compared with CABG. These findings were irrespective of the order in which LIMA-LAD graft and PCI were performed.

The only current randomized control trial comparing HCR and CABG was published in 2014 [19]. Two-hundred consecutive patients from a single institution with angiographically confirmed multi-vessel disease involving the proximal LAD and a significant (>70%) lesion in at least one major non-LAD epicardial vessel amenable to both PCI and CABG were randomized in a 1:1 fashion. The primary endpoint was the evaluation of the safety of HCR. The HCR group (n=98) utilized MIDCAB and cobalt chromium DES with a two-stage HCR with PCI performed within 36 h of initial MIDCAB, versus the conventional CABG group (n=102) in which 85.0% of the procedures were performed off-pump. Pre-operative characteristics were similar. Regarding HCR procedures, 6.1% patients were converted to CABG with no adverse early or late outcomes, and HCR was feasible in 93.9% of patients. At 1 year, the two groups had similar all-cause mortality (CABG 2.9% versus HCR 2%; p=NS) and MACE-free survival rates (CABG 92.2% versus HCR 89.8%; p log-rank =0.54). Larger studies are needed to power conclusions regarding long-term mortality data; however, this study suggests that HCR is feasible and safe.

Harskamp et al. recently published a study of practice patterns and clinical outcomes after HCR, in the United States, using the Society of Thoracic Surgeons Adult Cardiac Surgery Database from July 2011 to March 2013 [11]. This analysis demonstrated that HCR represented 0.48% (n=950; staged=809, concurrent=141) of the total CABG volume (n=198,622) over the studied time. HCR was performed in approximately one-third of participating centers (n=361). Interestingly, patients who underwent HCR had high-risk profiles but less extensive coronary disease. There was no statistically significant association between operative approach and operative mortality when comparing the HCR and conventional CABG treatment groups [11].

5. Conclusions

Hybrid coronary revascularization has emerged as a promising technique that combines the superior patency of the LIMA-LAD graft with the superior patency of DES to SVG grafts for non-LAD vessels. As with any new technique, ongoing research will benefit from standardized definitions as well as sub-classification for HCR procedures [20]. Current evidence also lacks direction as to which patient population benefits most from HCR. Current data supports HCR as a feasible alternative to CABG, however, the future of these techniques will rely on improved patient satisfaction, recovery, and financial feasibility. Current reported quality of life assessments 1 year post-operatively are remarkably better in patients undergoing HCR versus OPCAB [5]. Likely reasons include decreased post-operative pain and decreased length of intensive care and hospital stay with quicker return to work and normal activities. Cost analysis have been reported both equal and in favor of HCR; however, these analysis did not examine the hidden cost of construction of a cardiac hybrid operating room as well as training of personal [5]. Further studies are needed to firmly establish improved outcomes and financial benefits of HCR before this novel technique establishes itself as a widespread option in the algorithm of coronary revascularization.

Author details

Kendal M. Endicott[2] and Gregory D. Trachiotis[1,2*]

*Address all correspondence to: gregory.trachiotis@va.gov

1 Division of Cardiothoracic Surgery, Veterans Affairs Medical Center, Washington, DC, USA

2 Division of Cardiothoracic Surgery, The George Washington University, Washington, DC, USA

References

[1] Serruys PW, Morice MC, et al. Percutaneous Coronary Intervention versus Coronary-Artery Bypass Grafting for Severe Coronary Artery Disease. *N Engl J Med.* 2009;360:961-972.

[2] Popma JJ, Nathan S, et al. Hybrid Myocardial Revascularization: An Integrated Approach to Coronary Revascularization. *Catheterization and Cardiovascular Interventions.* 2010;75:S28-S34.

[3] Tatoulis J, Buxton BF, et al. Patencies of 2,127 Arterial to Coronary Conduits Over 15 Years. *Ann Thorac Surg.* 20004;77:93-101.

[4] Harskamp RE, Lopes RD, et al. Saphenous Vein Graft Failure after Coronary Artery Bypass Surgery: Pathophysiology, Management, and Future Directions. *Ann Surg.* 2013;257:824-833.

[5] Harskamp RE, Zheng Z, et al. Status Quo of Hybrid Coronary Revascularization for Multi-Vessel Coronary Artery Disease. *Ann Thorac Surg.* 2013;96:2268-2277.

[6] Brilakis ES, Rao SV, et al. Percutaneous Coronary Intervention in Native Arteries versus Bypass Grafts in Prior Coronary Artery Bypass Grafting Patients. *J Am Coll Cardiol Intv.* 2011;4:844-50.

[7] Green KD, Lynch DR, et al. Combining PCI and CABG: the Role of Hybrid Revascularization. *Curr Cardiol Rep*. 2013;15,351:1-8.

[8] Narasimhan S, Srinivas V, et al. Hybrid Coronary Revascularization. *Cardiology in Review*. 2011;19:101-107.

[9] Kiaii B, McClure S, et al. Simultaneous Integrated Coronary Artery Revascularization with Long-Term Angiographic Follow-Up. *J Thorac Cardiovasc Surg*. 2008;136:702-708.

[10] Bonatti JO, Zimrin D, et al. Hybrid Coronary Revascularization using Robotic Totally Endoscopic Surgery: Perioperative Outcoes and 5-Year Results. *Ann Thorac Surg*. 2012;94:1920-1926.

[11] Harskamp RE, Brennan, JM, et al. Practice Patters and Clinical Outcomes after Hybrid Coronary Revascularization in the United States: An Analysis from the Society of Thoracic Surgeons Adult Cardiac Database. *Circulation*. 2014;130:872-879.

[12] Shroyer AL, Grover FL et al.; The ROOBY Study Group. On-Pump versus Off-Pump Coronary-Artery Bypass Surgery. *N Engl J Med*. 2009;361:1827-1837.

[13] The Task Force on Myocardial Revascularization of the European Society of Cardiology (ESC) and the European Association for Cardio-Thoracic Surgery (EACTS): Guidelines on Myocardial Revascularization. *European Heart Journal*. 2010;31:2501-2505.

[14] Jokinen JJ, Werkkala K. Clinical Value of Intra-operative Transit-time Flow Measurement for Coronary Artery Bypass Grafting: a Prospective Angiography-Controlled Study. *Eur J Cardiothorac Surg*. 2011;39:918-923.

[15] Trachiotis GD. Value of Diastolic Flow with Transit-time Flow Meters in Coronary Artery Bypass Surgery. *Eur J Cardiothorac Surg*. 2011;39:424-437.

[16] Panoulas V, Colombo A. Hybrid Coronary Revascularization: Promising, But yet to Take Off. *J Am Coll Cardiol*. 2015;65:85-97.

[17] Leacche M, Byrne JG, et al. Comparison of 30-day Outcomes of Coronary Artery Bypass Grafting Surgery versus Hybrid Coronary Revascularization Stratified by SYNTAX and euroSCORE. *J Thorac Cardiovasc Surg*. 2013;145:1004-1012.

[18] Harskamp RE, Bagai A, et al. Clinical Outcomes after Hybrid Coronary Revascularization versus Coronary Artery Bypass Surgery: a Meta-analysis of 1,190 Patients. *Am Heart J*. 2014;166, 4:585-592.

[19] Gasior M, Zembala MO, et al. Hybrid Revascularization for Multivessel Coronary Artery Disease. *J Am Coll Cardiol Intv*. 2014;7:1277-1283.

[20] Harskamp RE, Bonatti, JO, et al. Standardizing Definitions for Hybrid Coronary Revascularization. *J Thorac Cardiovasc Surg*. 2014;147:556-560.

[21] Fihn SD, Gardin JM, et al. 2012 ACCF/AHA/ACP/AATS/PCNA/SCAI/STS Guideline for the diagnosis and management of patients with stable ischemic heart disease: a

report of the American College of Cardiology Foundation/American Heart Association Task Force on Practice Guidelines, and the American College of Physicians, American Association for Thoracic Surgery, Preventive Cardiovascular Nurses Association, Society for Cardiovascular Angiography and Interventions, and Society of Thoracic Surgeons. *Circulation*. 2012;126:e354-e471.

[22] Gosain P, Yamani N, et al. Hybrid Coronary Revascularization: A Systematic Review. *Cardiology in Review*. 2015;23:87-93.

[23] Shen L, Hu S, et al. One-Stop Hybrid Coronary Revascularization versus Coronary Artery Bypass Grafting and Percutaneous Coronary Intervention for the Treatment of Multivessel Coronary Artery Disease. *J Am Coll Cardiol*. 2013;61:2525-2533.

[24] Bachinsky WB. Abdelsalam M, et al. Comparative Study of Same Sitting Hybrid Coronary Artery Revascularization versus Off-Pump Coronary Artery Bypass in Multivessel Coronary Artery Disease. *J Interven Cardiol*. 2012;25:460-468.

[25] Halkos ME, Vassiliades TA, et al. Hybrid Coronary Revascularization versus Off-Pump Coronary Artery Bypass Grafting for the Treatment of Multivessel Coronary Artery Disease. *Ann Thorac Surg*. 2011;92:1695-1702.

[26] Vassiliades TA, Kilgo PD, et al. Clinical Outcomes after Hybrid Coronary Revascularization versus Off-Pump Coronary Artery Bypass. *Innovations*. 2009;4:299-306.

[27] Zhao DX, Leacche M, et al. Routine Intraoperative Completion Angiography after Coronary Artery Bypass Grafting and 1-Stop Hybrid Revascularization: Results from a Fully Integrated Hybrid Catheterization Laboratory/Operating Room. *J Am Coll Cardiol*. 2009;53:232-241.

[28] Reicher B, Poston RS, et al. Simultaneous "Hybrid" Percutaneous oronary Intervention and Minimally Invasive Surgical Bypass Grafting: Feasibility, Safety, and Clinical Outcomes. *Am Heart J*. 2008;155:661-667.

[29] Kon ZN, Brown EN, et al. Simultaneous hybrid coronary revascularization reduces postoperative morbidity compared with results from conventional off-pump coronary artery bypass. J Thorac Cardiovasc Surg. 2008;125:367-75.

Chapter 9

Mechanical Complications of Myocardial Infarction

Serena Mariani, Francesco Formica and Giovanni Paolini

Additional information is available at the end of the chapter

http://dx.doi.org/10.5772/61373

Abstract

Complications of acute myocardial infarction are different and life threatening. Prompt diagnosis and therapy are essential. In this, chapter we will analyse mechanical complications, such as ventricular free wall rupture, ventricular septal defect, papillary muscle rupture, ischaemic mitral regurgitation, left ventricle aneurysm, and cardiogenic shock.

Keywords: Mechanical complications, ventricular free wall rupture, ventricular septal defect, papillary muscle rupture, ischaemic mitral regurgitation, left ventricle aneurysm, cardiogenic shock, remodelling

1. Introduction

Complications of acute myocardial infarction are different and sometimes life threatening.

We can globally classify them in five categories: (1) ischaemic complications, which include infarct extension, recurrent infarction, and post infarction angina; (2) arrhythmic complications, in terms of atrial or ventricular arrhythmias, and sinus or atrioventricular node dysfunction; (3) embolic complications towards central nervous system or peripheral embolization; (4) inflammatory disturbances, such as pericarditis; (5) mechanical complications, as myocardial rupture, mitral valve dysfunction, ventricular aneurysms and cardiogenic shock up to heart failure.

Since the last years of the eighteenth century, many physicians discovered these clinical entities, firstly during autopsy, and progressively by doing pioneristic surgical efforts, starting by suturing heart wounds, and gradually trying to apply similar techniques on the infarcted heart.

Mechanical complications of myocardial infarction are direct consequences of anatomopathological changes occurring in ischaemic cardiac tissue. After a coronary occlusion, there is a lack in perfusion and in oxygen supply that cause functional, morphological, and biochemical alterations. In the first 30 minutes from the occlusion, reversible changes happen; macroscopically and microscopically there are no grossly damages yet, but myofibrils start to relax, and cells start to suffer. After half an hour, ischaemic necrosis begins, and the irreversible damage occurs. Complete necrosis of myocardial cells requires at least 2–4 hours, or longer, depending on the presence of collateral circulation, persistent or intermittent coronary arterial occlusion, pre-conditioning, and individual demand for oxygen and nutrients. The principal mechanism is coagulative necrosis, with neutrophil infiltration, oedema, and loss of myofibrils. After 6–12 hours, loss of vitality is complete. In one week, macrophagic phagocytosis and collagen disruption begin, and tissue becomes weaker; that is the most dangerous step in which heart ruptures are more frequent [1, 2, 3].

The irreversible damage starts at a subendocardic level, and when the ischemia is widespread, necrosis moves forward, involving the adjacent tissue both in width and in thickness. If coronary flow is promptly restored while the damage is still reversible yet, the cells' vitality could be preserved. On the other hand, reperfusion damage could be present by generating free oxygen radicals and apoptosis activators.

After a couple of weeks, granulation tissue and neoangiogenesys begin, up to the formation of a scar in about two months from myocardial infarction. Remodelling of myocardial tissue is the final step; both infarcted and non-infarcted regions change in dimensions, thickness, and shape, with hypertrophy and dilatation of the myocardial wall, and with the possible formation of an aneurysm. Remodelling could be seen as a sort of haemodynamic compensation; nevertheless, degenerative changes in myocardial tissue may cause a depression in regional and global contractility, with a final lack in myocardial function [1, 2, 3].

As we will discuss, on a clinical level, signs and symptoms of mechanical complications of myocardial infarction may vary according to the seriousness of the damage, going from rare asymptomatic medical cases, through plainly symptomatic patients showing classical chest pain, up to more frequent catastrophic, and even sudden onset with cardiogenic shock. Because of these, a prompt diagnosis is important. While ECG may demonstrate the presence of an infarction and help locate the ischaemic lesion, transthoracic echocardiography with Doppler is the modality of choice for bedside diagnosis, capable of detecting heart ruptures, as well as valve defects or ventricular motion abnormalities. Its immediate availability and the detailed information it provides are fundamental in the management of these patients, helping in the decision-making process. The use of other diagnostic tools, such as angiography, is subdued to haemodynamic stability of the patient [3].

As far as therapy is concerned, most of all mechanical complications of myocardial infarction require an urgent surgical approach. Meanwhile, initial management with medical therapy should be administered immediately, in order to improve systemic and coronary perfusion, and stabilise the haemodynamic status. Supplement oxygen and mechanical ventilatory support while necessary should be provided, as well as analgesic therapy, in order to control pain and reduce sympathetic tone; crystalloid infusion should be administered when hypotension and relative hypovolemia is present, together with inotropic agents. Many more pharmacologic agents are useful, depending on every different clinical presentation, but the positioning of an intra-aortic-balloon pump (IABP) is always a support of choice in order to

http://dx.doi.org/10.5772/61373

reduce cardiac workload and increase supply of oxygen by increasing coronary perfusion during diastole and reducing the after-load during systole [4].

Survival depends primarily upon the rapid recognition of each complication and upon an immediate therapy. Even if operative mortality remains high, surgery is the essential tool to avoid a fatal outcome.

In this chapter, we will analyse mechanical complications of myocardial infarction, such as ventricular free wall rupture, ventricular septal defect, papillary muscle rupture, ischaemic mitral regurgitation, left ventricle aneurysm, and cardiogenic shock. We will also deal with therapies for heart failure, and make a brief digression upon strategies against myocardial remodelling.

2. Left ventricular free wall rupture

The first description of left ventricular free wall rupture appeared in 1647 by William Harvey, but until 1970, with operations managed by the teams of Hatcher and FitzGibbon, no successful surgery was done [5, 6].

Left ventricular free wall rupture (LVFWR) is the most frequent presentation of myocardial rupture: it occurs up to ten times more frequently than septal or papillary muscle rupture, and mostly hits the lateral midventricular wall along the apex to base axis (the incidence of right ventricular free wall rupture is very low, roughly 0.44%). Free wall rupture may occur at any time after myocardial infarction, most frequently after 3–7 days, when coagulative necrosis, neutrophil infiltration, and tissue lysis make myocardium weaker. Moreover, an increase in wall tension may overcome the tensile strength of the weakened wall. However, at least 1/4 of heart rupture occurs within the first 24 hours. Interstitial oedema, damage to collagen network and myocyte apoptosis are proposed mechanisms [7].

The real incidence of this complication is unknown, although the reported incidence is increasing (1–4%) among patients surviving hospital admissions due to an increment of the availability of non-invasive diagnostic tools. Free wall rupture accounts for 6–17% of in-hospital mortality [8]. The National Registry of Myocardial Infarction (NRMI) shows an elevated incidence of in-hospital mortality among patients treated with thrombolytic therapy (12.1%) than patients who were not treated (6.1%) [9]. In the Thrombolysis in Myocardial Infarction Phase II (TIMI II) trial, 16% of patients died within 18 hours of therapy. Moreover, patients who were treated with PTCA had an incidence of free wall rupture lower than that of patients receiving thrombolytic therapy [10].

Risk factors are age (usually over 60 years old), gender (female), a history of hypertension, and the absence of ventricular hypertrophy. Moreover, LVFWR occurs mostly after an ST elevation myocardial infarction (STEMI), and in areas lacking of fibrosis (that means in patients without history of previous angina or myocardial infarction). These last associations suggest that the size of necrosis and the absence of collateral blood flow (with lack of previous ischaemic symptoms) are important determinants in the aetiology of heart rupture [8].

To understand the clinical presentation of the LVFWR, it is worthy to speak about the morphological pattern of rupture. Pathologically, Perdigao and associates described four types of ruptures: the type I, or direct rupture, is a single dissection of the wall in only one direction and without dissection or blood infiltration (Fig. 1); type II is represented by a multiple dissection, with a multicanalicular trajectory and an extensive haemorrhagic infiltration of neighbouring tissue (Fig. 2); in type III, rupture is protected either by an intracardiac thrombus or by adhesions on the epicardial side (Fig. 3); type IV is characterised by an incomplete rupture, that doesn't cross the thickness of the ventricular wall, creating an intramural haematoma [12]. However, Becker and van Mantgem proposed a different classification that could be connected to the clinical presentation: acute, subacute, and chronic [13]. The acute rupture (also called "blow-out" rupture, corresponding to Perdigao type I-II) is characterized by a massive haemopericardium (Fig. 4); the presentation is dramatic, with sudden and recurrent or persistent chest pain and a rapid deterioration into electro-mechanical dissociation caused by pericardial tamponade. A severe jugular venous destention and cyanosis may be present. Death occurs within a few minutes. When the rupture area is smaller, and temporarily sealed by thrombus or pericardial adhesions, a subacute onset happens (also called “ooze” rupture or Perdigao type III, and occurs in 30–40% of cases). Clinical presentation may involve the gradual onset of signs and symptoms of cardiac tamponade. A variety of other signs may be present, such as arrhythmias, a severe hypotension, syncope, and, eventually, cardiogenic shock, but also malaise and nausea for few days.

A chronic rupture occurs when the leakage of blood is slow and when surrounding pressure on the epicardium temporarily controls the haemorrhage, with the formation of a false aneurysm (or pseudoaneurysm). This is a rare entity and usually occurs within three months after myocardial infarction. Clinical presentation, in this case, is represented by congestive heart failure, recurrent or persistent chest pain, ventricular arrhythmias, and even emboliza-tion [14].

Perdigao type IV (intramural haematoma) has no different presentation from the usual infarction.

Perdigao	**Becker and van Mantgem**		
Type I	Acute (“blow-out”) rupture	Single dissection of the wall, in only one direction and without dissection or blood infiltration	Fig. 1
Type II		Multiple dissection, with a multicanalicular trajectory and an extensive haemorrhagic infiltration of neighbouring tissue	Fig 2
Type III	Subacute (“ooze”) rupture	Rupture is protected either by an intracardiac thrombus or by adhesions on the epicardial side	Fig. 3
	Chronic rupture (pseudoaneurysm)	Pressure on the epicardium temporarily controls the haemorrhage	
Type IV		Intramural haematoma	

Table 1. Nema

http://dx.doi.org/10.5772/61373

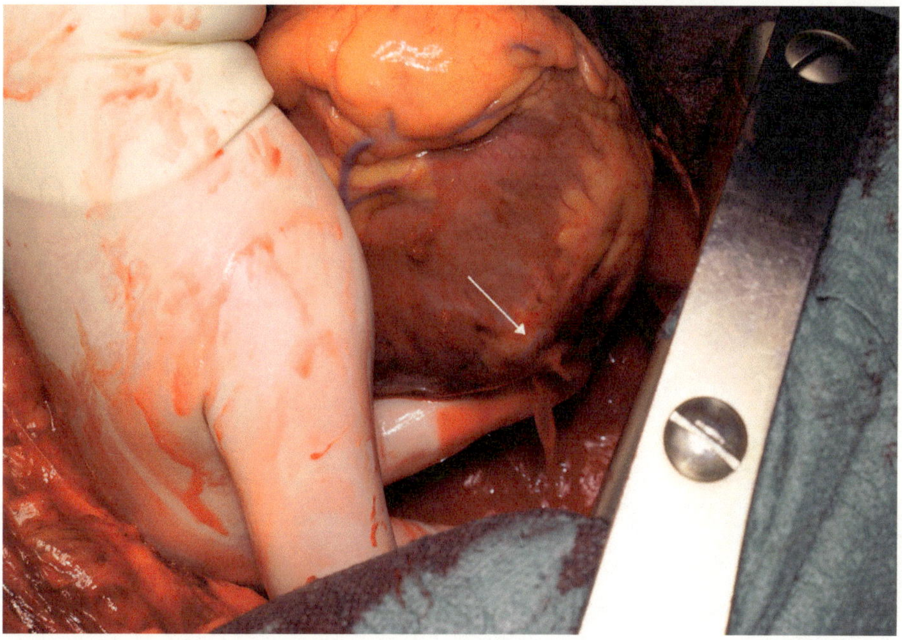

Figure 1. Perdigao type I, a single dissection of ventricular free wall

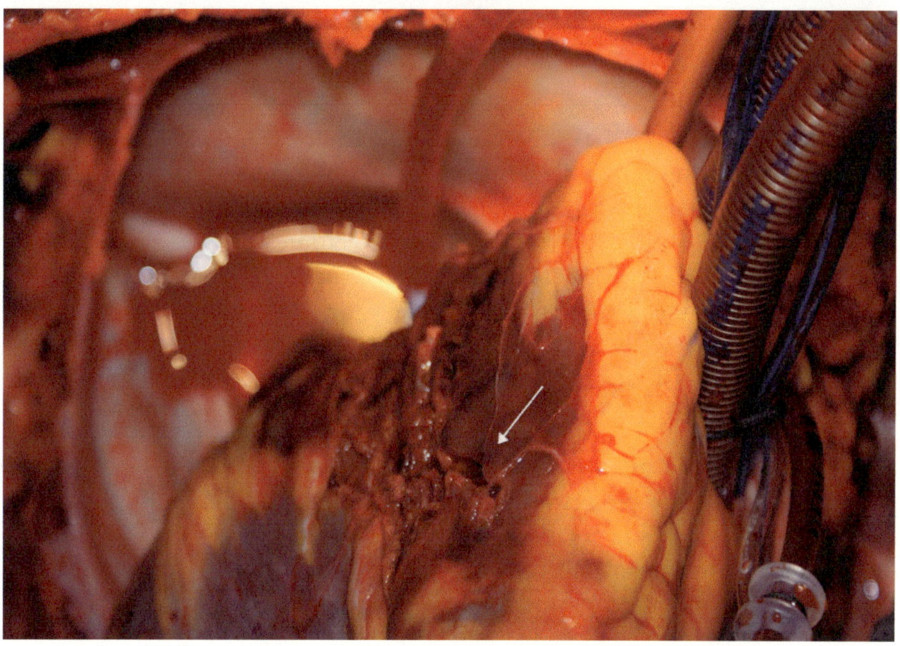

Figure 2. Perdigao type II, multicanalicular trajectory of rupture

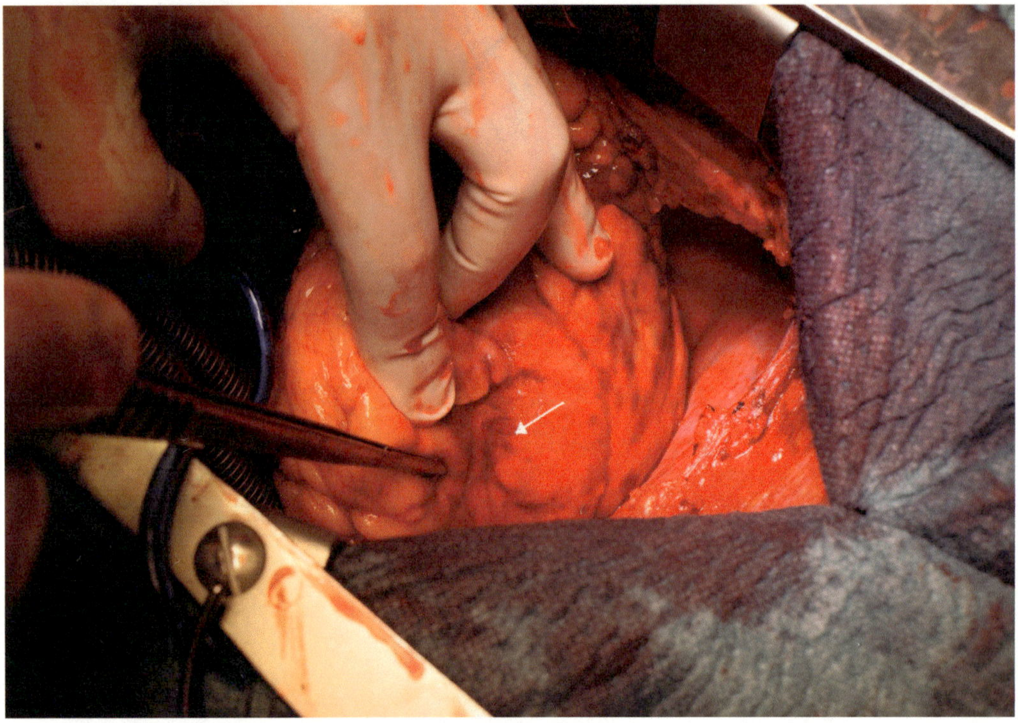

Figure 3. Perdigao type III, rupture is sealed by pericardial adhesions

Early diagnosis is improved by the use of transthoracic echocardiography, the fastest and most useful diagnostic test, with a high diagnostic sensitivity (≥ 70%) and specificity (> 90%). The most frequent finding is the presence of a pericardial effusion (> 5 mm), high-density intra-pericardial echoes, right atrial or right ventricular wall compression with tamponade, and, in 50% of cases, visible wall defects [15]. The role of the invasive diagnostic tools is still unclear and depends on the haemodynamic stability of the patient. Most of the time, the definitive diagnosis is made at surgery. Generally, when Perdigao type I, II, III, and IV are non-haemodynamically stable they require a surgical approach. Type IV in haemodynamically stable patients can be treated conservatively [11, 17, 18, 19].

The first objective of treatment is to reach haemodynamic stability. Rapid infusions of crystalloid along with inotropic agents may help to achieve this; pericardiocentesis may be carried out prior to surgery and not only may confirm a haemorrhagic effusion, but also may decrease the threat of tamponade. Placement of IABP should be done [20].

Surgical repair of the rupture site is the definitive treatment, and it can be administered in different ways and with different techniques. Traditional and standard repair involves performing infartectomy (including the area hit by the rupture) and reconstructing the ventricle or close the damage with simple pledgeted suture (Fig. 5), with or without cardio-

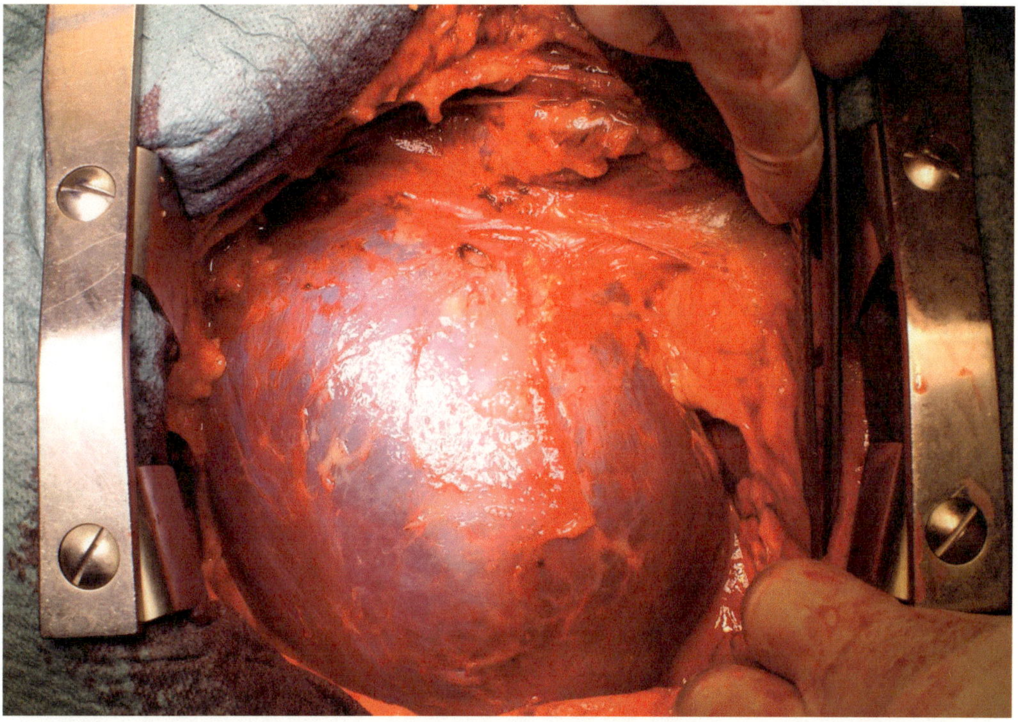

Figure 4. Haemopericardium

pulmonary bypass. Both techniques have a shortcoming: in the first case, a ventricular cavity distortion may damage the ventricular function; on the other hand, stitches are placed in a necrotic—and so weaker—tissue. Different authors heave recently reported newer surgical strategies, usually performed in the presence of oozing or sealed rupture (type III), by using different biological materials such as pericardium (Fig. 6) and newer acellular xenogeneic extracellular matrix patches, and non-biological patches made of polyethylene terephthalate polyester fibre (Dacron) or polytetrafluoroethylene fluoropolymer resin (Teflon). Suturless techniques with fibrin tissue-adhesive collagen fleece, and Gelatin-Resorcin Formaldehyde glue are described [12, 16, 21, 22, 23].

In the matter of chronic rupture, the treatment of choice is still surgery, but obviously the timing depends on the balance between risks and benefits. Pseudoaneurysm can be repaired by the closure of the neck or by using a patch (similar to true aneurysm). Percutaneous approaches (by using the Amplatzer™ occluder) are described as well [24].

The mortality rate is significantly high. It is strictly linked to the preoperative haemodynamic condition of patient and to a prompt diagnosis.

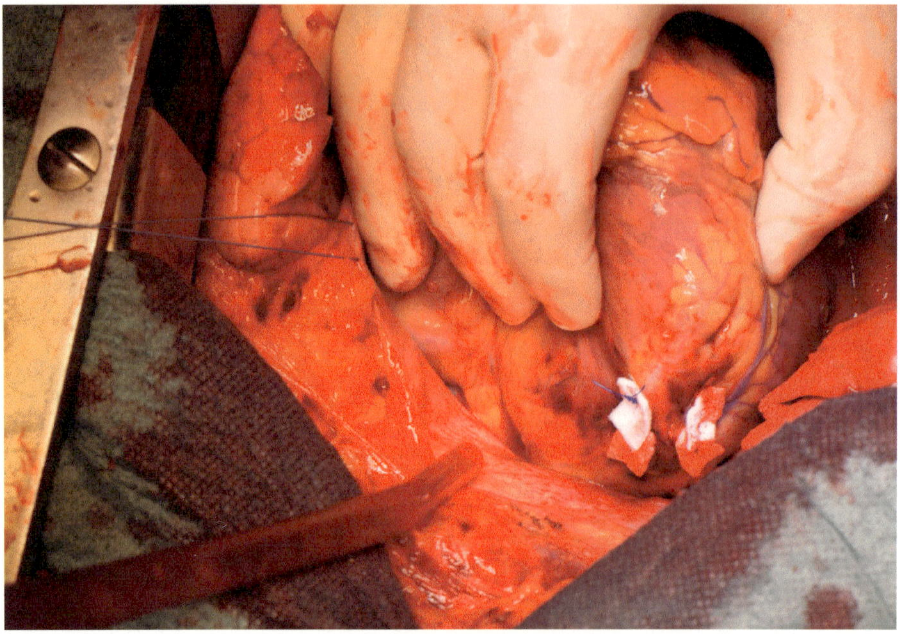

Figure 5. The damage has been closed with simple pledgeted suture

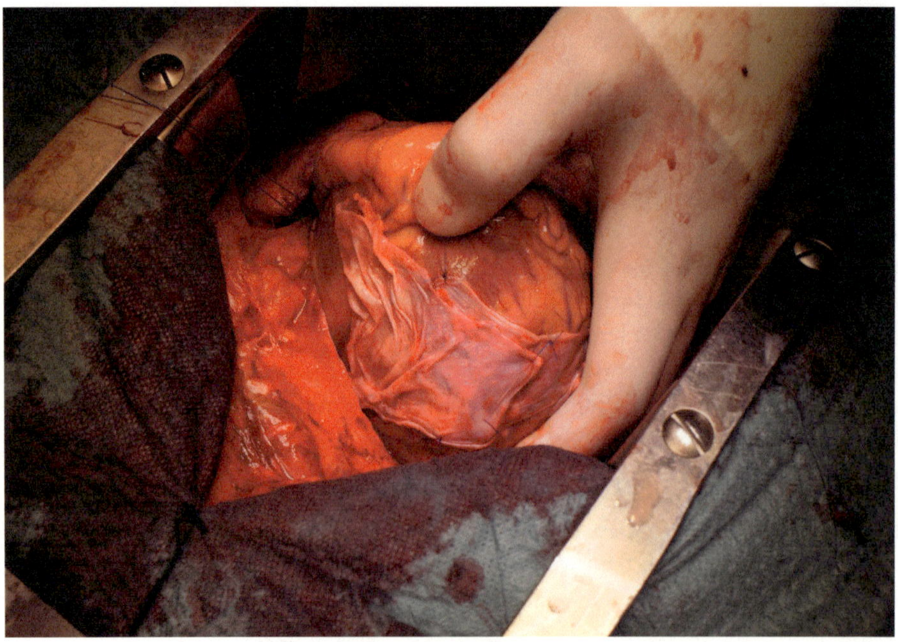

Figure 6. The damage has been sealed by using a pericardial patch

http://dx.doi.org/10.5772/61373

3. Interventricular septal rupture

Ventricular septal defect (VSD), firstly described by Latham in 1845 [25], is a serious complication of myocardial infarction that is little less frequent than free wall rupture. Its incidence has been estimated between 1% and 2% of all myocardial infarctions even if the advent of reperfusion therapy has decreased this value below 0.5%. However, the mortality is still high, with 60–70% of patients dying within the first 2 weeks, and less than 10% survives after 3 months [26].

As for free wall rupture, risk factors for septal rupture include advanced age, hypertension, and no previous myocardial infarction or angina.

The acute rupture occurs 3–7 days after a huge transmural infarction, with the weakening of the septal wall, but the median decrease below 24 h with the use of thrombolysis. Late rupture is possible (as long as 2 weeks). Pathophysiologically, this results in a left-to-right shunt with diversion of blood flow towards pulmonary circulation. Systemic vasoconstriction in response to peripheral hypotension and hypoperfusion worsens the shunt. As a consequence, low cardiac output and cardiogenic shock occur [2].

Classification of the defect are of three types: type I ruptures show an abrupt tear in the wall of normal thickness; in type II, the infarcted myocardium erodes before the rupture, and is covered by thrombus; type III shows perforation of an aneurysm grown after infarct healing. Moreover, defects can be classified in two other categories: simple and complex. Multiple defects may be present in 5–11% of cases, and are probably caused by infarct extension. Simple rupture is a discrete lesion, with holes located at a similar level in both ventricles and in a linear path. This is the typical pattern of an anterior infarction and usually hits the part in which the septum meets the free wall. On the other hand, inferior infarction usually leads to a complex type, which presents a meandering dissection path between ventricles and extensive haemorrhage in the nearby tissue that occurs near the base of the heart. Midseptal defects are rare and are usually elicited from the occlusion of a perforating artery [4].

In both cases, rupture may vary in size from mm to cm. This determines the magnitude of left-to-right shunting, influencing the clinical presentation (from asymptomatic to cardiogenic shock), and the likelihood of survival. Signs and symptoms may include recurrent chest pain and dyspnoea, but even a precipitous onset of haemodynamic compromise characterised by hypotension and biventricular failure (often predominantly right-sided failure), up to cardiogenic shock is possible. At physical examination, a harsh and loud pansystolic murmur at the left lower sternal border is present in over 90% of cases. A palpable thrill can be detected in up to 50% of patients [27].

ECG shows changes associated to myocardial infarction and may help to correlate the localization of infarction with the type of septal rupture.

Historically, the gold standard diagnostic tool was right cardiac catheterization using a Swan-Ganz catheter, useful also to differentiate among other clinical entities (mitral ischaemic regurgitation and papillary muscle rupture). In septal rupture, it is easy to find oxygen saturation step-up between the right atrium and pulmonary artery greater than 9% (in papillary rupture, giant V-waves in pulmonary artery wedge pressure are shown). Nowadays, the use of echocardiography (both transthoracic and transesophageal) has almost replaced this diagnostic tool. Doppler may easily and accurately identify the location, the size, and the presence of the shunt, indeed, with 100% specificity and 100% sensitivity. It may also assess the ventricles function and estimate the right ventricle systolic pressure. The use of angiography is debatable; it can provide important information about coronary lesions, but, on the other hand, may delay the surgical treatment [28].

Kirklin and colleagues reveal that nearly 25% of patients with post infarction septal rupture and no surgical intervention died within the first 24 hours, 50% died within 1 week, 65% within 2 weeks, 80% within 4 weeks [28]; only 7% lived longer than one year. In the GUSTO-I trial, the 30-day mortality rate was lower in patients treated with surgical repair than in patients treated only medically (47% vs. 94%). The same results for the 1-year mortality rate (53% vs. 97%) [29]. In the SHOCK trial, the in-hospital mortality rate was higher in patients with cardiogenic shock due to septal rupture (87.3%) than in patients with cardiogenic shock from all other causes (59.2% with pure left ventricle failure and 55.1% with acute mitral regurgitation) [30].

The optimal approach varies with the clinical presentation. Medical therapy is considered to be a support tool in the offing of surgery, and is usually managed with the use of pharmacologic support with vasodilators (which reduce afterload, thereby decreasing left ventricular pressure and the left to right shunt), inotropic agents (which may increase the cardiac output), diuretics, and IABP. In patients with cardiogenic shock, death is inevitable in the absence of urgent surgical intervention. Delayed elective surgical repair is feasible in patients with heart failure without shock, but an unpredictable and rapid deterioration is always lurking in general; adverse outcomes are correlated with advanced age and a lengthy delay between septal rupture and operation [28].

The surgical approach has been performed since 1959 when Cooley and associates performed the first successful surgical repair through a right ventriculotomy with incision of right ventricular outflow tract [31]. Disadvantages of this approach were suboptimal exposure and failure to eliminate the bulging segment of infarcted left ventricular wall. Later, Heimbecker [32] and colleagues developed a different technique, performing a left ventriculotomy. Nowadays, multiple techniques are described. Apical amputation is simpler, but apical defects are rare. This technique was proposed in the 1970s by Daggett [33]. After the resection, the ventricular free walls are linked using Teflon strips. Other techniques involve infarct exclusion and defect closure with a patch (biological or synthetic) using both stitches and glues [34].

Preservation of the geometric configuration of the ventricles is an important target, together with the closure of the defect.

Even a percutaneous approach has been considered, mostly in order to close contingent residual defects (residual defects are present in about 28% of survived patients) or sometimes used for the acute stabilization of critically ill patients. However, no long-term outcome data about this mini-invasive technique are available [35].

Despite continuous advances in surgical approaches, operative mortality remains high (20–50%), with no clear differences between different techniques (Fig. 7–13) [34].

http://dx.doi.org/10.5772/61373

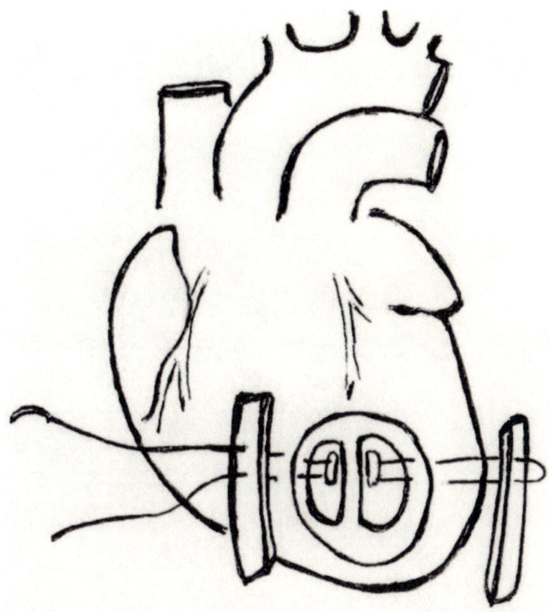

Figure 7. Anterior repair of VSD [Adapted from Chikwe J, Beddow E, Glenville B. Cardiothoracic Surgery. Oxford University Press 2006]

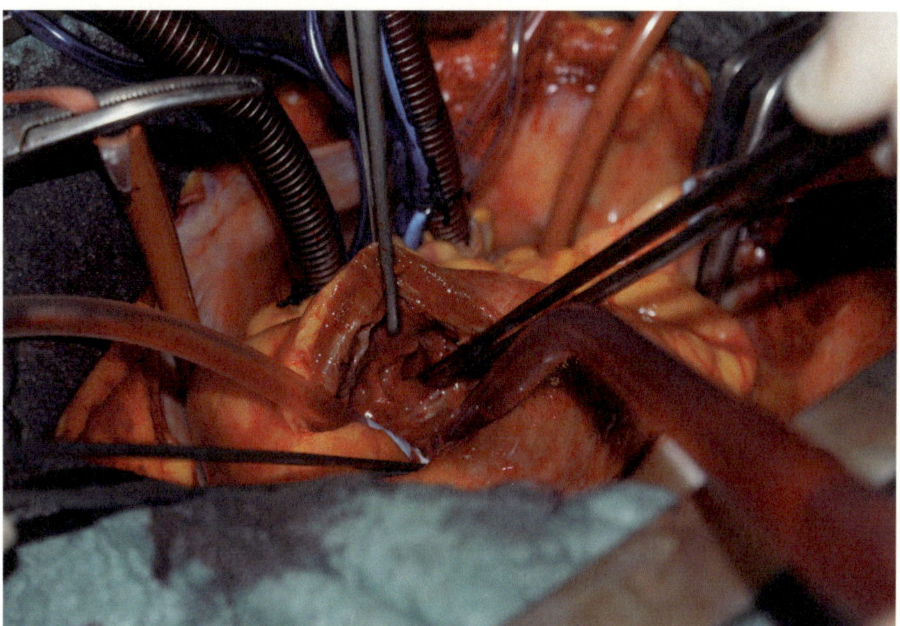

Figure 8. VSD, anterior surgical approach

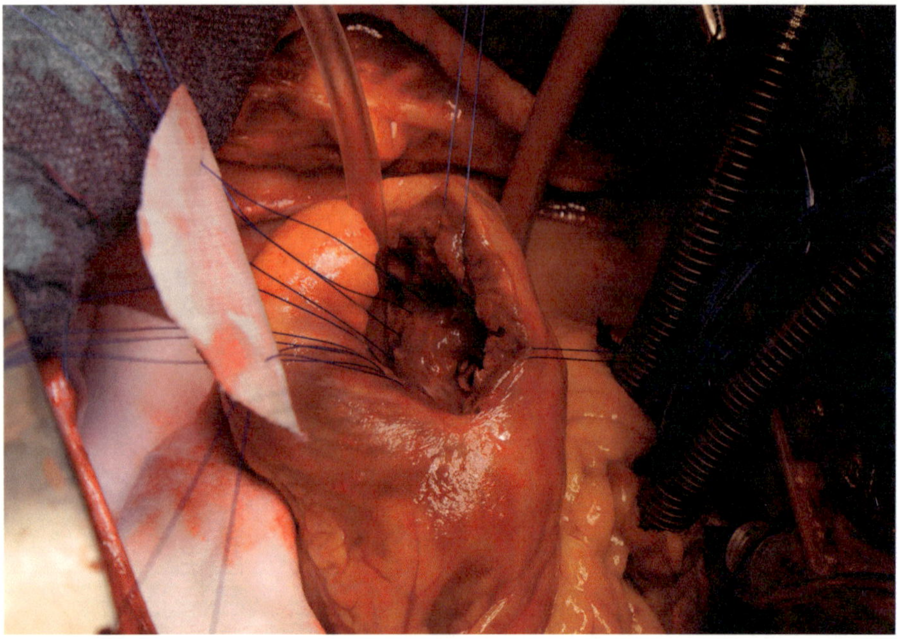

Figure 9. VSD closure with synthetic patch

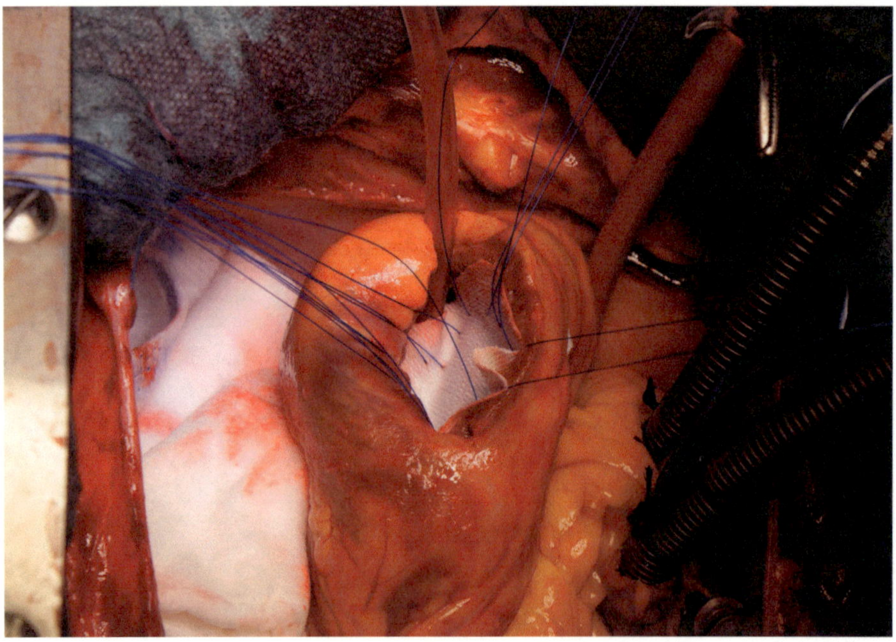

Figure 10. VSD closure with synthetic patch

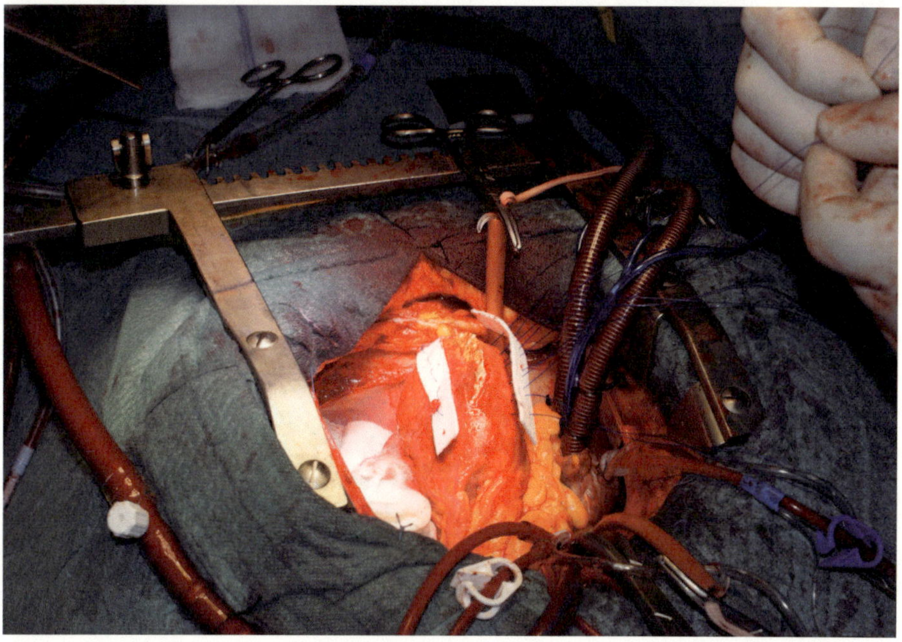

Figure 11. Ventricular free walls are linked using Teflon strips

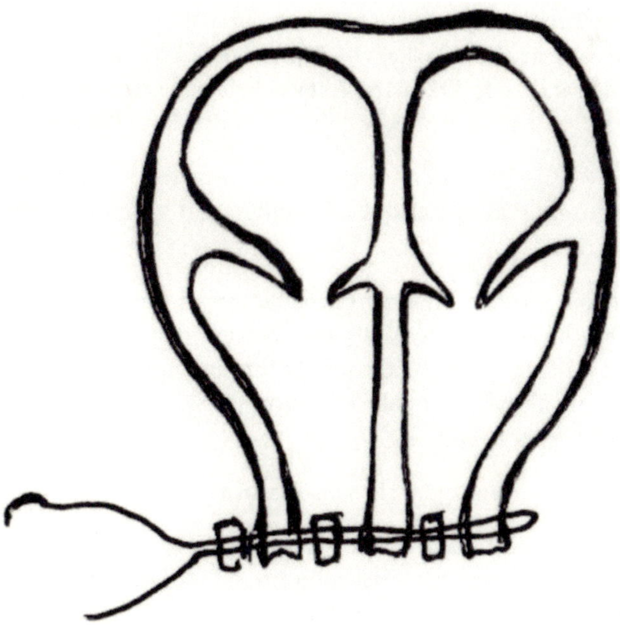

Figure 12. Apical resection [Adapted from Chikwe J, Beddow E, Glenville B. Cardiothoracic Surgery. Oxford University Press 2006]

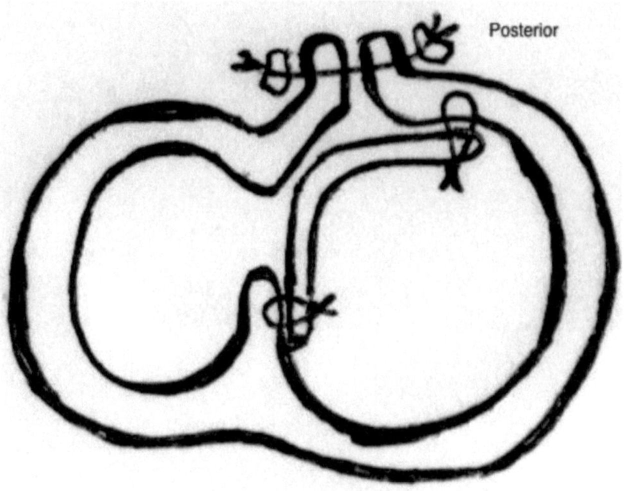

Figure 13. Posterior repair of VSD [Adapted from Chikwe J, Beddow E, Glenville B. Cardiothoracic Surgery. Oxford University Press 2006]

4. Papillary muscle rupture

Papillary muscle rupture (PMR) is a rare entity and occurs in about 1% of patients with acute myocardial infarction. It accounts for 5% of infarct-related deaths. Mortality may be as high as 50% in the first 24 h, and up to 80% in the first week, when only medical treatment is applied. Timing of rupture stays in a range between 1 and 14 days, but 80% occurs in 7 days [36].

Rupture of papillary muscles results from infarction of the muscle itself and leads to an ischaemic mitral regurgitation by lack of leaflet tethering (Carpentier type II, see next chapter for further information).

PMR is most common with an inferior myocardial infarction, and the posteromedial papillary muscle is most often involved (6 to 12 times more frequently than anterolateral papillary muscle); that's because of its single blood supply through the posterior descending coronary artery (anterolateral papillary has a dual blood supply, instead, from the left anterior descending and left circumflex arteries) [36, 37, 39].

Among risk factors, there is, once again, the absence of a previous infarction in medical history.

PMR may be complete, with a massive mitral regurgitation and rapid onset of symptoms up to hemodynamic collapse and death, or partial, with a moderate to severe mitral regurgitation. Clinical presentation may vary according to the completeness of rupture, but usually presents dyspnoea, hypotension, acute pulmonary oedema, and cardiogenic shock. At the physical examination, a soft murmur without thrill may be present, even if the absence of new heart murmur does not exclude the diagnosis.

The gold standard in diagnosis is Doppler transthoracic and transesophageal echocardiography, with the evidence of a tear in papillary tissue and the flail of mitral leaflet leading to severe mitral regurgitation (Fig. 14, 15). Left ventricular function is usually hyperdynamic as a result of ventricular contraction against the low impedance left atrium. Haemodynamic monitoring with a Swan-Ganz catheter can reveal large (> 50 mmHg), early V waves in the pulmonary capillary wedge pressure, and no increase in oxygen saturation from right atrium to right ventriculum (useful to conduct differential diagnosis with septal rupture) [36, 37, 38].

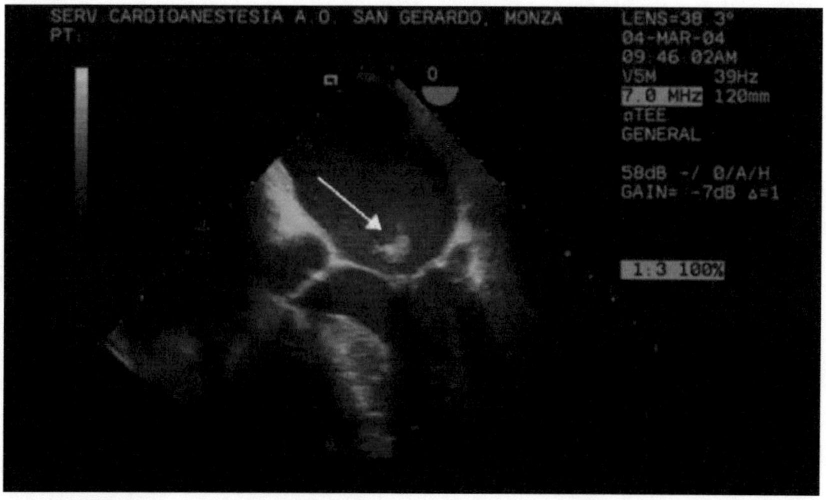

Figure 14. Echo findings in complete papillary muscle rupture

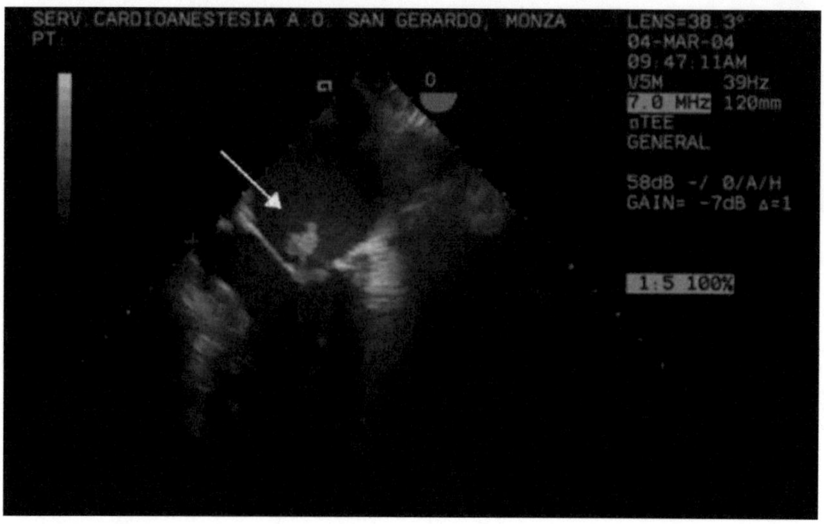

Figure 15. Echo findings in complete papillary muscle rupture

The only real treatment for papillary muscle rupture is surgery, although it is high risk (operative mortality up to 20–25%) [37]. Medical therapy could be performed in order to reach a hemodynamic stability prior to emergency surgery, and includes aggressive afterload reduction in order to decrease the regurgitant fraction by using nitrates, sodium nitroprusside, diuretics, and IABP.

The surgical technique depends upon the location and the completeness of the rupture. With partial PMR, some surgeons prefer to stabilise the patient and delay surgery for 6–8 weeks after myocardial infarction to avoid operating on the necrotic myocardial tissue. However, an acute intervention in patients that cannot be stabilized must be considered. A surgical repair of the papillary muscle head is really rare, but possible, with pledgeted sutures and the addition of glue to strengthen the repair. Mitral valve repair rather than replacement should be attempted when there is no papillary muscle necrosis [36, 37].

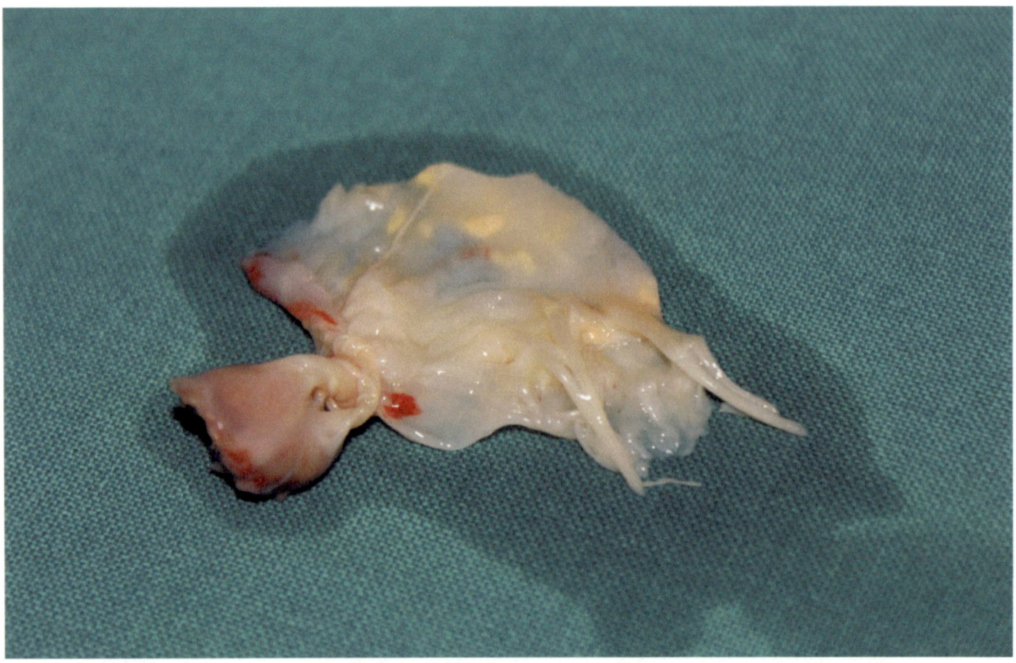

Figure 16. The excised mitral valve showing complete rupture of the papillary muscle

5. Ischaemic mitral regurgitation

Ischaemic mitral regurgitation (IMR) is a functional entity that occurs in 8% to 50% of patients after myocardial infarction. Unlike the structural mitral regurgitation, here the valve leaflets and valvular apparatus are normal, even if the coexistence of coronary artery disease and non-ischaemic mitral disease has led to a poor understanding of this clinical entity [40].

http://dx.doi.org/10.5772/61373

Carpentier described three general types of mitral regurgitation according to different pathophysiologic mechanisms: type I, in which there is a normal leaflet motion, and regurgitation is caused by annular dilatation from ischemia of adjacent ventricular wall or by leaflet perforation; type II, in which we can find an increased leaflet motion, with a prolapse of valve leaflet (in this case, regurgitation is caused either by papillary muscle rupture or in papillary muscle elongation due to chronic ischemia, and usually lead to an asymmetric leak); type IIIa, with leaflet restriction during systole and diastole (not seen in ischaemic mitral regurgitation); type IIIb, leaflet restriction only during systole caused by a dysfunction of ventricular wall, dilated after ischaemic injury, with systolic tethering of papillary muscle (as a consequence, there's a failure in mitral coaptation).

IMR could be acute or chronic, but both result from ischemia of ventricular wall and missed coaptation. The remodelling secondary to acute and chronic ischemia remains the principal mechanism for IMR and depends on apical tethering and an excessive tenting volume, which cause coaptation failure of the mitral leaflets. Mild-to-moderate mitral regurgitation is often clinically silent and detected on Doppler echocardiography performed during the early phase of myocardial infarction.

Risk factors are advanced age, female sex, large infarct, multivessel coronary artery disease, and, unlike other mechanical complications, history of a previous myocardial infarction or recurrent ischemia.

The acute onset of severe IMR is a life-threatening complication and arises from a few hours to weeks after myocardial infarction; in this case, a sudden volume overload is imposed on the left ventricle, increasing preload and a small increase in total stroke volume. Acute mitral regurgitation usually results from the rupture of papillary muscles or chordae tendineae: haemodynamic deterioration is sudden, because no compensatory structural changes in atrium and ventricle are possible. Pulmonary congestion, as well as cardiogenic shock, may occur. Clinical features include pulmonary oedema, chest pain, and dyspnoea. A new pan-systolic murmur can be detected, best heard at the apex [40, 44].

Chronic IMR occurs as a consequence of ventricular dilatation secondary to ischaemic ventricular remodelling (both regional or global), with papillary muscle displacement and failure of leaflet coaptation. During chronic onset of the disease, the left atrium and ventricle may develop an offsetting hypertrophy and dilatation. Enlargement of the left atrium allows volume overload, but may cause arrhythmias, such as atrial fibrillation, and the formation of thrombi. Until systolic dysfunction prevents effective ventricular contraction, patients are asymptomatic. After that, exertional dyspnoea and fluid retention may be present [40].

The gold standard diagnostic tool is echocardiography, both transthoracic and transeosophageal, which assess mitral valve apparatus, the mechanism of regurgitation, and the ventricular function [3, 15]

Medical therapy may have a supportive role in case of acute onset of mitral regurgitation, while in chronic cases it is useful in decreasing the regurgitant volume and improve ventricular function by using ACE-inhibitors, and to reduce remodelling by using beta-blockers. Most patients with acute mitral regurgitation are managed with percutaneous coronary intervention

(PCI) or thrombolysis. Surgery is usually reserved for acute and severe cases, which do not ameliorate after these approaches, and for chronic patients symptomatic for coronary disease.

Repair versus replacement of the mitral valve is still debatable. Mitral valve repair is generally preferred whenever possible based on valve pathology and patient stability: it avoids long-term anticoagulation, decreases infective endocarditis risk, and provides greater leaflet durability. Among repairs, different techniques are available, but annuloplasty with prosthetic ring is the gold standard [41, 42]. On the other hand, valve replacement is usually reserved for situations where the valve cannot be reasonably repaired, or when repair is unlikely to be tolerated clinically. Moreover, it being a faster procedure is better in high-risk surgical candidates. Mitral valve replacement could be managed by using the chordal-sparing techniques, a range of procedures that permit the resuspension of chordae and the preservation of subvalvular anatomy [43].

Percutaneous approaches are available, but often limited to patients with lots of comorbidity and a poor surgical outcome [40].

6. Left ventricular true aneurysm

The earliest reports of a ventricular aneurysm appeared in 1757, during an autopsy managed by Galeati and Hunter; but the first surgical approach to this pathology was performed in 1942 by Beck.

A true aneurysm is the result of the gradual thinning and the expansion of the scarred left ventricular wall after transmural infarction. This is a different entity from a pseudoaneurysm, which does not contain all the three layers of the myocardium and is frequently lined by pericardium and mural thrombus [45, 47, 49].

The 85% of true aneurysm is located anterolaterally, near the apex of the heart. Two types of true aneurysm are present: a traditional aneurysm, namely a region of myocardium with an abnormal diastolic contour and a systolic dyskinesia, with a paradoxic bulging; and a functional aneurysm, in which bulging is not present, but is characterised by large areas of akinesia, that affects ventricular function. They originate from two distinct phases of myocardial infarction. First, an early expansion phase defined as the deformation or stretch of infarcted myocardium during the first week after the ischaemic injury: wall thinning due to the degradation of collagen matrix and dilatation lead to an augmentation in both systolic and diastolic wall stress, following LaPlace law, and to a greater request of oxygen supply. Fibre stretching is progressive until fibrosis and scarring. Increased diastolic stretch, elevated catecholamines and stimulation of natriuretic peptides may demonstrate increased fibre shortening and myocardial hypertrophy as adaptive changes. The second phase is constituted by late remodelling. Here, the aneurysm is composed of scar tissue; systolic and diastolic ventricular dysfunctions are present, in fact aneurysm does not contract nor distend (this impairs diastolic filling and increases left ventricular end-diastolic pressure). Mechanism of compensation such as chamber dilatation, hypertrophy, and changes in ventricular geometry lead to a poor contractile function, and eventually heart failure [46, 48]

http://dx.doi.org/10.5772/61373

The incidence of true aneurysm is 10–35% after transmural myocardial infarction, even if it may result from trauma, Chagas' disease, sarcoidosis, or may be congenital as well. Risk factors seem to be the presence of a previous infarction in medical history and a decreased ejection fraction (less than 50%).

Clinical presentation often involves angina (in more than 60% of patients, three-vessels coronary disease is present), dyspnoea, and symptoms of congestive heart failure. Atrial and ventricular arrhythmias may occur in the scar tissue, producing palpitations, syncope, and even sudden death. A mural thrombus is often found (50%) [43, 44, 45, 50, 51, 52, 53].

Even if echocardiography is a useful diagnostic tool capable of identifying false aneurysm and assessing ventricular function, angiography and left ventriculography is the gold standard, estimating the size of aneurysm and evaluating cardiac function and kinesis, as well as coronary status. Tomographic three-dimensional echocardiography and magnetic resonance imaging are the most reliable means of evaluating left ventricular volume. Positron emission tomography (PET) can be helpful in an early phase to differentiate true aneurysm from hibernating myocardium with reversible dysfunction. Even magnetic resonance imaging can be useful, but cannot assess coronary anatomy.

Medical therapy aims to minimise the remodelling of the left ventricle: both in acute and chronic heart failure; ACE inhibitors may reduce ventricular wall stress, as well as ventricular dilatation. Beta-blockers do the same. Nitrates may reduce hypertrophy, but it seems they don't affect mortality.

Anticoagulation with warfarin is indicated for patients with a mural thrombus. Patients should be treated initially with intravenous heparin, with a target aPTT of 50–70 seconds. Warfarin is started simultaneously, and the INR target is 2–3 for a period of 3 to 6 months. The use of anticoagulation without the presence of a thrombus is controversed. Anticoagulation should be reinitiated if a new thrombus develops, and an echocardiographic follow up must be done [54].

Asymptomatic patients with a small aneurysm may be treated medically. However, an aneurysm that occupies more than 25% of the ventricular surface may significantly affect the global function. When refractory heart failure or ventricular arrhythmias are present, as well in the presence of a huge aneurysm, surgery is indicated.

Resection of the aneurysm may be followed by conventional closure or newer techniques to maintain LV geometry. In the plication technique, a direct closure of the aneurysm without excision is performed; this is usually done for very small aneurysms without internal thrombus [55]. Another conventional strategy, the linear repair, was first introduced by Cooley in 1958. In this technique, the incision is extended round the aneurysm leaving a rim of scar tissue and buttressed mattress sutures are placed successively. With this technique, changing ventricular geometry is possible [55].

Other newer techniques aim to maintain ventricular geometry by using the external patch (procedure performed by Daggett) or inverted T closure of ventriculotomy (as done by Komeda) [56], or circular patch technique for posterior aneurysms [57]. Finally, endoaneurysmorraphy, a procedure proposed by Jatene, Dor, and Cooley, positions an endocardial patch in order to preserve both normal ventriculum and septal geometry [58, 59, 60].

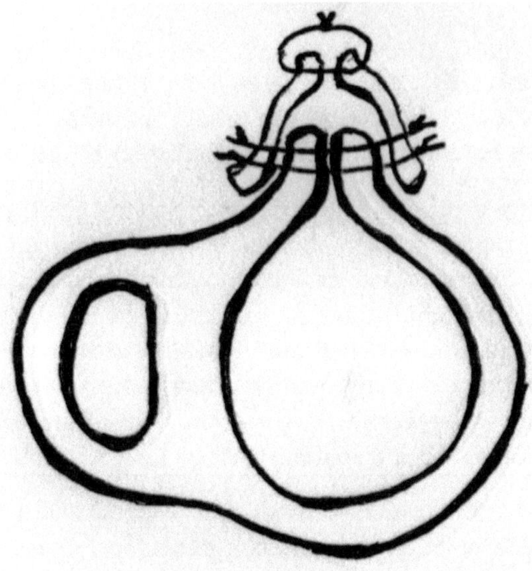

Figure 17. Traditional aneurismectomy: Linear closure [Adapted from Chikwe J, Beddow E, Glenville B. Cardiothoracic Surgery. Oxford University Press 2006]

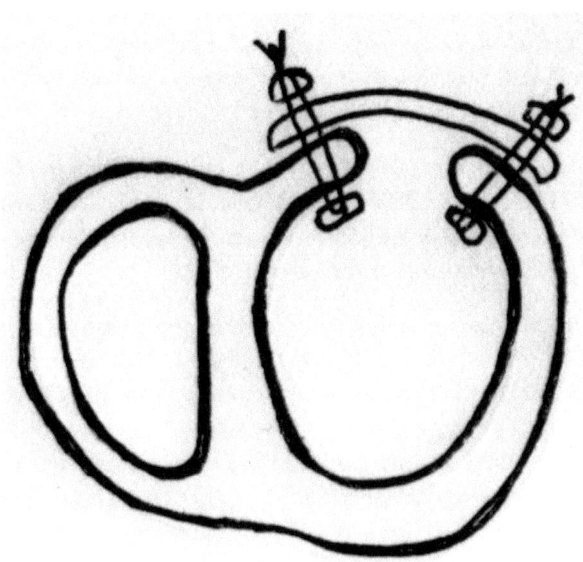

Figure 18. Traditional aneurismectomy: Patch closure [Adapted from Chikwe J, Beddow E, Glenville B. Cardiothoracic Surgery. Oxford University Press 2006]

http://dx.doi.org/10.5772/61373

7. Cardiogenic shock and heart failure

Cardiogenic shock is a clinical syndrome characterised by end-organ hypoperfusion, due to a rapid worsening of ventricular function.

It occurs in 5–8% of hospitalised patients with STEMI, and 12% of these cases are caused by a mechanical complication of myocardial infarction. Cardiogenic shock may also occur in 2.5% of non-coronary cases: any cause of acute, severe left or right ventricular dysfunction such as acute myopericarditis, tako-tsubo cardiomyopathy, hypertrophic cardiomyopathy, acute valvular regurgitation caused by endocarditis or chordal rupture due to trauma or degenerative disease, as well as aortic dissection, severe aortic or mitral insufficiency. Moreover, cardiac tamponade or massive pulmonary embolism may lead to this kind of shock [60, 61, 62, 63, 64].

Risk factors are directly related to the principal trigger. In the context of myocardial infarction, risk factors may include older age, hypertension, diabetes mellitus, multivessel coronary artery disease, prior myocardial infarction or angina, anterior location of infarction, prior diagnosis of heart failure, STEMI, and left bundle-branch block.

Considering the ischaemic aetiology of cardiogenic shock, pathological mechanism starts with the ischaemic injury of myocite, with loss of effective contractility, and a systolic and diastolic dysfunction. A decrease in cardiac output leads to a decrease in systemic and coronary perfusion. A vicious cycle originates, with the worsening of hypoperfusion and the increasing of infarcted regions of myocardium. To compensate the decrease in stroke volume and cardiac output, sympathetic tone is increased, eliciting tachycardia, systemic vasoconstriction, and increased contractility of the healthy non-ischaemic myocardium. This results in an increase in the cardiac workload and oxygen consumption. When these compensatory mechanisms cannot meet the increased demand, there's once again a progression in myocardial injury. Even systemic inflammation may contribute to myocardial dysfunction, decreasing systemic perfusion. The spiral worsening of ventricular function and a subsequent shock was thought to occur after the loss of at least 40% of the left ventricular mass [60].

The definition of cardiogenic shock includes haemodynamic parameters, such as persistent hypotension (systolic blood pressure < 90 mmHg, with severe reduction in cardiac index < 1.8 L/min/m^2), elevated filling pressure, and pulmonary capillary wedge pressure < 15 mmHg. Signs and symptoms include cool and sweaty extremities, cyanosis, decreased urine output, and/or alteration in mental status. Haemodynamic abnormalities go from mild hypoperfusion to profound shock, and the short-term outcome is directly related to the severity of the haemodynamic derangement [60, 61, 62, 63, 64].

The diagnosis is usually made with invasive haemodynamic monitoring using pulmonary artery catheterisation (Swan-Ganz catheter); however, Doppler echocardiography may help to confirm the elevation of the left ventricle filling pressures, and may assess mechanical causes of shock above all. ECG confirms ischaemic aetiology.

Therapies should not be delayed. On the pharmacological side, no drugs have been shown to improve survival, but they are fundamental in supporting and stabilising the patients prior to the definitive therapy. Support includes inotropic and vasopressor agents, which should be used in the lowest possible doses (higher vasopressor doses are associated with poorer survival due to a combination between hemodynamic derangement and direct toxic effects).

IABP has long been a mainstay of mechanical therapy for cardiogenic shock [66, 67, 68, 69]. It improves coronary and peripheral perfusion via diastolic balloon inflation and augments left ventricular performance via systolic balloon deflation with an acute decrease in afterload. Nowadays, the reported efficacy of this mechanical support in studies has been variable; some studies, such as the IABP-SHOCK II trial have downgraded IABP, showing no significant differences in treatment groups [71]. Despite this fact, IABP remains in wide use, driven by substantial anecdotal evidence as well as meta-analytic results [70].

In the vicious cycle that characterises cardiogenic shock, revascularisation fulfills an important role, increasing the likelihood of survival with good quality of life (in the randomized SHOCK trial, a 13% increase in 1-year survival in patients assigned to early revascularisation was found) [30]. Mechanical reperfusion may be obtained with a percutaneous approach (angioplasty with or without stenting) or with surgical approach (coronary artery bypass grafting). The optimal revascularisation strategy for patients with multivessel coronary artery disease and cardiogenic shock is not clear. At large, immediate coronary artery bypass surgery is the preferred method of revascularisation when severe triple-vessel or left main disease is present, and should be performed when mechanical complications coexist. Percutaneous coronary intervention of the infarct-related artery is recommended in the case of single or double-vessel disease, or when surgery is not possible [60, 65]. In the STICH (Surgical Treatment for Ischaemic Heart Failure) trial, the addition of coronary artery bypass surgery to medical therapy reduced the most common modes of death (sudden death and fatal pump failure events), with beneficial effects principally seen after two years [72].

Temporary mechanical circulatory support may theoretically interrupt the vicious spiral of ischaemic damage, and allow for recovery of stunned and hibernating myocardium. This kind of support involves circulation of blood through a device that drains venous blood and returns it to the systemic arteries with pulsatile or continuous flow after passing a membrane oxygenator. The major limitations of temporary mechanical circulatory support are device-related complications and irreversible organ failure.

It is possible to distinguish between two main classes of devices with short-term and long-term support. Short-term devices are usually placed in patients with acute heart failure, with a refractory cardiogenic shock and/or mechanical complications of myocardial infarction.

Veno-arterial extra-corporeal membrane oxygenation (VA-ECMO) assists both ventricles and provides a continuous flow with maintenance of a pulsatile arterial pressure unless the circulation is completely supported by the cardio pulmonary bypass device. This pump may be beneficial in cases of severe cardiogenic shock refractory to other pharmacological and mechanical support measures, although its use has not been tested in randomised clinical trials. In a recent meta-analysis, it is shown that VA-ECMO provides acceptable short-term survival for adult patients with cardiogenic shock and stable long-term survival outcomes at up to 3 years. These benefits, however, must be considered alongside the significant associated risks in the decision to institute this type of haemodynamic support [73, 74].

http://dx.doi.org/10.5772/61373

Other short term supports are axial flow pumps, with pumps positioned across the aortic valve to provide active support by transvalvular left ventricle assistance, placed with percutaneous or peripheral surgical approach (e. g., The Impella Recover® - Impella CardioSystems GmbH, Aachen, Germany), and the left atrial-to-femoral arterial left ventricular assist devices, with percutaneously inserted transseptal and arterial cannulae connected to a centrifugal pump (e. g., The Tandem HeartTM pVAD - Cardiac Assist Technologies, Inc., Pittsburgh, PA, USA) [75].

Studies have shown that these mechanical supports may reverse haemodynamic and metabolic parameters in cardiogenic shock more effectively than with standard IABP treatment alone.

However, when end-stage heart failure occurs, cardiac transplantation remains the gold standard, even if the lack of suitable donor organs significantly limits this therapeutic option.

Implantation of a long-term ventricular assist device as a bridge to transplantation or as a destination therapy is an established life-sustaining treatment option for select patients [76, 77, 78, 79].

8. New therapeutic strategies against myocardial remodelling

As seen in the beginning of this chapter, at the bottom of any mechanical complication after a myocardial infarction is the process that starts with an ischaemic injury and finishes with the remodelling of the myocardial tissue. As a result of myocite apoptosis, fibrous tissue deposition and the formation of a myocardial scar, heart failure occurs [2].

Although modest cardiomyocyte turnover occurs in the adult heart, it is insufficient for the restoration of a normal contractile function after substantial cardiomyocyte loss, and even if this cardiac remodelling can be slowed or sometimes reversed by intense pharmacological therapy (thrombolysis, ACEi, beta-blockers, and statins), this process is often progressive.

Several studies aim to find new therapeutic strategies for daily practise against myocardial remodelling. Many of them focused on biochemical patterns occurring during the remodelling process, principally on the ischaemic-reperfusion injury, by searching strategies against the generation of reactive oxygen species (ROS) in the ischaemic myocardium, or by interacting with complex cytokines pathways [80].

On the other hand, stem cells therapy seems to be another new approach to the problem of remodelling. Replacement and regeneration of functional cardiac muscle after an ischaemic insult co

uld be achieved by either stimulating proliferation of endogenous mature cardiomyocytes (reinitiating mitosis) or resident cardiac stem cells or by implanting exogenous donor-derived or allogeneic cardiomyocytes. New strategies may consist of transplanted bone marrow-derived cardiomyocyte or endothelial precursors, foetal cardiomyocytes, and skeletal myoblasts [81, 82, 83, 84].

Author details

Serena Mariani, Francesco Formica* and Giovanni Paolini

*Address all correspondence to: francesco_formica@fastwebnet.it

Cardiac Surgery Clinic, Department of Surgery and Translational Medicine, School of Medicine, University of Milan-Bicocca, San Gerardo Hospital, Monza (MB), Italy

References

[1] Thygesen K, Alpert JS, Jaffe AS, Simoons ML, Chaitman BR, White HD: The Writing Group on behalf of the Joint ESC/ACCF/AHA/WHF Task Force for the Universal Definition of Myocardial Infarction - Third Universal Definition of Myocardial Infarction. *JACC. 2012;60(16):1581-98.*

[2] Schoen FJ. The heart. In: Kumar V, Abbas AK, Fausto N. *Robbins and Cotran Pathologic Bases of Disease, 7th edition. 2006;575-585.*

[3] Marques JS, Jorge C, Feija A, Diogo AN. Acute myocardial infarction complication diagnosed by three-dimensional echocardiography. *European Journal of Echocardiography. 2011;12:E29.*

[4] Harmony R. Reynolds HR, Hochman JS. Heartbreak. *European Heart Journal. 2010;31:1433-1435.*

[5] Hatcher CR Jr, Mansour K, Logan WD Jr, et al. Surgical complications of myocardial infarction. *Am Surg. 1970;36(3):163-170.*

[6] FitzGibbon GM, Hooper GD, Heggtveit HA. Successful surgical treatment of postinfarction external cardiac rupture. *J Thorac Cardiovasc Surg. 1972;63(4):622-630.*

[7] Figueras J, Cortadellas J, Soler-Soler J. Left ventricular free wall rupture: Clinical presentation and management. *Heart. 2000;83:499e504.*

[8] Kumar Mishraa P, Pathib V, Murdaya A. Post myocardial infarction left ventricular free wall rupture. *Interactive CardioVascular and Thoracic Surgery 6. 2007;39-42.*

[9] Becker RC, Gore JM, Lambrew C, Weaver WD, Rubison RM, French WJ. A composite view of cardiac rupture in the United States National Registry of Myocardial Infarction. *J Am Coll Cardiol. May 1996;27(6):1321-6.*

[10] Kleiman NS, Terrin M, Mueller H, Chaitman B, Roberts R, Knatterud GL. Mechanisms of early death despite thrombolytic therapy: Experience from the Thrombolysis in Myocardial Infarction Phase II (TIMI II) study. *J Am Coll Cardiol. May 1992;19(6):1129-35.*

[11] Wehrens XHT, Doevendans PA. Cardiac rupture complicating myocardial infarction. *Int J Cardiol. 2004;95:285e92.*

[12] Perdigao C, Andrade A, Ribeiro C. Cardiac rupture in acute myocardial infarction: Various clinico-anatomical types in 42 recent cases observed over a period of 30 months. *Arch Mal Coeur Vaiss. 1987;80(3):336-334.*

[13] Becker AE, van Mantgem JP. Cardiac tamponade: A study of 50 hearts. *Eur J Cardiol. 1975;3(4):349-358.*

[14] Van Tassel RA, Edwards JE. Rupture of heart complicating myocardial infarction: Analysis of 40 cases including nine exemples of left ventricular false anurysm. *Chest. 1972;61(2):104-106.*

[15] Nihoyannopoulos P, Kisslo, editors. *Echocardiography. 2009. doi: 10.1007/978-1-84882-293-1.*

[16] Holubeca T, Caliskana E, Bettex D, Maisano F. Repair of post-infarction left ventricular free wall rupture using an extracellular matrix patch. *Oxford University Press on behalf of the European Association for Cardio-Thoracic Surgery. 2015.*

[17] Mantovani V, Vanoli D, Chelazzi P, Leporel V, Ferrarese S, Sala A. Post-infarction cardiac rupture: Surgical treatment. *European Journal of Cardio-thoracic Surgery 22. 2002;777-780.*

[18] Chen SSM, Ruengsakulrach P, Dick RJL, Buxton BF. Post-infarct left ventricular free wall rupture—not always a lethal complication of acute myocardial infarction. *Heart Lung and Circulation. 2004;13:26-30.*

[19] Mundth ED. Rupture of the Heart Complicating Myocardial Infarction. *Circulation. 1972;46:427-429.*

[20] Reardon MJ, Carr CL, Diamond A, Letsou GV, Safi HJ, Espada R, Baldwin JC. Ischemic left ventricular free wall rupture: Prediction, diagnosis, and treatment. *Ann Thorac Surg. 1997;64:1509-13.*

[21] Iemura J, Oku H, Otaki M, Kitayama H, Inoue T, Kaneda T. Surgical strategy for left ventricular free wall rupture after acute myocardial infarction. *Ann Thorac Surg. 2001;71:201-4.*

[22] Canovasa SJ, Limb E, Horneroa F, Monteroa J. Surgery for left ventricular free wall rupture: patch glue repair without extracorporeal circulation. *European Journal of Cardio-thoracic Surgery. 2003;23:639-641.*

[23] Fujimatsu T, Oosawa H, Takai F, Aruga M, Ogiwara F, Mawatari E, Sakurai S. Patch-and-Glue sutureless repair for blowout rupture after myocardial infarction: Report of two cases. *Ann Thorac Cardiovasc Surg. 2008;14(1).*

[24] Harrison W, Ruygrok PN, Greaves S, Wijesinghe N, Charleson H, Wade C, Devlin G. Percutaneous closure of left ventricular free wall rupture with associated false aneurysm to prevent cardioembolic stroke. *Heart, Lung and Circulation. 2008;17:243-263.*

[25] Latham PM. Lectures on subjects connected with clinical medicine comprises disease of the heart. *London: Longman Rees; 1845.*

[26] Deja MA, Szostek J, Widenka K, Szafron B, Spyt TJ, Hickey MSJ, Sosnowski AW. Post infarction ventricular septal defect: can we do better? *European Journal of Cardio-thoracic Surgery. 2000;18:194-201.*

[27] Lemery R, Smith HC, Giuliani ER, Gersh BJ. Prognosis in rupture of the ventricular septum after acute myocardial infarction and role of early surgical intervention. *Am J Cardiol. 1992;70(2):147-151.*

[28] Agnihotri AK, Madsen JC, Daggett WM. Surgical treatment for complications of acute myocardial infarction: postinfarction ventricular septal defect and free wall rupture. In: Cohn LH, Edmunds LH Jr. *Cardiac Surgery in the Adult. 2003;681-734.*

[29] Crenshaw BS, Granger CB, Birnbaum Y, Pieper KS, Morris DC, Kleiman NS. Risk factors, angiographic patterns, and outcomes in patients with ventricular septal defect complicating acute myocardial infarction. GUSTO-I (Global Utilization of Streptokinase and TPA for Occluded Coronary Arteries) Trial Investigators. *Circulation. Jan 4-11 2000;101(1):27-32.*

[30] Menon V, Webb JG, Hillis LD, et al. Outcome and profile of ventricular septal rupture with cardiogenic shock after myocardial infarction: a report from the SHOCK Trial Registry. SHould we emergently revascularize Occluded Coronaries in cardiogenic shock? *J Am Coll Cardiol. Sep 2000;36(3 Suppl A):1110-6.*

[31] Cooley DA, Belmonte BA, Zeis LB, Schnur S. Surgical repair of ruptured interventricular septum following acute myocardial infarction. *Surgery. 1957;41-930.*

[32] Heimbacker RO, Legmire G, Chen C. Surgery for massive myocardial infarction. An experimental study of emergency infartectmoy with a preliminar report on the clinical application. *Circulation. 1968;37(Suppl 4):II3-I1.*

[33] Daggett WM, Buckley MJ, Akins CW. Improved results of surgical management of postinfarction ventricular septal rupture. *Ann Surg. 1982;196(3):269-277.*

[34] Miyajima M, Kawashima T, Saito T, Yokoyama H, Ohori K, Kuwaki K, Sasaki A, Higami T. Delayed closure of postinfarction ventricular septal rupture. *Ann Thorac Cardiovasc Surg. 2010; 16(2).*

[35] Ari H, Melek M, Ari S, Doganay K, Cosar Oztas S. Percutaneous closure of post-myocardial infarction ventricular septal rupture in patients with ventricular septal rupture and apical thrombus: First case in literature. *International Journal of Cardiology. 2015;182:487-490.*

[36] Bouma W, Wijdh-den Hamer IJ, Klinkenberg TJ, Kuijpers M, Bijlevelda A, van der Horst ICC, Erasmus ME, Gorman III JH, Gorman RC, Mariani MA. Mitral valve repair for post-myocardial infarction papillary muscle rupture. *European Journal of Cardio-Thoracic Surgery. 2013;44:1063-1069.*

[37] Bouma W, Wijdh-den Hamer IJ, Koene BM, Kuijpers M, Natour E, Erasmus ME, Jainandunsing JS, van der Horst ICC, Gorman III JH, Gorman RC, Mariani MA. Long-term survival after mitral valve surgery for post-myocardial infarction papillary muscle rupture. *Journal of Cardiothoracic Surgery. 2015;10:11.*

[38] Ming Ming Sim. Giant V wave in an obscured acute mitral regurgitation due to rupture of the papillary muscle. *A712 JACC. March 17 2015;65(Issue 10S).*

[39] Ranganthan N, Burch GE. Gross morphology and arterial supply of the papillary muscles of the left ventricle of man. *Am Heart J. 1969;77(4):506-516.*

[40] Connell JM, Worthington A, Chen FY, Shernan SK. Ischemic mitral regurgitation mechanisms, intraoperative echocardiographic evaluation, and surgical considerations. *Anesthesiology Clin. 2013;31:281-298.*

[41] Formica F, Corti F, Sangalli F, Greco P, Ferro O, Colagrande L, Paolini G. Mitral valve annuloplasty with a semirigid annuloplasty band in ischemic mitral regurgitation: Early results. *Journal of Cardiovascular Medicine. 2007;8:499-503.*

[42] Calafiore AM, Iacò AL, Clemente D, Refaie R, Romano S, Asif M, Penco M, Di Mauro M. Repair or prosthesis insertion in ischemic mitral regurgitation: Two faces of the same medal. *IJC Heart & Vessels. 2014;3:32-36.*

[43] Talwar S, Jayanthkumar HV, Kumar AS. Chordal preservation during mitral valve replacement: Basis, techniques and results. *IJTCVS. 2005;21:45-52.*

[44] Thompson CR, Buller CE, Sleeper LA, Antonelli TA, Webb JG, Jaber WA, Abel JG, Hochman JS. Cardiogenic shock due to acute severe mitral regurgitation complicating acute myocardial infarction: a report from the SHOCK Trial Registry. *J Am Coll Cardiol. 2000;36:1104-9.*

[45] Aguiar J, del Mar Barba M, Alba Gil J, Caetano J, Ferreira A, Nobre A, Cravino J. Aneurisma do ventrículo esquerdo e diagnóstico diferencial com pseudoaneurisma. *Rev Port Cardiol. 2012. doi:10.1016/j.repc.2012.04.001.*

[46] Sutton MG, Sharpe N. Left ventricular remodeling after myocardial infarction: Pathophysiology and therapy. *Circulation. 2000;101(25):2981-2988.*

[47] Kumar Das A, Wilson GM, Furnary AP. Coincidence of true and false left ventricular Aneurysm. *Ann Thorac Surg. 1997;64:831-4.*

[48] Forman MB, Collins HW, Kopelman HA, Vaughn WK, Perry JM, Virmani R, Freisinger GC. Determinants of left ventricular aneurysm formation after anterior myocardial infarction: A clinical and angiographic study. *JACC. December 1986;8(6): 1256-62.*

[49] Tikiz H, Atak R, Balbay Y, Genc Y, Kutuk E. Left ventricular aneurysm formation after anterior myocardial infarction: clinical and angiographic determinants in 809 patients. *International Journal of Cardiology. 2002;82:7-14.*

[50] Heatlie GJ, Mohiddin R. Left ventricular aneurysm: Comprehensive assessment of morphology, structure and thrombus using cardiovascular magnetic resonance. *Clinical Radiology. 2005;60:687-692.*

[51] Chao HH, Lu MJ, Hung CR. Spontaneous rupture of left ventricular true aneurysm. *Ann Thorac Surg. 2005;80:1106-8.*

[52] Arsan S, Akgun S, Turkmen M, Kurtoglu N, Yildirim T. Delayed rupture of a postinfarction left ventricular true aneurysm. *Ann Thorac Surg. 2004;77:1813-5.*

[53] Hirota M, Omoto T, Ishikawa N, Fukuzumi M, Ohno M, Tedoriya T. Surgical strategy for subepicardial aneurysm: Two case reports. *Ann Thorac Cardiovasc Surg. 2010;16:291-293.*

[54] Kutty RS, Jones N, Moorjani N. Mechanical complications of acute myocardial infarction. *Cardiol Clin. 2013;31:519-531. doi:10.1016/j.ccl.2013.07.004.*

[55] Mills NL, Everson CT, Hockmuth DR. Technical advances in the treatment of left ventricular aneurysm. *Ann Thorac Surg. 1993;55(3):792-800.*

[56] Komeda M, David TE, Malik A, et al. Operative risks and long-term result of operation for left ventricular aneurysm. *Ann Thorac Surg. 1992;53(1):22-28;discussion 8-9.*

[57] Glower DD, Lowe JE. Left ventricular aneurysm. In: Cohn LH, Edmunds LH Jr. *Cardiac Surgery in the adult.* New York: Mc-Graw Hill; 2003:771-788.

[58] Jatene AD. Left ventricular aneurismectomy. Resection or reconstruction. *J Thorac Cardiovasc Surg. 1985;89(3):321-331*

[59] Dor V, Saab M, Coste P, et al. Endoventricular patch plasties with septal exclusion for repair of ischemic left ventricle: Technique, results and indications from a series of 781 cases. *Jpn J Thorac Cardiovesc Surg. 1998;46(5):389-398.*

[60] Cooley DA, Frazier OH, Duncan JM, et al. Intracavitary repair of ventricular aneurysm and regional dyskinesia. *Ann Surg. 1992;215(5):417-423; discussion 23-24.*

[61] Reynolds HR, Hochman JS. Cardiogenic shock current concepts and improving outcomes. *Circulation. 2008;117:686-697.*

[62] Hochman JS, Buller CE, Sleeper LA, Boland J, Dzavik V, Sanborn TA, Godfrey E, White HD, Lim J, LeJemtel T. Cardiogenic shock complicating acute myocardial infarction—Etiologies, management and outcome: A Report from the SHOCK Trial Registry. *JACC. September 2000;36 (3 Suppl A):1063-70.*

[63] Kaminski KA, Tycinska AM, Stepek T, Szpakowicz A, Oledzka E, Dobrzycki S, Musiał WJ. Natural history and risk factors of long-term mortality in acute coronary syndrome patients with cardiogenic shock. *Advances in Medical Sciences. 2014;59:156-160.*

[64] Morici N, Sacco A, Paino R, Oreglia JA, Bottiroli M, Senni M, Nichelatti M, Canova P, Russo C, Garascia A, Kulgmann S, Frigerio M, Oliva F. Cardiogenic shock: How to

overcome a clinical dilemma. Unmet needs in Emergency Medicine. *International Journal of Cardiology. 2015. doi:10.1016/j.ijcard.2015.02.111.*

[65] Babaev A, Frederick PD, Pasta DJ, Every N, Sichrovsky T, Hochman JS. Trends in management and outcomes of patients with acute myocardial infarction complicated by cardiogenic shock. *JAMA. July 27 2005;294(4).*

[66] Goldberg RJ, Gore JM, Alpert JS, Osganin V, de Groot J, Bade J, Chen Z, Frid D, Dalen JE. Cardiogenic shock after acute myocardial infarction. Incidence and mortality from a community-wide perspective, 1975 to 1988. *N Eng J Med. 1991;325:1117-22.*

[67] Jensen JK, Thayssen P, Antonsen L, Hougaard M, Junker A, Pedersen KE, Jensen LO. Influence of cardiogenic shock with or without the use of intra-aortic balloon pump on mortality in patients with ST-segment elevation myocardial infarction. *IJC Heart & Vasculature. 2015;6:19-24.*

[68] Trost JC, Hillis LD. Intra-aortic balloon counterpulsation. *Am J Cardiol. 2006;97:1391e8.*

[69] White JM, Ruygrok PN. Intra-aortic balloon counterpulsation in contemporary practice – where are we? *Heart, Lung and Circulation. 2015;1-7.*

[70] Cassese S, de Waha A, Ndrepepa G, Ranftl S, King L, Schomig A, Kastrati A. Intra-aortic balloon counterpulsation in patients with acute myocardial infarction without cardiogenic shock. A meta-analysis of randomized trials. *Am Heart J. 2012;164:58-65.e1.*

[71] Thiele H, Schuler G, Neumann F-J, Hausleiter J, Olbrich H-G, Schwarz B, Hennersdorf M, Empen K, Fuernau G, Desch S, de Waha S, Eitel I, Hambrecht R, Bohm M, Kurowski V, Lauer B, Minden H-H, Figulla H-R, Braun-Dullaeus RC, Strasser RH, Rochor K, Maier SKJ, Mollmann H, Schneider S, Ebelt H, Werdan K, Zeymer U. Intraaortic balloon counterpulsation in acute myocardial infarction complicated by cardiogenic shock: Design and rationale of the Intraaortic Balloon Pump in Cardiogenic Shock II (IABP-SHOCK II) trial. *Am Heart J. 2012;163:938-45.*

[72] Carson P, Wertheimer J, Miller A, O'Connor CM, Pina IL, Selzman C, Sueta C, She L, Greene D, Lee KL, Jones RH, Velazquez EJ. The STICH Trial (Surgical Treatment for Ischemic Heart Failure). *JCHF. 2013;1(5):400-408. doi:10.1016/j.jchf.2013.04.012.*

[73] Formica F, Avalli L, Colagrande L et al. Extracorporeal membrane oxygenation to support adult patients with cardiac failure: predictive factors of 30-day mortality. *Interact Cardiovasc Thorac Surg. 2010 May;10(5):721-6.*

[74] Pujara D, Sandoval E, Simpson L, Mallidi HR, Singh SK. The State of the Art in Extra Corporeal Membrane Oxygenation. *Semin Thoracic Surg, http://dx.doi.org/10.1053/j.semtcvs.2015.02.004.*

[75] Thiele H, Smalling RW, Schuler GC. Percutaneous left ventricular assist devices in acute myocardial infarction complicated by cardiogenic shock. *European Heart Journal. 2007;28:2057-2063.*

[76] White CW, Chelvanathan A, Zieroth S, Cordova-Perez F, Menkis AH, Freed DH. Can long-term ventricular assist devices be safely implanted in low-volume, non-heart transplant centres? *Canadian Journal of Cardiology. 2013;29:983-989.*

[77] McIlvennan CK, Matlock DD, Narayan MP, Nowels C, Thompson JS, Cannon A, Bradley WJ, Allen LA. Perspectives from mechanical circulatory support coordinators on the pre-implantation decision process for destination therapy left ventricular assist devices. *Heart & Lung. 2015;1e6.*

[78] Morris RJ, Shore ED. Pro: LVAD: Patient's desire for termination of vad therapy should be challenged. *Journal of Cardiothoracic and Vascular Anesthesia. October 2013;27(50):1048-1050.*

[79] Hirose H, Amano A, Yoshida S, Nagao T, Sunami H, Takahashi A, Nagano N. Surgical management of unstable patients in the evolving phase of acute myocardial infarction. *Ann Thorac Surg. 2000;69:425-8.*

[80] Florian A, Ludwig A, Rosch S, Yildiz H, Klumpp S, Sechtem U, Yilmaz A. Positive effect of intravenous iron-oxide administration on left ventricular remodelling in patients with acute ST-elevation myocardial infarction – A cardiovascular magnetic resonance (CMR) study. *International Journal of Cardiology. 2014;173:184-189.*

[81] Sheu Jiunn-Jye, Lee Fan-Yen, Yuen Chun-Man, Chen Yi-Ling, Huang Tien-Hung, Chua Sarah, Chen Yung-Lung, Chen Chih-Hung, Chai Han-Tan, Sung Pei-Hsun, Chang Hsueh-Wen, Sun Cheuk-Kwan, Yip Hon-Kan, Combined Therapy with Shock Wave and Autologous Bone Marrow-Derived Mesenchymal Stem Cells Alleviates Left Ventricular Dysfunction and Remodeling through Inhibiting Inflammatory Stimuli, Oxidative Stress & Enhancing Angiogenesis in a Swine Myocardial Infarction Model. *International Journal of Cardiology. 2015. doi:10.1016/j.ijcard.2015.03.044.*

[82] Itescu S, Schuster MD, Kocher AA. New directions in strategies using cell therapy for heart disease. *J Mol Med. 2003;81:288-296. doi:10.1007/s00109-003-0432-0.*

[83] Chen J, Guo R, Zhou Q, Wang T. Injection of composite with bone marrow-derived mesenchymal stem cells and a novel synthetic hydrogel after myocardial infarction: A protective role in left ventricle function. *Kaohsiung Journal of Medical Sciences. 2014;30:173e180.*

[84] Zhong Ye, Bi-Li Zhang, Xian-Xian Zhao, Yong-Wen Qin, Hong Wu, Jiang Cao, Jian-Liang Zhang, Jian-Qiang Hu, Xing Zheng, Rong-Liang Xu. Intracoronary infusion of bone marrow-derived mononuclear cells contributes to longstanding improvements of left ventricular performance and remodelling after acute myocardial infarction: A meta-analysis. Heart, Lung and Circulation. 2012;21:725-733.

Section 3

Prevention of Coronary Heart Disease

Chapter 10

Diabetes and Coronary Artery Disease – Pathophysiologic Insights and Therapeutic Implications

David Fridman, Amgad N. Makaryus, John N. Makaryus, Amit Bhanvadia, Erion Qaja, Alina Masters and Samy I. McFarlane

Additional information is available at the end of the chapter

http://dx.doi.org/10.5772/61875

Abstract

Cardiovascular disease is the leading cause of morbidity and mortality among people with diabetes worldwide, accounting for 60% of all deaths in diabetics. Despite advances in our pathophysiologic understanding of diabetic co-morbidities and measures to help counter these, diabetics still remain at increased risk for cardiovascular disease complicating our overall approach to management. Diabetics, in particularly type 2, are often fraught with additional risk factors contributing to their overall propensity for developing cardiovascular disease. These include, but are not limited to, obesity, dyslipidemia, poor glycemic control, lack of physical activity, and hypertension. In response to this, research driven guidelines focusing on primary prevention have continued to arise with new clinical targets and goals substantially changing our approach with the diabetic population. It is important to note early on, type 1 diabetics carry a higher risk of cardiovascular disease for which the pathophysiology is only recently being elucidated. The underlying relationship between cardiovascular events and risk factors is, however, not well understood. For this reason, management approaches to risk reduction have been extrapolated from experience in type 2 diabetes mellitus. The purpose of this chapter is to present the conclusions of current literature pertaining to blood pressure and blood glucose control, cholesterol management, aspirin therapy, and lifestyle modification. We present a synthesis of the new guidelines, and clinical targets, including preventative measures for subclinical cardiovascular disease for the contemporary management of patients with diabetes mellitus.

Keywords: Diabetes, atherosclerosis, coronary artery disease, glycemic control, antidiabetic medications

1. Introduction

1.1. Diabetes and cardiovascular risk: Scope of the problem

Cardiovascular disease (CVD) is the major cause of morbidity and mortality in the diabetic population which is rapidly expanding around the globe and is increasing due to the rising epidemic of obesity and increasing sedentary lifestyle along with poor dietary habits.[1] The cardiovascular events associated with type 2 diabetes and the high incidence of other macro-vascular complications, such as strokes and amputations, are major causes of illnesses and a large economic burden. Heart disease and strokes account for over 2/3 of mortality in the diabetic population who are 2–4 times more likely to have atherosclerotic heart disease compared to non-diabetic individuals. In fact, diabetes itself is considered a cardiovascular risk equivalent and the diabetic population is less likely to survive when they develop CVD, compared to their non-diabetic counterparts. While the additional risk diabetes confers cannot be completely eliminated, large benefit is seen when multiple risk factors and associated comorbid conditions are addressed globally in this patient population and addressed specifically with respect to treatment targets and goals.

1.2. Risk factors for cardiovascular disease in diabetes

Risk factors for increased CVD among people with diabetes include traditional ones such as insulin resistance, hypertension, dyslipidemia, central obesity, and cigarette smoking. Non-traditional risk factors include microalbuminuria, increased inflammation, oxidative stress, hyperuricemia, hypercoagulable states, endothelial dysfunction, decrease nitric oxide function, increase vascular reactivity and permeability, increased glycated end products, as well as stimulation of the renin angiotensin aldosterone (RAAS) system.

Modifiable Risk Factors	Non-modifiable Risk Factors
Overweight/obesity	Family history of diabetes or premature coronary disease
Sedentary lifestyle	Latino/Hispanic, Non-Hispanic black, Asian American, Native American, or Pacific Islander ethnicity
Hypertension	History of gestational diabetes
Elevated LDL-C and/or triglycerides and/or low HDL-C	History of infant delivery birth weight "/>9 pounds
Psychiatric illness	Polycystic ovarian syndrome
IGT, IFG	Age
HDL-C, high-density lipoprotein cholesterol; LDL-C, low-density lipoprotein cholesterol; IFG, impaired fasting glucose; IGT, impaired glucose tolerance	
Adapted from Diabetes Care Volume 38, Supplement 1, January 2015 [2]	

Table 1. Modifiable and non-modifiable risk factors associated with type 2 diabetes mellitus and cardiovascular disease

http://dx.doi.org/10.5772/61875

1.3. Hypertension

Hypertension is the most common comorbid disease associated with diabetes. It has been found to increase the risk of nephropathy, retinopathy, left ventricular hypertrophy, and cardiovascular events.[3] Prevention of these vascular complications is a worldwide priority as the prevalence of diabetics by 2030 is estimated to be approximately 350 million.[4] As a result, blood pressure (BP) management is arguably one of the more critical aspects of the care of the patient with diabetes. The current 2015 American Diabetes Association (ADA) recommendations are for all diabetics to achieve a systolic blood pressure (SBP) of <140 and a diastolic blood pressure (DBP) of <90. This has been revised to reflect the most recent high-quality evidence that exists to support a goal of DBP, 90 mmHg. Although, it has been traditionally recommended that diabetics achieve a blood pressure of less of 130/80, there is insufficient evidence to justify the benefit of this value.[5] While hypertension therapy is not the main focus of this chapter, it is important to realize that lifestyle therapy for hypertension should be offered to all patients as a reasonable first intervention; this includes weight loss, increased physical activity, and a Dietary Approaches to Stop Hypertension (DASH)–style diet. If despite this the patient is unable to achieve the goal BP pharmacological therapy should comprise a regimen that includes either an angiotensin converting enzyme (ACE) inhibitor or angiotensin receptor inhibitor (ARB)–either of which are effective in preventing the development or progression of microalbuminuria which reduces the incidence of new or worsening nephropathy.[6]

2. Hyperglycemia and cardiovascular risk

Hyperglycemia, even in the non-diabetic range such as impaired fasting glucose and/or impaired glucose tolerance (collectively classified as pre-diabetes) is associated with increased risk of coronary artery disease. This has been shown in several trials and also evidence exists that glycemic control is associated with decreased coronary artery disease. For example, the landmark United Kingdom Diabetes Perspective Study (UKPDS) showed a graded risk reduction in myocardial infarction among the diabetic population with 14% decreased risk for every 1% decrease in A1C. Glucose control is important and associated with decreased microvascular complications such as diabetic nephropathy, retinopathy, as well as neuropathy, with about 30% risk reduction with each 1% decrease in A1C, as evidenced from large trials in type 1 DM such as Diabetes Complication (DCCT) in type 1 diabetes and from UKPDS study in type 2 diabetes in patient with new onset/early onset diabetes.[7]

Long term follow up of these cohorts also provided evidence of decreased macrovascular disease such as in the Epidemiology of Diabetes Interventions and Complications (EDIC), a follow up of the DCCT trial where intensive blood glucose control reduced risk of any CVD event by 42% and the risk of nonfatal myocardial infarction, stroke, or death from cardiovascular causes by 57%.[8] However, tight glycemic control has been shown to be associated with increased mortality among high-risk population. In the large randomized controlled trial, ACCORD (Action to Control Cardiovascular Risk in Diabetes), tight control of blood glucose to a hemoglobin A1C of 6.4%, compared to 7.5% in the control group, was associated with a

22% increased mortality leading to premature termination of the study protocol. Furthermore, there was increased risk of hypoglycemia requiring assistance and an average of 10 kg weight gain in the period of 3.5 years of follow up. This study, as well as others, triggered a Position Statement by the American Diabetes Association (ADA) and the European Association for the Study of Diabetes (EASD) calling for an individualized patient approach with less stringent glycemic control for patients with established vascular complications, as well as those with longer diabetes duration and increased risk of hypoglycemia such as those with CKD and the elderly with long standing diabetes and neuropathy.

2.1. Cardiovascular disease in the high-risk diabetic sub-population

Diabetes disproportionately affects minority populations such as blacks, Hispanics, Native Americans, and South Asians. In these populations, the prevalence of diabetes is much higher compared to Whites and they are disproportionately affected by diabetes complications including chronic kidney disease, strokes, and coronary artery disease.

Premenopausal women with diabetes lose the estrogen protective effects that are partially mediated through nitric oxide and women with diabetes have worse outcomes compared to men when presented with acute coronary syndrome. Despite advances in the diagnosis and treatment of acute coronary syndrome, and through improved medical therapies such as revascularization, improved survival among men and women without diabetes as well as men with diabetes has been observed, but evidence suggests worse prognosis for women with diabetes remains.

2.2. Screening for cardiovascular disease

Screening of asymptomatic patients with high CVD risk is not recommended, as there have been no trials that demonstrate improved outcomes even in the setting of angiographically defined coronary disease. One of the largest trials to address this concern was the Detection of Ischemia in Asymptomatic Diabetics (DIAD) study. DIAD randomized 1,123 subjects into two categories: those who would and would not be screened with stress myocardial perfusion imaging (MPI). Despite abnormal myocardial perfusion imaging in more than one in five patients, cardiac events were lower than expected and equivalent in screened versus unscreened patients.[9] Furthermore, trials including the COURAGE and BARI 2D have shown no difference between revascularization and optimal medical therapy in patients who are effected by stable coronary disease supporting a less invasive approach to management.[10,11] The favorable cardiac outcomes among asymptomatic diabetics can likely be attributed to guideline-driven management of cardiac risk factors. Therefore, the current standard of care for type 2 diabetes should focus on the reduction of cardiovascular risk factors with avoidance of indiscriminate screening.

2.3. Type I diabetes mellitus

Type I diabetes is a challenging clinical entity. It deserves separate mention as its management has lagged in success when compared to type II diabetes.

Type I diabetes is associated with an increased risk of early death with acute diabetes-related complications responsible for the majority of younger deaths and cardiovascular disease the main cause for older patients.[12,13,14] CVD occurs much earlier in type I diabetics than in the general population—often after 2 decades of disease. This can occur as early as 30 years of age disease rates of >3% per year.[15] Poor glycemic control has correlated to cardiovascular risk (Table 2), however, the success rates of achieving optimal A1c levels is far from ideal. In two national registries, only 13% to 15% of patients with type 1 diabetes met a target A1c level of <7%.[16,13] The difficulty partially lies in dietary/insulin regimen adherence and risks of tight blood sugar control (absolute risk of severe hypoglycemia increasing with tighter control).[6]

Mean HbA1c	Death from any cause	Death from cardiovascular disease
≤ 6.9%	2.36 (95%CI: 1.97–2.83)	2.92 (95%CI: 2.07–4.13)
7.0%–7.8%	2.38 (95%CI: 2.02–2.80)	3.39 (95%CI: 2.49–4.61)
7.9%–8.7%	3.11 (95%CI: 2.66–3.62)	4.44 (95%CI: 3.32–5.96)
8.8%–9.6%	3.65 (95%CI: 3.11–4.30)	5.35 (95%CI: 3.94–7.26)
≥ 9.7%	8.51 (95%CI: 7.24–10.01)	10.46 (95%CI: 7.62–14.37)

Adapted from Lind et al [11].

Table 2. Adjusted hazard ratios for death from any cause and death from cardiovascular disease among individuals with type 1 diabetes vs control according to the glycated hemoglobin

Even when target glycemic control is achieved, the risk of death from cardiovascular causes is more than twice the risk in the general population and poor glycemic control portends a risk ten times higher.[17] The issue is complicated by several components highlighted by the Scottish Registry Linkage Study. Unlike type 2 diabetics, type 1 diabetics generally do not suffer from obesity and hypertension/dyslipidemia rates are not in excess of the general population.[18] At this time, there is no clear explanation for the additional risk. It is postulated that earlier onset and severely altered glucose homeostasis produces a variety of oxidative stressors promoting a milieu of underlying vascular disease. This may be especially true in the preadolescent years where subclinical disease manifests, priming the cardiovascular system for accelerated atherosclerosis despite the best efforts at achieving glycemic control later in life.[19] The term coined, *metabolic memory*, has been used to denote this theoretical process. The phenomenon gained support after a significant trend was noted at the conclusion of the DCCT and follow-up EDIC trial in regards to microvascular complications, e.g. nephropathy, retinopathy. In summary, the DCCT trial ended with a transition of participants to an intensive insulin regimen secondary to successful glycemic control and reduction in microvascular complications with this method. Interestingly, as the same patients were followed, those originally on the standard insulin regimen continued to have higher incidences of microvascular disease when compared to their counterpart. This occurred despite achieving near equivalent A1c levels.[20,21,22] The notion of early vascular stress portending a worse prognosis was also echoed in a recent Cochrane review where findings concluded that tight control reduced the risk of developing microvascular diabetes complications (the risk for macrovascular complications was less clear secondary to the younger patient population they examined), but the impact became weaker once complications manifested.[23] Furthermore, during the EDIC study, macrovascular relationship became more apparent. Those participants who initially were under the intensive regimen experienced a 42% reduction in CVD events after 17 years. The ongoing EDIC showed these benefits persisted up to 10 years after the end of the DCCT.[7,24,25,26] These findings are promising as more effort is being placed at identifying subjects and initiating treatment earlier. Early therapy stands to eliminate or reduce a large amount of complications; however, longer-term studies are still needed to realize the full potential. It is also still unclear why cardiovascular complications start so early in the disease history when, presumably, only mild hyperglycemia exists.

3. Multifactorial therapy: A comprehensive evidence based approach

Over the past two decades, diabetes management has evolved substantially as epidemiologic and therapeutic based research has broadened our understanding of this complex disease. As a general principle, diabetes magnifies many of the indolent cardiovascular risk factors for morbidity and mortality amongst non-diabetic patients. As the population of diabetics increases, there is a growing effort to acknowledge the risks and lessen them to the best of our abilities. This begins with addressing modifiable risk factors for late complications in patients which includes hyperglycemia, hypertension, and dyslipidemia—all of which increase the risk of a poor outcomes.

Intensive treatment of multiple cardiovascular risk factors can have a major impact among patients with diabetes. Reduction in glycosylated hemoglobin values, systolic and diastolic blood pressure, fasting serum cholesterol and triglyceride levels, and urinary albumin excretion rate all have their value in reducing cardiovascular morbidity and mortality. Up until the turn of the century, numerous randomized trials investigated the effect of intensified intervention involving a single risk factor in patients with type 2 diabetes demonstrating benefits in terms of both macrovascular and microvascular complications in kidneys, eyes, and nerves.[27,28,29,30,31] This formed the basis of American Diabetes Association recommendations for many years which were finally bolstered by the landmark publication, Steno-2 study, which investigated a multifactorial, goal directed strategy involving lifestyle modification and pharmacologic management addressing all major metrics. An unrivalled 50% reduction in the risk of macro and micro-vascular events was demonstrated in those who received intensive treatment.[32] Since this study, several further trials have replicated these findings and have shown that the benefit of aggressive lifestyle and multi-drug therapy is effective and should be coupled with timely screening to confer a life-long benefit.[33,34,35]

3.1. Dietary management

Diet is one of the most important behavioral aspects of diabetes treatment, slowing and potentially preventing the rate of developing complications. Basic principles of nutritional management have evolved over the past decade from a generalized approach to an individualized one in the form of medical nutrition therapy (MNT). This approach takes scientific evidence, individual goals and abilities into consideration to formulate lifestyle changes that can be maintained. It is monitored and guided by a dietician or nutritionist with regular follow up. Goals of MNT that apply to individuals with diabetes include achieving and maintaining (1) blood glucose levels in the normal range or as close to normal as is safely possible, (2) a lipid and lipoprotein profile that reduces the risk for vascular disease, (3) blood pressure levels in the normal range or as close to normal as is safely possible, (4) to prevent, or at least slow, the rate of development of the chronic complications of diabetes by modifying nutrient intake and lifestyle to address individual nutrition needs, taking into account personal and cultural preferences and willingness to change, and (5) the pleasure of eating by only limiting food choices when indicated by scientific evidence.[36] By the mid-90's diet directed research had bolstered this involved form of dietary intervention with promising results. Randomized controlled trials of MNT have reported decreases in HbA1c (A1C) of 1% in type 1 diabetics and 1–2% in type 2 diabetics, depending on the duration of diabetes. After initiation of MNT, improvements were apparent in 3–6 months.[10,37,38]

3.2. Lipid management

Both types of diabetes associated with a substantially increased risk of atherosclerotic vascular disease, identification of treatments for the prevention of major occlusive vascular events is a public-health priority.[39,40,41] The most recent meta-analyses have underscored the importance of lipid management and have changed the medical communities general approach to risk reduction in the diabetic community. There appears to be an approximately linear relationship between the absolute reductions in LDL cholesterol achieved in these trials and the proportional reductions in the incidence of major vascular events.[42,43] The implications of this is far reaching. What used to be a categorical approach with a goal cholesterol level in mind has broadened considerably. In all patients with diabetes over the age of 40 years moderate intensity statin treatment should be considered, in addition to lifestyle therapy (Table 3). If the patient falls under a 'high-risk' category—those with acute coronary syndromes or previous cardiovascular events, LDL cholesterol > 100mg/dL, high blood pressure, currently smoking and/or overweight should have more aggressive therapy with high doses of statins.[44,45] This strategy should be coupled with medical nutritional therapy.

3.2.1. Aspirin therapy

In general, patients with or without diabetes, who have known occlusive vascular disease, stand to benefit from long-term antiplatelet therapy with aspirin, reducing the yearly risk of serious vascular events. The benefits of antiplatelet therapy substantially exceed the risk of major bleeding events and it is therefore widely accepted as means of secondary prevention. For primary prevention, however, the balance is less clear with no single trial demonstrating a clear benefit.[46,47] In order to reconcile the uncertainty regarding primary prevention the American Diabetes Association performed a meta-analysis that added data from additional trials performed specifically in patients with diabetes to the data from the subgroups of

Age	Risk factors	Recommended statin dose*	Monitoring with lipid panel
< 40 years	None CVD risk factor(s)** Overt CVD***	None Moderate or high High	Annually or as needed to monitor for adherence
40-75 years	None CVD risk factors Overt CVD	Moderate High High	As needed to monitor adherence
>75 years	None CVD risk factors Overt CVD	Moderate Moderate or high High	As needed to monitor adherence

* Moderate-Intensity Statin Therapy: Atorvastatin 10-20 mg, Rosuvastatin 5-10 mg, Simvastatin 20-40 mg, Pravastatin 40-80 mg, Lovastatin 40 mg. High-Intensity Statins Therapy: Atorvastatin 80 mg, Rosuvastatin 20-40 mg

**CVD risk factors include LDL cholesterol $100 mg/dL (2.6 mmol/L), high blood pressure,

smoking, and overweight and obesity.

***Overt CVD includes those with previous cardiovascular events or acute coronary syndromes.

Adapted from Diabetes Care Volume 38, Supplement 1, January 2015 [2]

Table 3. Recommendations for statin treatment in people with diabetes

patients with diabetes from the six trials included in the ATT (Antiplatelet Trialists' Collaboration Collaborative) meta-analysis. They concluded that aspirin appears to produce a modest-sized reduction in MI and stroke in patients with diabetes, but current evidence remains inconclusive. This was partially rectified by recent 14 trial meta-analysis which found a significant net benefit, but the authors still concluded inconclusiveness in regards to diabetic patients.[48,49,50]

In 2010, a position statement of the ADA, the American Heart Association, and the American College of Cardiology Foundation recommended physicians consider aspirin therapy (75–162 mg/day) as a primary prevention strategy in those with type 1 or type 2 diabetes at increased cardiovascular risk (10-year risk >10%). This includes most men aged >50 years or women aged >60 years who have at least one additional major risk factor (family history of CVD, hypertension, smoking, dyslipidemia, or albuminuria). However, aspirin was no longer recommended for those at low CVD risk (women under age 60 years and men under age 50 years with no major CVD risk factors; 10-year CVD risk under 5%) as the low benefit is likely to be outweighed by the risks of significant bleeding.[27]

3.3. Anti-diabetic medications and cardiovascular disease

Several classes of antidiabetic medications are currently available and effectively decreased hyperglycemia; however, concern regarding increased CVD risk was raised with the publication of the famous metanalysis by Nissen et al (2007) and showed rosiglitazone to be associated with a significant increase in the risk of myocardial infarction and with an increase in the risk of death from cardiovascular causes that had borderline significance. This study eventually, as well as other concerns, led to the withdrawal of the medication from the European Union as well as severe restriction that amounted to effective withdrawal in the United States as well. These findings also prompted the FDA to require cardiovascular safety data prior to approval of new diabetes drugs in the USA. Currently, evidence available regarding cardiovascular safety and even protective effects for metformin either neutral or uncertain effects of others agents due to lack of long-term safety data.

4. Global control of cardiovascular risk in the diabetic population

The estimation and categorization of cardiovascular risk requires close attention to the risks being explored (Table 4). While certain CVD risks are modifiable such as smoking, obesity, hypertension and dyslipidemia, others are non-modifiable such as family history of premature coronary artery disease. Despite evidence for improved CVD outcomes with control of CVD risk factors, data from our group (McFarlane et al., 2002, 2005) conducted at multiple centers in the USA, among various ethnic groups and practice settings, showed largely suboptimal control of glycemia, blood pressure, and cholesterol and also demonstrated gender disparity in the outcomes of diabetic care. For these reasons, a multifactorial targeted and evidence based approach as detailed in this chapter needs to be employed for the appropriate and adequate management of these diabetic patients at risk for cardiovascular disease.

Modifiable Risk Factors	Non-Modifiable Risk Factors
Hypertension	Age
Diabetes	Sex
Dyslipidemia	Race/Ethnicity
Tobacco Use	Family history of premature CAD
Poor dietary habits (high fat, high carbohydrate)	
Sedentary lifestyle	
Obesity (particularly central distribution)	
microalbuminuria	
Increased inflammation	
Stimulation of RAAS	

CAD= Coronary artery disease

RAAS = Renin Angiotensin Aldosterone System

Table 4. Risk Factor Categorization

Author details

David Fridman[1], Amgad N. Makaryus[1,2], John N. Makaryus[1], Amit Bhanvadia[3], Erion Qaja[4], Alina Masters[3] and Samy I. McFarlane[3*]

*Address all correspondence to: smcfarlane@downstate.edu

1 North Shore-LIJ Health System, Hofstra NSLIJ School of Medicine, Manhasset, NY, USA

2 Department of Cardiology, NuHealth, Nassau University Medical Center, East Meadow, NY, USA

3 Division of Endocrinology, Department of Medicine, SUNY Downstate Medical Center, Brooklyn, NY, USA

4 Wyckoff Heights Medical Center, Brooklyn, NY, USA

References

[1] Global Atlas on Cardiovascular Disease Prevention and Control. Mendis S, Puska P, Norrving B editors. World Health Organization (in collaboration with the World Heart Federation and World Stroke Organization), Geneva 2011.

[2] Cardiovascular disease and risk management. Diabetes Care. 2015;38 Suppl:S49–57.

[3] Buse JB, Ginsberg HN, Bakris GL, et al.; American Heart Association; American Diabetes Association. Primary prevention of cardiovascular diseases in people with diabetes mellitus: a scientific statement from the American Heart Association and the American Diabetes Association. Diabetes Care 2007;30:162–172

[4] Wild, G Roglic, A Green, R Sicree, H King. Global prevalence of diabetes; estimates for year 2000 and projections for 2030. Diabetes Care, 21 (2004), pp. 1047–1053

[5] James PA, Oparil S, Carter BL, et al. 2014 evidence-based guideline for the management of high blood pressure in adults: report from the panel members appointed to the Eighth Joint National Committee (JNC 8). JAMA. 2014;311(5):507–20.

[6] Patel A, Macmahon S, Chalmers J, et al. Effects of a fixed combination of perindopril and indapamide on macrovascular and microvascular outcomes in patients with type 2 diabetes mellitus (the ADVANCE trial): a randomised controlled trial. Lancet. 2007;370(9590):829–40.

[7] The effect of intensive treatment of diabetes on the development and progression of long-term complications in insulin-dependent diabetes mellitus. The Diabetes Control and Complications Trial Research Group. N Engl J Med. 1993;329(14):977–86.

[8] Epidemiology of Diabetes Interventions and Complications (EDIC). Design, implementation, and preliminary results of a long-term follow-up of the Diabetes Control and Complications Trial cohort. Diabetes Care. 1999;22(1):99–111.

[9] Young LH, Wackers FJ, Chyun DA, et al. Cardiac outcomes after screening for asymptomatic coronary artery disease in patients with type 2 diabetes: the DIAD study: a randomized controlled trial. JAMA. 2009;301(15):1547–55.

[10] Boden WE, O'Rourke RA, Teo KK, et al.; COURAGE Trial Research Group. Optimal medical therapy with or without PCI for stable coronary disease. N Engl J Med 2007;356:1503–1516 67.

[11] BARI 2D Study Group; Frye RL, August P, et al. A randomized trial of therapies for type 2 diabetes and coronary artery disease. N Engl JMed 2009;360:2503–2515

[12] Laing SP, Swerdlow AJ, Slater SD, et al. The British Diabetic Association Cohort Study, I: all-cause mortality in patients with insulin-treated diabetes mellitus. Diabet Med 1999;16:459–65

[13] Skrivarhaug T, Bangstad HJ, Stene LC, Sandvik L, Hanssen KF, Joner G. Longterm mortality in a nationwide cohort of childhood-onset type 1 diabetic patients in Norway. Diabetologia 2006;49:298–305

[14] Secrest AM, Becker DJ, Kelsey SF, Laporte RE, Orchard TJ. Cause-specific mortality trends in a large populationbased cohort with long-standing childhood-onset type 1 diabetes. Diabetes 2010;59:3216–22.

[15] Secrest AM, Becker DJ, Kelsey SF, Laporte RE, Orchard TJ. Cause-specific mortality trends in a large population-based cohort with longstanding childhood-onset type 1 diabetes. Diabetes 2010;59:3216–3222

[16] Swedish National Diabetes Register.Annual Report 2012 (https:/ / www .ndr .nu/ pdf/Annual_Report_NDR_2012 .pdf).

[17] Lind M, Svensson AM, Kosiborod M, et al. Glycemic control and excess mortality in type 1 diabetes. N Engl J Med. 2014;371(21):1972–82.

[18] Livingstone SJ, Looker HC, Hothersall EJ, et al. Risk of cardiovascular disease and total mortality in adults withtype 1 diabetes: Scottish registry linkage study. PLoS Med 2012;9(10):e1001321

[19] Mameli C, Mazzantini S, Ben nasr M, Fiorina P, Scaramuzza AE, Zuccotti GV. Explaining the increased mortality in type 1 diabetes. World J Diabetes. 2015;6(7):889–95.

[20] Writing Team for the Diabetes Control and Complications Trial/Epidemiology of Diabetes Interventions and Complications Research Group 2002 Effect of intensive therapy on the microvascular complications of type 1 diabetes mellitus. *JAMA* 287:2563–2569

[21] Writing Team for the Diabetes Control and Complications Trial/Epidemiology of Diabetes Interventions and Complications Research Group 2003 Sustained effect of intensive treatment of type 1 diabetes mellitus on development and progression of diabetic nephropathy: the Epidemiology of Diabetes Interventions and Complications (EDIC) study. *JAMA* 290:2159–2167

[22] Ceriello A, Ihnat MA, Thorpe JE. Clinical review 2: The "metabolic memory": is more than just tight glucose control necessary to prevent diabetic complications?. J ClinEndocrinolMetab. 2009;94(2):410–5.

[23] Fullerton B, Jeitler K, Seitz M, Horvath K, Berghold A, Siebenhofer A. Intensive glucose control versus conventional glucose control for type 1 diabetes mellitus. Cochrane Database Syst Rev. 2014;2:CD009122.

[24] The Diabetes Control and Complications Trial (DCCT)/Epidemiology of DiabetesInterventions and Complications (EDIC) Research Group. Beneficial effects ofintensive therapy of diabetes during adolescence: outcomes after the conclusionof the diabetes control and complications trial (DCCT). J Pediatr 2001;139:804–12.

[25] Diabetes Control and Complications Trial/Epidemiology of Diabetes Interventionsand Complications Research Group. Prolonged effect of intensive therapyon the risk of retinopathy complications in patient with type 1 diabetes mellitus:10 years after the Diabetes Control and Complications Trial. Arch Ophthalmol2008;126(12):1707–15.

[26] White NH, Sun W, Cleary PA, et al, for the DCCT-EDIC Research Group. Effect ofprior intensive therapy in type 1 diabetes on 10-year progression of retinopathyin the DCCT/EDIC: comparison of adults and adolescents. Diabetes 2010;59(5):1244–53.

[27] UK Prospective Diabetes Study (UKPDS) Group. Intensive blood-glucose control with sulphonylureas or insulin compared with conventional treatment and risk of complicationsin patients with type 2 diabetes (UKPDS 33). Lancet 1998;352:837–53.

[28] Tight blood pressure control and risk of macrovascular and microvascular complications in type 2 diabetes: UKPDS 38. BMJ 1998;317:703–13.

[29] Pyörälä K, Pedersen TR, Kjekshus J, Færgeman O, Olsson AG, Thorgeirsson G. Cholesterol lowering with simvastatin improves prognosis of diabetic patients with coronary heart disease: a subgroup analysis of the Scandinavian Simvastatin Survival Study (4S). Diabetes Care 1997;20:614–20.

[30] Ravid M, Lang R, Rachmani R, Lishner M. Long-term renoprotective effect of angiotensin-converting enzyme inhibition in non-insulin-dependent diabetes mellitus: a 7-year follow-up study. Arch Intern Med 1996;156:286–9.

[31] The Heart Outcomes Prevention Evaluation Study Investigators. Effects of an angiotensin- converting–enzyme inhibitor, ramipril, on cardiovascular events in high-risk patients. N Engl J Med 2000;342:145–53.

[32] Gaede P, Vedel P, Larsen N, Jensen GV, Parving HH, Pedersen O. Multifactorial intervention and cardiovascular disease in patients with type 2 diabetes. N Engl J Med. 2003;348(5):383–93.

[33] Gaede P, Lund-andersen H, Parving HH, Pedersen O. Effect of a multifactorial intervention on mortality in type 2 diabetes. N Engl J Med. 2008;358(6):580–91.

[34] Wu WX, Ren M, Cheng H, et al. Prevention of macrovascular disease in patients with short-duration type 2 diabetes by multifactorial target control: an 8-year prospective study. Endocrine. 2014;47(2):485–92.

[35] Gaede P, Lund-andersen H, Parving HH, Pedersen O. Effect of a multifactorial intervention on mortality in type 2 diabetes. N Engl J Med. 2008;358(6):580–91.

[36] Franz, Marion J., et al. "Evidence-based nutrition principles and recommendations for the treatment and prevention of diabetes and related complications." *Diabetes care* 25.1 (2002): 148–198.

[37] Bantle, John P., et al. "Nutrition recommendations and interventions for diabetes: a position statement of the American Diabetes Association." *Diabetes care* 31 (2008): S61-S78.

[38] Franz MJ, Monk A, Barry B, et al. Effectiveness of medical nutrition therapy provided by dietitians in the management of non-insulin-dependent diabetes mellitus: a randomized, controlled clinical trial. J Am Diet Assoc. 1995;95(9):1009–17.

[39] MJ Garcia, PM McNamara, T Gordon, WB KannellMorbidity and mortality in diabetics in the Framingham population: sixteen year follow-up study. Diabetes, 23 (1974), pp. 105–111

[40] Pyörälä, M Laakso, M Uusitupa. Diabetes and atherosclerosis: an epidemiologic view. Diabetes Metab, 3 (1987), pp. 464. 46

[41] Stamler, O Vaccaro, JD Neaton, D Wentworth. Diabetes, other risk factors, and 12-yr cardiovascular mortality for men screened in the multiple risk factor intervention trial.Diabetes Care, 16 (1993), pp. 434 pp.

[42] Mihaylova B, Emberson J, Blackwell L, et al. The effects of lowering LDL cholesterol with statin therapy in people at low risk of vascular disease: meta-analysis of individual data from 27 randomised trials. Lancet. 2012;380(9841):581–90.

[43] Baigent C, Keech A, Kearney PM, et al. Efficacy and safety of cholesterol-lowering treatment: prospective meta-analysis of data from 90,056 participants in 14 randomised trials of statins. Lancet. 2005;366(9493):1267–78.

[44] Taylor F, Huffman MD, Macedo AF, et al. Statins for the primary prevention of cardiovascular disease. Cochrane Database Syst Rev 2013;1:CD004816

[45] Carter AA, Gomes T, Camacho X, Juurlink DN, Shah BR, Mamdani MM. Risk of incident diabetes among patients treated with statins: population based study. BMJ 2013;346:f2610

[46] Antiplatelet Trialists' Collaboration Collaborative overview of randomised trials of antiplatelet therapy—I: prevention of death, myocardial infarction, and stroke by prolonged antiplatelet therapy in various categories of patients. BMJ. 1994;308:81–106.

[47] Antithrombotic Trialists' Collaboration Collaborative meta-analysis of randomised trials of antiplatelet therapy for prevention of death, myocardial infarction, and stroke in high risk patients. BMJ. 2002;324:71–86.

[48] Baigent C, Blackwell L, Collins R, et al. Aspirin in the primary and secondary prevention of vascular disease: collaborative meta-analysis of individual participant data from randomised trials. Lancet. 2009;373(9678):1849–60.

[49] Pignone M, Alberts MJ, Colwell JA, et al. Aspirin for primary prevention of cardiovascular events in people with diabetes. J Am CollCardiol. 2010;55(25):2878–86.

[50] Xie M, Shan Z, Zhang Y, et al. Aspirin for primary prevention of cardiovascular events: meta-analysis of randomized controlled trials and subgroup analysis by sex and diabetes status. PLoS ONE. 2014;9(10):e90286.

Chapter 11

Obesity and Heart Diseases, a Worsened Epidemic in Recent Decades

Jian-Lin Wu and Chi-Wen Juan

Additional information is available at the end of the chapter

http://dx.doi.org/10.5772/61044

Abstract

Overweight and obesity are major risk factors for a number of chronic diseases, including diabetes, cardiovascular diseases and metabolic diseases. Obesity induces serious heart diseases such as hypertension, heart failure, and coronary disease by multiple mechanisms. The endothelial dysfunction and artherosclerosis induced by obesity lead to the result of coronary artery disease. In addition, obesity is a substantial public health crisis worldwide, and internationally, with the prevalence increasing rapidly in numerous industrialized nations. Worldwide, 39% of adults aged 18 years and over were overweight in 2014, and 13% were obese. The first choice of treatment is weight loss by life-style modification, such as diet and exercise. Medication and surgery are for moderate obese patients with comorbidity. How to find the appropriate method of weight losing is the most important issue.

Keywords: obesity, definition, coronary artery diseases, treatment, weight loss

1. Introduction

Obesity has become one of the most important public health issues due to the increased prevalence of the comorbidities associated with obesity. Recommendations, guidelines, and consensus statements for the definition and classification of obese children, adolescents, and adults have been published by many famous journal in these decades. Generally speaking, obesity is not only a major risk factors for a number of chronic diseases which mentioned above, but also a chronic disease that is increasing in prevalence in adults, adolescents, and children, and is now considered to be a global epidemic.

The fundamental cause of obesity and overweight is an energy imbalance between calories consumed and calories expended. People travel on transportation, rather than walking, and so many people work in offices, where they are sitting still for most of the day. A sedentary lifestyle lowers calories expenditure. Eating excess calories with less consumption promotes weight gain. Of all sedentary behaviors, long-time TV watching appears to be the most predictive of obesity risk. In the Nurses' Health Study, after adjustment for age, smoking, exercise level, and dietary factors, every 2-hour increment spent watching TV was associated with a 23% (95% CI 17-30 %) increase in obesity[1].

2. Definition and classification

- Overweight and obesity refer to a weight above the "normal" range.

We use body mass index (BMI)[BMI = body weight (in kg) ÷ height squared, in meters], which is currently used as the most accurate and reliable way of measuring how overweight an adult(18 years and older) is. For most people, an ideal BMI is between 18.5 and 24.9kg/m^2. The classification is as follows:

- Underweight—BMI <18.5 kg/m^2.
- Normal weight—BMI ≥18.5–24.9 kg/m^2.
- Overweight—BMI ≥25.0–29.9 kg/m^2.
- Obesity—BMI ≥30 kg/m^2.
  - Obesity class I—BMI of 30.0–34.9 kg/m^2.
  - Obesity class II—BMI of 35.0–39.9 kg/m^2.
  - Obesity class III—BMI ≥40 kg/m^2. This type of obesity is also referred to as severe, extreme, or massive obesity.

Unfortunately, a strung healthy fitness instructor may be mistaken for an obese adult if we only use BMI to screen overweight and obesity. Because BMI cannot well describe the central fat accumulation in the abdomen, we use waist circumference as another measurement of obesity, especially abdominal obesity, and it provides risk information that is not accounted by BMI.A waist circumference of ≥40inches (102 cm, 90cm for Asian) for men and ≥35inches (88 cm, 80cm for Asian) for women is considered elevated and indicative of increased cardio-vascular and metabolic disease risk [2].

Screening measures by BMI with waist circumference can identify adults at increased risk for morbidity and mortality, particularly in the BMI range 25–35 kg/m^2 [3].

For children, the different normal ranges of BMI are classified by age [4, 5]. A growing consensus supports the following definitions for children between 2 and 18 years of age

- Underweight—BMI <5th percentile for age and sex

http://dx.doi.org/10.5772/61044

- Normal weight—BMI between the 5th and the 85th percentile for age and sex
- Overweight—BMI between the 85th and the 95th percentile for age and sex
- Obese—BMI ≥95th percentile for age and sex
- Severe obesity—BMI ≥120% of the 95th percentile values, or a BMI ≥35 kg/m^2 (whichever is lower) [6, 7, 8]. This corresponds to approximately the 99th percentile, or BMI Z-score ≥2.33 (e.g., 2.33 standard deviations above the mean) [8, 9, 10]. Some authors distinguish an additional subgroup with more severe obesity with BMI ≥140% of the 95th percentile values or a BMI ≥40 kg/m^2, which corresponds to class III obesity in adults [7, 8].

3. Prevalence

- Adults

Based on data collected for the National Health and Nutrition Examination Survey (NHANES) between 2011 and 2012, the measured prevalence of obesity in adults in the United States is 34.9% [11]. The age-adjusted prevalence of class III obesity (BMI ≥40), sometimes referred to as severe obesity, was 6.3% in 2009–2010 [12].Worldwide, 36.9% of men and 38% of women estimated to have a BMI ≥25 kg/m^2 [13,14]. In 2013, reported prevalence rates of obesity (BMI of ≥30 kg/m2) included 20% of men and 21.7% of women in Belgium, 25% of men and women in the United Kingdom, 21% of men and 33% of women in Mexico, and 13.5% of men and 42% of women in South Africa [13,15].

- Children

Worldwide, 42 million children under the age of 5 years were overweight or obese in 2013.In the United States, the percentage of age of children aged 6–11 years in the United States who were obese increased from 7% in 1980 to nearly 18% in 2012. Similarly, the percentage of age of adolescents aged 12–19 years who were obese increased from 5% to nearly 21% over the same period [16, 17].For example, Childhood obesity has more than doubled in children and quadrupled in adolescents in the past 30 years.

By reported data, the worldwide prevalence of obesity more than doubled between 1980 and 2014.Before, obesity was considered a high-income country problem due to stereotype about the relationship between money, the increased intake of energy-dense foods, and increase in physical inactivity. In fact, overweight and obesity are now on the rise in low- and middle-income countries, particularly in urban settings. In developing countries, the rate of increase of childhood overweight and obesity has been more than 30% higher than that of developed countries.

Changes in dietary and physical activity patterns are often the result of environmental and technical changes associated with economic development and lack of supportive policies in sectors such as health, urban planning, food processing, distribution, marketing, and education.

4. Pathogenesis and its related coronary artery disease

Obesity has many causes, each of which has a variable genetic component. At one extreme are the kinds of obesity caused by single-gene mutations. At the other extreme are the kinds of obesity caused by various diseases in subjects in whom obesity would otherwise not occur. The followings focus on obesity caused by single-gene defects, the genetic susceptibility to obesity, and the pathogenetic mechanisms that operate within this genetic framework to cause differences in total body fat content and in regional fat distribution.

Genetic disorders of obesity

- Prader–Willi syndrome

The Prader–Willi syndrome is a neurodegenerative disorder that is caused by genetic abnormalities of the long (q) arm of chromosome 15 (15q11-q13).Affected infants have poor muscle tone and feed poorly at birth. Later their appetite becomes voracious and they become obese, have behavior problems (irritability, tantrums), delayed development, short stature, and, later, hypogonadotropic hypogonadism.

- Bardet–Biedl syndrome

The Bardet–Biedl syndrome is an autosomal recessive disorder characterized by obesity and several other abnormalities, including microorchidism in men, intellectual disability (mental retardation), retinal dystrophy, polydactyly, renal malformations (particularly calyceal abnormalities), and polyuria and polydipsia[18]. The primary cilia dysfunction is considered as a key defect in this syndrome [19].

Genetic models of obesity

- Leptin gene

The Lep gene codes for a protein called leptin [20]. Leptin-deficient mice have hyperphagia, insulin resistance, hyperinsulinemia, and infertility. In human, leptin is produced in fat cells and to a lesser degree in the gut [20]. It acts on leptin receptors (LEPRs), which are widely distributed and account for its pleiotropic effects on energy homeostasis, neuroendocrine function, and immune function [21].Food intake is reduced by systemic leptin administration in normal-weight experimental animals, but the response decreases as the animals become obese. The resistance to the action of leptin has been related to blunting the negative feedback signal to brain to reduce energy intake.

- Leptin receptor gene

The Leptin receptor (LEPR) deficiency has a relationship with human obesity. In a study, 3% with severe, early-onset obesity had nonsense or missense LEPR mutations. Normal linear growth, but reduced adult height as adults and increased serum leptin concentrations were also observed [22, 23].

http://dx.doi.org/10.5772/61044

- Agouti gene

The Agouti gene defect causes the Agouti-signaling protein overexpressed in many tissues. The Agouti protein competes with melanocyte-stimulating hormone (MSH) for a melanocortin-4 receptor in the hypothalamus that modulates food intake. MSH inhibits food intake. Food over-intake results from the blockage of MSH pathway by the agouti protein [24].

Other factors associated with the development of obesity, such as body fact distribution, diet, lifestyle, drugs, and endocrine disorders, have promote the dysregulation of fat and glucose metabolism. Now scientists understand that fat, especially intra-abdominal fat, has significant impact on blood pressure and blood lipid levels and interferes with the ability to use insulin effectively.

Obesity and coronary artery disease

In the past two decades, the growing development in vascular biology has been elucidating the nature of atherosclerotic lesions: they correspond to a series of cellular and molecular inflammatory responses [25, 26].

The coronary endothelial dysfunction is considered an early stage of the coronary arteriosclerosis. Arteriosclerosis develops through the influence of stress conditions to the endothelium, such as obesity, aging, systemic arterial high blood pressure,hypercholesterolemia, diabetes, and tobacco addiction. These factors damage the endothelium and induce an inflammatory reaction on the vascular wall. Such reaction increases the secretion of primary proinflammatory cytokines, such as interleukin (IL)-1 and tumor necrosis factor-alpha (TNF-α) [27, 28].

In fact, adipose tissue is considered not only a deposition of triacylglycerol and free fatty acids but also an important endocrine and paracrine organ, which produces several proinflammatory substances [29]. An excess of adipose tissue indicates that obesity is being regarded as a source of proinflammatory mediators that contribute to vascular injury, insulin resistance, and atherogenesis. The adipokines, which play an important role of endothelium dysfunction and arteriosclerosis, include C-reactive protein (CRP), TNF-α, angiotensinogen, resistin, leptin, IL-6, and plasminogen activator inhibitor-1 (PAI-1).

Main inflammatory markers in obesity

- C-reactive protein (CRP): The CRP is an acute phase protein (APP) synthesized in the liver and regulated by the circulating levels of IL-6. Recently, high levels of CRP in plasma were considered as independent predictors of coronary artery disease [30]. Circulating plasma levels of CRP are high in obese and are directly related to the amount of body fat, estimated by means of body mass index, visceral obesity, abdominal circumference, insulin resistance, metabolic syndrome, and diabetes mellitus [31].

- The CRP participates directly in the process of atherogenesis and modulates the endothelial function. It also induces the expression of several molecules (intercellular adhesion molecule-1 (ICAM-1), vascular cell adhesion molecule-1 (VCAM-1), monocyte chemoattractant protein-1 (MCP-1), and selectins). It acts as regulator of the production of nitric oxide in the endothelium and coordinates the production and secretion of several cytokines, increasing the proinflammatory activity of several adipokines [32].

- TNF-α: High amounts of secretion of inflammatory cytokine produced by obese individuals and by insulin-resistant patients not only give rise, but spread the formation of atherosclerotic lesion. The TNF-α participates in the acceleration of atherogenesis by inducing the expression of VCAM-1, ICAM-1, MCP-1, and E-selectin. It also reduces the bioavailability of nitric oxide in endothelial cells and impairs endothelium-dependant vasodilation, promoting the endothelial dysfunction. Besides this, it causes apoptosis in endothelial cells, contributing for endothelial injury [33].
- Resistin: It is a hormone specific of the adipose tissue recently discovered, which directly induces the insulin resistance in muscles and liver. The resistin induces the expression of messenger RNA producer of endothelin-1 in endothelial cells, thus contributing to endothelial dysfunction. It also significantly increases the expression of the cellular adhesion molecule VCAM-1 and the MCP-1, hey factors in formation of early atherosclerotic lesion [34]. It was recently demonstrated the proinflammatory action of resistin in smooth muscle cells: it induces the proliferation of such cells, suggesting the action of these hormones is restenosis of coronary lesions in patients with diabetes [35].
- Angiotensinogen: It is a precursor of angiotensin II, expressed and produced in adipocytes. The angiotensin II directly stimulates the expression of ICAM-1, VCAM-1, MCP-1, and M-CSF in vascular cells. The increased production of angiotensinogen by the adipose tissue is associated with high blood pressure and angiogenesis, both related to endothelial dysfunction. Similarly, the angiotensin II acts in the formation of oxygen-derived free radicals, decreasing the availability of nitric oxide and causing damages to the vascular tissue [36].
- Adiponectin: Opposed to what happens to other adipokines already referred to, the levels of adiponectin are lower in obese patients, functioning as an inhibitor agent of the inflammatory process [37]. Clinical and experimental studies suggest that low levels of adiponectin contribute for the development of diseases related to obesity, including cardiovascular diseases [38]. Levels of adiponectin in plasma generally range from 3 to30 µg/ml in healthy individuals. In obese individuals, these levels are significantly reduced, with negative correlation between BMI and adiponectin levels in plasma [39]. The reason for the reduction of the levels of adiponectin in obese individuals seem to be related with proinflammatory cytokines, such as the IL-6, which, due to the fact they increase in obese individuals, may cause a reduction in the expression of the messenger RNA producer of adiponectin and its release by adipocytes [40]. In vascular levels, actions of the adiponectin comprise reduction in expression of ICAM-1, VCAM-1, and E-selectin.

5. Obesity and its related heart disease

Obesity increases total blood volume and cardiac output, and cardiac workload is greater in obesity. Typically, obese patients have a higher cardiac output but a lower level of total peripheral resistance at any given level of arterial pressure. With increased filling pressure and volume, overweight and obese individuals often develop left ventricular (LV) chamber dilation and the risk of left ventricular hypertrophy also increases [41]. In addition to LV structural abnormalities, obesity also leads to left atrial enlargement, both from increased circulating blood volume as well as abnormal LV diastolic filling [42]. These abnormalities not only increase the risk of heart failure, but may increase the risk of atrial fibrillation.

- Obesity and hypertension

A study [43] showed that activation of the sympathetic nervous system has been considered to have an important function in the pathogenesis of obesity-related hypertension. Plasma renin activity, angiotensinogen, angiotensin II, and aldosterone values display significant increase during obesity. Insulin resistance and inflammation may promote an altered profile of vascular function and consequently hypertension. Leptin and other neuropeptides are possible links between obesity and the development of hypertension.

The arterial pressure control mechanism of diuresis and natriuresis, according to the principle of infinite feedback gain, seems to be shifted toward higher blood pressure levels in obese individuals.

- Obesity and Heart failure

A study of 5,881 Framingham Heart Study participants [44] showed that during a 14-year follow-up, heart failure developed in 496 participants (258 women and 238 men). The crude cumulative incidence and the age-adjusted incidence rates of heart failure increased across categories of body mass index for both men and women. For every 1 kg/m^2 increment in BMI, the risk of heart failure increased 5% in men and 7% in women. In fact, a graded increase in the risk of HF was observed across all categories of BMI.

The strength of the association, the stepwise increase in the risk of heart failure across increasing categories of body mass index, the demonstration of a temporal sequence (with increased body mass index preceding the development of heart failure), and the consistency of results in multiple analyses suggest a causal relation between increased body mass index and heart failure.

Obesity and arrhythmias

- Atrial fibrillation (Af)

The mechanisms linking atrial fibrillation and obesity include: structural and electrophysiological atrial remodeling, metabolic factors, sympathovagal imbalance, clinical links (obstructive sleep apnea, cardiovascular comorbidities) and inflammation.

Based on a population-based cohort studies [45], obese individuals have an associated 49% increased risk of developing Af compared to non-obese individuals (relative risk 1.49, 95% confidence interval 1.36–1.64). The risk of atrial fibrillation increased in parallel with greater BMI in this cohort. Thus, Af evolves as yet another pathogenic factor by which obesity may increase cardiovascular and cerebrovascular events. In contrast, in the postcardiac surgery studies, obese individuals do not have an associated increased risk of developing Af compared to non-obese individuals (relative risk 1.02, 95% confidence interval 0.99–1.06) [45].

- Ventricular arrhythmias

The another commonly reported arrhythmias resulting from obesity is ventricular tachycardia. The main mechanisms leading to ventricular arrhythmia and sudden cardiac death in obese individuals include cardiomyopathy, metabolic factors, sympathetic hyperinnervation, obesity-induced electrophysiological remodeling, coronary heart disease as common comorbidity and radical weight reduction strategies. Electrocardiographic monitoring, including P wave and QT interval duration, are extremely important in obese patients [46].

A positive association between corrected QT (QTc) interval and BMI has been noted, and prolonged QTc has predicted increased mortality even in apparently healthy populations. Although a relationship between QTc and increased obesity has been noted in many studies, this is most evident in the severely obese [47]. The presence of late potentials may be related to some of the pathological changes noted with cardiomyopathy of obesity, including myocyte hypertrophy, fibrosis, and fat. Finally, obesity is associated with abnormalities in sympathovagal balance, leading to higher heart rate and reduced heart rate variability, known factors related with increased risk of sudden cardiac death (SCD).

Overwhelming evidence supports the importance of obesity in the pathogenesis and progression of heart diseases, with increased indexes of morbidity and mortality. If the obesity epidemic continues, human may soon witness an unfortunate end in life.

6. Evaluation

Determine etiology

Many factors contribute to obesity. However, most cases of obesity are related to factors such as a sedentary lifestyle and increased caloric intake [48].

To determine etiology, the medical history should include age at onset and duration of weight gain, any habit change and events associated with weight gain, previous weight loss attempts, change in dietary patterns, exercise, current and past medications, and history of smoking. Medications are a common cause of weight gain and obesity, in particular insulin, sulfonylureas, thiazolidinediones, and antipsychotics agent.

Physical examination should focus on the possible secondary cause of obesity, including thyroid goiter (hypothyroidism), proximal muscle weakness, purple striae, osteoporosis (Cushing's syndrome), and acne/hirsutism. The related vital sign change (e.g., Blood pressure and heart rate) and testing (e.g., laboratory tests) to assess other metabolic diseases associated with obesity are also important to evaluate overweight and obese individuals.

Assessment of risk

To assess an individual's risk for subsequent mortality, the degree of overweight (BMI) and the presence of abdominal obesity (waist circumference), cardiovascular risk factors, comorbidities, and other factors should be measured.

- Cardiovascular risk factors

Risk factors for CVD include high blood pressure (hypertension) and smoking, dysregulation of blood cholesterol (reduced levels of high-density lipoprotein [HDL] or elevated levels of low-density lipoprotein [LDL]), diabetes, sleep apnea, lack of exercise, family history of heart disease, and ethnic background. These risk factors should be managed independent of weight loss efforts.

- Comorbidities and other factor
  - Symptomatic osteoarthritis: The disease is associated with obesity that do not increase cardiovascular risk. The precise mechanism by which obesity leads to osteoarthritis remains unknown but is likely to be due to a combination of mechanical, humoral, and genetic factors. Weight loss has clear medical benefits for the obese patient and seems to be a logical way of relieving joint pain associated with degenerative arthritis [49].
  - Pregnancy: Women have more fat as a percent of body weight than men from puberty onward and tend to gain more fat during adult life than men. Being overweight increases the risk of complications for pregnant women and their babies. The higher a woman's BMI, the higher the risks. The increasing risks are in relation to: gestational diabetes and miscarriage, high blood pressure and preeclampsia, blood clots, and having a baby weighing more than 4 kg.
  - Age of onset: Children with a low birth weight and those whose weight rises more rapidly in the first 10 years are at high risk for diabetes as adults [50].

7. Treatment

The goal of treatment for obesity is to lose weight in order to improve your health, both physically and psychologically. For example, losing weight may help you to improve your self-esteem or help you to decrease the risk of coronary artery disease.

Types of treatment—Based on patient's measurements and medical history, doctor or nurse can determine what combination of weight loss treatments would work best. Treatments may include changes in lifestyle, exercise, dieting and, in some cases, weight loss medicines or weight loss surgery.

- Importance of weight loss

The importance of weight loss in obese subjects is that obesity is associated with many health risks, including hypertension, heart failure, coronary artery disease, dyslipidemia, and diabetes.The higher the BMI and waist circumference, the greater the risk.

One study indicated that overweight/obese women with obesity-related illness, who lost weight intentionally within 1 year, had significantly reduced mortality rates of 19–25%. In contrast, studies of overweight/obese diabetics irrespective of gender showed significant benefit of intentional weight loss on mortality in a meta-analysis, hazard ratios = 0.75 (0.67–0.83) [51].

- Treatment options

It is important to set goals when discussing a weight loss program with an individual patient. Many nervous patients have a weight loss goal of 40% or more below current weight, which is unrealistic. A realistic weight loss goal will make a better initial point. An initial weight loss goal of 5–7% of body weight is realistic for most individuals [52].A weight loss of more than 5% can reduce risk factors for cardiovascular disease, such as dyslipidemia, hypertension, and diabetes mellitus [53]. In trials comparing pharmacologic therapy with placebo, weight loss of 10–15% using both drug and behavioral intervention is considered a very good response, and weight loss exceeding 15% is considered an excellent response. Thus, the clinician and the patient need to come to a mutual understanding of the realities of weight loss.

Individuals with a BMI of 25–29.9 kg/m^2, who do not have risk factors for cardiovascular disease or other obesity related comorbidities, may be described as having low risk. They should receive counseling on prevention of weight gain. Individuals with a BMI between 25 and 29.9 kg/m^2 and with one or more risk factors for CVD (diabetes, hypertension, and dyslipidemia), or with a BMI of 30–34.9 kg/m^2, are at moderate risk. They should be counseled about weight loss interventions.

- Types of treatment

  - Changes in lifestyle: lifestyle modification is the most essential and gentle method of body weight loss. It is also physician's first choice. A comprehensive lifestyle intervention (combined diet, exercise, and behavioral treatment) is the most important strategy for weight management. The behavioral component facilitates adherence to diet and exercise regimens. It includes regular self-monitoring of food intake, physical activity, and body weight. Some behavioral components were used to help achieve these weight loss goals, including behavioral self-management training, individual case managers, group and/or individual sessions, individualized adherence strategies, and a network of training, feedback, and clinical support [54].

  - Exercise and dietary therapy: Exercise and dietary therapy remain essential to the treatment of obesity, even for patients who choose medications or surgery. In most studies, exercise modestly improves weight loss and show an association between higher levels of physical activity and lower rates of many chronic diseases, such as obesity [55]. The multicomponent exercise program should be designed to prevent the possibility of exercise injury and to fit individuals, who can receive a pre-exercise evaluation by physicians. A well-designed exercise program should include balanced training and flexibility, and aerobic exercise and high-intensity resistance training may be effective. The duration and the energy expenditure goal should also fit individuals.

The goal of dietary therapy is to reduce the calories consumed. Balanced low-calorie diets/portion-controlled diets with low-fat diets and low-carbohydrate diets are the components of the commonly used dietary therapy to reach the goal of calories restriction. However, the over- or rapid decrease of calories may lead to side effects such as mentioned below.

Weight loss medicines or weight loss surgery

Drug therapy is not the first choice, but it is recommended for patients with a BMI greater than 30 kg/m^2, or a BMI of 27–29.9 kg/m^2 if they have comorbid conditions, such as hypertension, heart failure, coronary artery disease, diabetes, etc.

- Orlistat, as the drug to alter fat digestion, has cardiovascular safety and beneficial effects on serum total cholesterol and low-density lipoprotein concentrations. The recommended dose for patients who are candidates for pharmacologic therapy is 120 mg three times per day. Orlistat does not alter the pharmacokinetics of many drugs. However, absorption of fat-soluble vitamins may be decreased by orlistat. Patients with orlistat therapy should be advised to take a multivitamin. For patients taking warfarin, a decrease in vitamin K may be related to a higher bleeding tendency.Reduction in the dose of warfarin with INR regular monitor are recommended.

- Lorcaserin, as the drug of serotonin agonist, is approved as an addition to a reduced-calorie diet and exercise for patients who are obese (BMI ≥30 kg/m^2) or overweight (BMI ≥27 kg/m^2) with at least one medical comorbidity, such as type 2 diabetes, hypertension, heart failure, dyslipidemia, or sleep apnea [56, 57]. Lorcaserin appears to have similar efficacy as and fewer adverse effects than orlistat, although long-term safety data are limited.

- Diabetes drugs, such as metformin, exenatide, and liraglutide, are suitable for diabetic patients with obesity. In one trial of patients with obesity and the metabolic syndrome, patients receiving metformin lost significantly more weight (1–2 kg) than the placebo group [58]. The weight loss efficacy of the other two drugs, as GLP-1 receptor agonists, has been reported in trials. In the United State, liraglutide is available for diabetic patients with body mass index (BMI) ≥30 kg/m^2 or ≥27 kg/m^{2}with at least one obesity related comorbidity.

- Combination drugs: Phentermine–topiramate combination was compared with placebo in 2487 adults with BMI of 27–45 kg/m^2 and two or more comorbidities [59]. After 1 year, mean weight loss was greater in those assigned to treatment (8–10% versus 1.4 kg with placebo [8–10% versus 1.2% of baseline bodyweight]). Unfortunately, the combination was less effective in further weight loss in the second year.

- Bariatric surgery is only considered for patients with BMI ≥40 kg/m^2 who have "failed" to lose weight with diet, exercise, and drug therapy.

- Risks of treatment—treatments for obesity can be divided according to the risk of side effects.

- The side effects of orlistat include intestinal borborygmi and cramps, flatus, fecal incontinence, oily spotting, and flatus with discharge.

- In clinical trials [44, 45], the most common side effect of lorcaserin was headache, experienced by about 18% of drug arm participants compared to 11% of placebo participants. The other side effects are as follows: upper respiratory tract infection (14.8% vs. 11.9%), sinusitis (7.2% vs. 8.2%), and nausea (7.5% vs. 5.4%).

- The most common adverse events verse placebo in these trials of phentermine–topiramate combination were dry mouth (13–21%vs. 2%), constipation (15–17% versus 6%), and paresthesia (14–21%vs. 2%) [59].

- The most common adverse effects of bariatric surgery were iron deficiency anemia and the need for reoperations.

8. Conclusion

The general consensus is that excess intake of calories from any source and physical inactivity, associated with a sedentary lifestyle, causes weight gain and obesity. The strong evidences from trials, studies, and guidelines have been reported that obesity and its related comorbidity increase the risk of mortality. The benefits of weight loss are also seen. However, it is not good enough to just decrease body weight.

A well-designed weight loss program for individuals includes the weight loss goal, preexercise evaluation, exercise program, diet therapy, and the adequate medication—"Right drug, Right does, Right population" for these obese patients with comorbidities.

Even though obesity increases prevalence year by year, we must look forward to the challenge of reversing this epidemic and have confidence in our future.

Appendices and nomenclatures

Waist circumference measurement sites:

1. Locate upper hip bone and top of right iliac crest.

2. Place measuring tape in horizontal plane around abdomen at iliac crest.

3. Ensure tape in sung but does not compress the skin.

4. Tape should be parallel to floor.

5. Record measurement at the end of a normal expiration.

Author details

Jian-Lin Wu[1] and Chi-Wen Juan[1,2*]

*Address all correspondence to: juanchiwen@yahoo.com.tw

1 Department of Family Medicine, Kuang Tien General Hospital, Taichung, Taiwan

2 Department of Nursing, Hung Kuang University, Taichung, Taiwan

References

[1] Hu FB, Li TY, Colditz GA, et al. Television watching and other sedentary behaviors in relation to risk of obesity and type 2 diabetes mellitus in women. JAMA 2003; 289: 1785.

[2] Jensen MD, Ryan DH, Apovian CM, et al. 2013 AHA/ACC/TOS guideline for the management of overweight and obesity in adults: a report of the American College of Cardiology/American Heart Association Task Force on Practice Guidelines and The Obesity Society. Circulation 2014; 129:S102.

[3] Jensen MD, Ryan DH, Apovian CM, et al. 2013 AHA/ACC/TOS guideline for the management of overweight and obesity in adults: a report of the American College of Cardiology/American Heart Association Task Force on Practice Guidelines and The Obesity Society. Circulation 2014; 129:S102.

[4] Ogden CL, Carroll MD, Kit BK, Flegal KM. Prevalence of childhood and adult obesity in the United States, 2011–2012. JAMA 2014; 311(8):806–814.

[5] Strauss RS, Pollack HA. Epidemic increase in childhood overweight, 1986–1998. JAMA 2001; 286: 2845.

[6] Kelly AS, Barlow SE, Rao G, et al. Severe obesity in children and adolescents: identification, associated health risks, and treatment approaches: a scientific statement from the American Heart Association. Circulation 2013; 128: 1689.

[7] Skinner AC, Skelton JA.Prevalence and trends in obesity and severe obesity among children in the United States, 1999–2012. JAMA Pediatr 2014; 168: 561.

[8] Kelly AS, Barlow SE, Rao G, et al. Severe obesity in children and adolescents: identification, associated health risks, and treatment approaches: a scientific statement from the American Heart Association.Circulation 2013.

[9] Flegal KM, Wei R, Ogden CL, et al. Characterizing extreme values of body mass index-for-age by using the 2000 Centers for Disease Control and Prevention growth charts.Am J ClinNutr 2009;90:1314.

[10] Gulati AK, Kaplan DW, Daniels SR. Clinical tracking of severely obese children: a new growth chart. Pediatrics 2012; 130: 1136.

[11] Ogden CL, Carroll MD, Kit BK, Flegal KM. Prevalence of childhood and adult obesity in the United States, 2011–2012. JAMA 2014; 311: 806.

[12] Centers for Disease control and Prevention, Overweight and Obesity. http://www.cdc.gov/obesity/data/adult.html (accessed on September 09, 2013)

[13] Ng M, Fleming T, Robinson M, et al. Global, regional, and national prevalence of overweight and obesity in children and adults during 1980–2013: a systematic analysis for the Global Burden of Disease Study 2013. Lancet 2014; 384: 766.

[14] Swinburn BA, Sacks G, Hall KD, et al. The global obesity pandemic: shaped by global drivers and local environments. Lancet 2011; 378: 804.

[15] International Association for the Study of Obesity http://www.iaso.org/resources/world-map-obesity/ (accessed on February 06, 2014).

[16] Ogden CL, Carroll MD, Kit BK, Flegal KM. Prevalence of childhood and adult obesity in the United States, 2011–2012. JAMA 2014; 311(8):806–814.

[17] Skinner AC, Skelton JA. Prevalence and trends in obesity and severe obesity among children in the United States,1999–2012.JAMA Pediatr 2014.

[18] Parfrey PS, Davidson WS, Green JS.Clinical and genetic epidemiology of inherited renal disease in Newfoundland. Kidney Int 2002; 61: 1925.

[19] Marion V, Stoetzel C, Schlicht D, et al. Transient ciliogenesis involving Bardet–Biedl syndrome proteins is a fundamental characteristic of adipogenic differentiation. ProcNatlAcadSci U S A 2009; 106: 1820.

[20] [20]Dardeno TA, Chou SH, Moon HS, et al.Leptin in human physiology and therapeutics. Front Neuroendocrinol 2010; 31: 377.

[21] Procaccini C, Jirillo E, Matarese G. Leptin as an immunomodulator. Mol Aspects Med 2012; 33: 35.

[22] Clément K, Vaisse C, Lahlou N, et al. A mutation in the human leptin receptor gene causes obesity and pituitary dysfunction. Nature 1998; 392: 398.

[23] Farooqi IS, Wangensteen T, Collins S, et al. Clinical and molecular genetic spectrum of congenital deficiency of the leptin receptor. N Engl J Med 2007; 356: 237.

[24] Mountjoy KG. Functions for pro-opiomelanocortin-derived peptides in obesity and diabetes.Biochem J 2010; 428: 305.

[25] Rocha VZ, Libby P.Obesity,inflammation,and atherosclerosis.Nat Rev Cardiol. 2009; 6 (6): 399–409.

[26] Serrano CV Jr, Souza JA, Paiva MSMO. Fatoresdesencadeantes da instabilização da placaateroscler ótica.RevSocCardiol Estado de São Paulo.2001; 4: 724–32.

[27] Fernandes JL, Soeiro A, Ferreira CB, Serrano CV Jr. Síndromescoronáriasagudas e inflamação. Rev SocCardiol Estado de São Paulo.2006; 3: 178–87.

[28] Serrano CV Jr, Souza JA, Heinisch RH.Aagressão vascular no desencadeamento das síndromesisquêmicasmiocárdicasinstáveis. In: Nicolau JC, Marin JA.(eds.). Síndromesisquêmicasmiocárdicasinstáveis. São Paulo: Atheneu; 2001. p. 25–36.

[29] Mazurek T, Zhang L, Zalewski A. Human epicardial adipose tissue is a source of inflammatory mediators.Circulation.2003;108;2460–6.

[30] Ridker PM. Clinical application of C-reactive protein for cardiovascular disease detection and prevention.Circulation.2003; 107: 363–9.

[31] Pasceri V, Willerson JT, Yeh ET. Direct proinflammatory effect of C-reactive protein on human endothelial cells. Circulation 2000; 102: 2165–8.

[32] Lemieux I, Pascot A, Prud'home D, Alméras N, Bogaty P, Nadeau A, et al. Elevated C-reactive protein: another component of the atherothrombotic profile of abdominal obesity. Arterioscler ThrombVasc Biol.2001; 21:961–7.

[33] Hotamisligil G, Arner P, Caro JF, Atkinson RL, Spiegelman BM. Increased adipose tissue expression of tumor necrosis factor-alpha in human obesity and insulin resistence. J Clin Invest.1995; 95: 2409–15.

[34] Steppan CM, Bailey ST, Bhat S, Brown EJ, Banerjee RR, Wright CM, et al. The hormone resistin links obesity to diabetes. Nature.2001; 409: 307–12.

[35] Calabro P, Samudio I, Willerson JT, Yeh ET. Resistin promotes smooth muscle cell proliferation through activation of extracellular signal-regulated kinase 1/2 and phosphatidylinositol 3-kinase pathways. Circulation.2004; 10: 3335–40.

[36] Tham DM, Martin-McNulty B, Wang YX, Wilson DW, Vergona R, Sullivan ME, et al. Angiotensin II is associated with activation of NF-B-associated genes and downregulation of PPARs. Physiol Genomics.2002; 11: 21–30.

[37] Hopkins T, Ouchi N, Shibata R, Walsh K. Adiponectin actions in the cardiovascular system. Cardiovasc Res.2007; 74: 11–8.

[38] Arita Y, Kihara S, Ouchi N, Takahashi M, Maeda K, Miyagawa J, et al. Paradoxical decrease of an adipose-especific protein, adiponectin, in obesity. BiochemBiophys Res Commun.1999; 270: 79–83.

[39] Ouchi N, Kihara S, Funahashi T. Obesity, adiponectin and vascular inflammatory disease. CurrOpin Lipidol.2003; 14: 561–6.

[40] Ouchi N, Kihara S, Arita Y, Okamoto Y, Maeda K, Kuriyama H, et al. Adiponectin, an adipocyte-derived plasma protein, inhibits endothelial NFkappaB signaling through a cAMP-dependent pathway. Circulation.2000; 102: 1296–301.

[41] Carl J. Lavie, MD, Richard V. Milani, MD, Hector O. Ventura, MD. Obesity and Cardiovascular Disease: Risk Factor, Paradox, and Impact of Weight Loss doi:10.1016/j.jacc.2008.12.068.

[42] Alpert MA. Obesity cardiomyopathy: pathophysiology and evolution of the clinical syndrome Am J Med Sci 2001; 321: 225–236.

[43] Kotsis VI, Stabouli S, Papakatsika S, Rizos Z, Parati G. Mechanisms of obesity-induced hypertension. Hypertens Res. 2010 May; 33(5):386–93. doi: 10.1038/hr.2010.9.

[44] Kenchaiah S, Evans JC, Levy D, et al. Obesity and the risk of heart failure N Engl J Med 2002; 347: 305–313.

[45] Wanahita N, Messerli FH, Bangalore S, et al. Atrial fibrillation and obesity—results of a meta-analysis Am Heart J 2008; 155: 310–315.

[46] [46]Mozos I.Arrhythmia risk and obesity.J Mol Genet Med 2014: S1.

[47] el-Gamal A, Gallagher D, Nawras A, et al. Effects of obesity on QT, RR, and QTc intervals. Am J Cardiol 1995;75: 956–959.

[48] Tsai AG, Wadden TA. In the clinic: obesity. Ann Intern Med 2013; 159:ITC3.

[49] Sridhar MS, Jarrett CD, Xerogeanes JW, Labib SA.Obesity and symptomatic osteoarthritis of the knee. J Bone Joint Surg Br. 2012 Apr; 94(4):433–40. doi: 10.1302/0301-620X.94B4.27648.

[50] [50]Bhargava SK, Sachdev HS, Fall CH, et al. Relation of serial changes in childhood body-mass index to impaired glucose tolerance in young adulthood.N Engl J Med 2004; 350:865.

[51] Poobalan AS, Aucott LS, Smith WC, et al. Long-term weight loss effects on all cause mortality in overweight/obese populations. Obes Rev 2007; 8:503.

[52] National Institutes of Health, National Heart, Lung,and Blood Institute. The Practical Guide: Identification, Evaluation, and Treatment of Overweight and Obesity in Adults. NIH Publication Number 00-4084, October 2000. http://www.nhlbi.nih.gov/guidelines/obesity/prctgdc.pdf (accessed on December 05, 2011).

[53] Diabetes Prevention Program (DPP) Research Group. The Diabetes Prevention Program (DPP): description of lifestyle intervention. Diabetes Care 2002; 25:2165.

[54] Douketis JD, Macie C, Thabane L, Williamson DF. Systematic review of long-term weight loss studies in obese adults: clinical significance and applicability to clinical practice. Int J Obes (Lond) 2005; 29:1153.

[55] Physical Activity Guidelines Advisory Committee.Physical Activity Guidelines Advisory Committee Report, 2008.US Department of Health and Human Services, Washington, DC, 2008.

[56] FDA News and Events: FDA approves Belviq to treat some overweight or obese adults (accessed on June 29, 2012). http://www.fda.gov/NewsEvents/Newsroom/PressAnnouncements/ucm309993.htm?utm_campaign=Google2&utm_source=fdaSearch&utm_medium=website&utm_term=lorcaserin&utm_content=4

[57] FDA Highlights of Prescribing Information: BELVIQ (lorcaserin hydrochloride) tablets, for oral use (accessed on September 17, 2012). http://www.accessdata.fda.gov/drugsatfda_docs/label/2012/022529lbl.pdf

[58] Fontbonne A, Charles MA, Juhan-Vague I, et al. The effect of metformin on the metabolic abnormalities associated with upper-body fat distribution. BIGPRO Study Group. Diabetes Care 1996; 19: 920.

[59] Gadde KM, Allison DB, Ryan DH, et al. Effects of low-dose, controlled-release, phentermine plus topiramate combination on weight and associated comorbidities in overweight and obese adults (CONQUER): a randomised, placebo-controlled, phase 3 trial. Lancet 2011; 377: 1341.

Chapter 12

Prevention of Coronary Artery Disease through Diet

Oguzhan Yildiz, Melik Seyrek and Kemal Gokhan Ulusoy

Additional information is available at the end of the chapter

http://dx.doi.org/10.5772/61339

Abstract

Our understanding of the potential role of diet in the prevention and risk reduction of coronary artery disease (CAD) has evolved in the past 100 years. Data on trends in food consumption and ecological studies are the early evidences that showed associations between prevalence and fat intake across and within countries. The last 50 years of epidemiology and clinical trials have focused on the efficiency of nutritional interventions in the prevention of CAD.

The original diet-heart hypothesis was very simple: Cholesterol is a constituent of atherosclerotic plaque. This hypothesis was based on the differences in average population serum cholesterol levels and population rates of CAD mortality. The Seven Country study was the first to show that the intake of saturated fat varied considerably by region and populations, with the greatest intake of saturated fat were found to have the highest serum cholesterol levels. Follow-up studies confirmed that these study groups also had the highest incidence of CAD. Thus, it was thought that there was a direct relation between cholesterol in diet, cholesterol in blood, and cholesterol in the plaque and its clinical complications such as myocardial infarction (MI). These findings stimulated further inquiry to determine whether altering the diet could decrease serum cholesterol levels and, thereby, decrease the incidence of CAD. Nearly all clinical trials in the 1960s, 1970s, and 1980s compared usual diets with those characterized by low total fat, low saturated fat, low dietary cholesterol, and increased polyunsaturated fats. Actually, these diets did reduce cholesterol levels. However, they did not reduce the incidence of MI and CAD mortality. With accumulating evidence, we have now moved away from a focus on total fat and cholesterol to the importance of considering the content of fat and total calories in the diet. In other words, the type of fat, rather than the total or the ratio or balance between the saturated and certain unsaturated fats may be the determinant. Recent meta-analyses of intervention studies confirm the beneficial effects of replacing saturated with polyunsaturated fatty acid on CAD risk. Additionally, recent studies indicate that dietary patterns consistent with the traditional Mediterranean-style diets (MedD) with a strong focus on veggies, fruits, fish, whole grain, and olive oil are effective in preventing CAD to a degree greater than low-fat diets and equal to or greater than the benefit observed in statin trials. Recent secondary prevention studies have convincingly demonstrated the benefit of diets that closely followed the MedD in reducing re-infarction and clinical manifestations of CAD.

In conclusion, CAD is still a significant problem and a growing health concern worldwide. Although mortality rates from CAD have decreased due to advances in pharmacological treatments, the prevalence of cardiovascular risk factors continue to increase. The importance of diet as a key modifiable risk factor in CAD is undisputable. Nutritional interventions have proven that a complicated set of many nutrients interact to influence CAD risk. Therefore, recent guidelines consider diet as a whole and combine nutrient and energy recommendations into a healthy pattern that is nutrient dense and energy balanced.

Keywords: CAD prevention, reducing cholesterol, low-fat diets, Mediterranean diet

1. Introduction

Unfortunately, coronary artery disease (CAD) is the leading cause of morbidity and mortality worldwide despite costly aggressive drug and surgical interventions as a *first line* strategy [1]. However, these therapies fail to address the origin of the problem, that is, the most proximal risk factors for progression of atherosclerotic CAD, including poor-quality diet patterns, physical inactivity, obesity, and cigarette smoking [1, 2]. Consistent evidence from landmark epidemiological studies supports the concept that these risk factors contribute nearly 80% of population-attributable risk of cardiovascular diseases (CVD) [3-4]. Accordingly, a healthy lifestyle modification may afford close to 80% protection from CAD [5]. Therefore, lifestyle managements to reduce cardiovascular risk are of superior importance as stated in population-based strategies for cardiovascular prevention such as 2012 European guidelines [6] and the 2013 American College of Cardiology (ACC)/American Heart Association (AHA) guidelines [7].

Research on the origin of CAD has been ongoing for approximately a century [8]. From the beginning, diet played a paramount role in research on the cause of CAD. At the same time, one of the great interests was explaining differences in the incidence of CAD among populations. In the early 1900s, evidence from cross-cultural studies indicated some associations between diet and cholesterol. However, systemic associations between diet, cholesterol, and CAD were made almost after half a century. In the 1950s, cross-cultural studies indicated that endemic diets had important impact on the variation of CAD across populations [9]. Thus, it was thought that there was a direct relation between cholesterol in diet, cholesterol in blood, and cholesterol in the plaque, and its clinical complications such as myocardial infarction (MI). The findings of cross-cultural studies stimulated further inquiry to determine whether altering the diet could decrease serum cholesterol levels and, thereby, decrease the incidence of CAD. Nearly all clinical trials in the 1960s, 1970s, and 1980s compared usual diets with those characterized by low total fat, low saturated fat, low dietary cholesterol, and increased polyunsaturated fats. Actually, these diets did reduce cholesterol levels. However, they did not reduce the incidence of MI and CAD mortality. Secondary prevention trials in the 1990s, together with primary prevention approaches in the 2000s, indicate that dietary patterns consistent with the traditional Mediterranean-style diets (MedD) with a strong focus on veggies, fruits, fish, whole grain, and olive oil are effective in preventing CAD to a degree greater than low-fat diets and equal to or greater than the benefit observed in statin trials. With accumulating evidence, we have now moved away from a focus on total fat and cholesterol to the importance of considering the content of fat and total calories in the diet. In other words, the type of fat, rather than the total or the ratio or balance between the saturated and certain unsaturated fats may be the determinant. Recent meta-analyses of intervention studies confirm the beneficial effects of replacing saturated with polyunsaturated fatty acid on CAD risk. Nutritional interventions have proven that a complicated set of many nutrients interact to influence CAD risk. Therefore, recent guidelines consider diet as a whole and combine nutrient and energy recommendations into a healthy pattern that is nutrient dense and energy balanced.

This chapter begins with early studies and interventions for prevention of CAD through diet, and it continues with recent clinical trials. In the next section, we will focus on the newer "whole diet" approach, consistent with the traditional MedD, which has proven to be successful in preventing CAD. Finally, we will summarize the current state of knowledge on dietary fats and prevention of CAD by foods.

2. Diets to prevent CAD: From early studies to recent trials

2.1. Early clues that diet may prevent CAD

In 1908, A.I. Ignatowski was first to observe that cholesterol-rich food promoted atherosclerosis in rabbits [10]. Then, as reported by Finking and Hanke, Nikolai N. Anichkov showed in 1913 that cholesterol-enriched diet led to atheromatous changes such as fatty streaks and advanced atheromatous plaques in the vascular wall of rabbits that are similar to the lesions in humans with coronary atherosclerosis [11]. During the ensuing decades, atherosclerosis moved from a laboratory curiosity to a major public health concern.

Starting in the 1950s, research on atherosclerosis gained more credibility and support, as a multidisciplinary community of clinical investigators accomplished new research programs dedicated to unraveling the puzzle about pathophysiological origins and treatment of CAD. In 1952, Kinsell reported that intake of vegetable oil instead of animal fats resulted in a striking decrease in serum cholesterol and phospholipid levels [12]. Groen et al. found out that intake of vegetarian diets decreased serum cholesterol levels [13].

The first study on the variation in the occurrence of CAD across populations was published in 1916 by the Dutch physician De Langen, who observed that cholesterol levels of Dutch immigrants in the former Dutch Indies were approximately twice as high as those of native Javanese [14]. He hypothesized for the first time that differences in diet patterns could be associated difference in average population cholesterol levels. However, the first systemic association between diet, cholesterol, and CAD waited until the 1950s.

2.2. The first systemic association between diet, cholesterol, and CAD: The diet-heart hypothesis

In 1957, Angel Keys cited extensive epidemiological evidence that indicate a sequence of etiologic relations existed between the saturated fat content of the diet, serum cholesterol concentrations, and the development of CAD [9]. These observations, based on the differences in average population serum cholesterol levels and population rates of CAD mortality, played a pivotal role for the development of diet-heart hypothesis: Dietary saturated fat, and in some versions, dietary cholesterol, raise blood cholesterol, which in turn leads to coronary atherosclerosis [9]. In 1957, Keys et al. began the Seven Countries Study by surveying 12,763 men aged 40 to 59 years formed 16 cohorts in seven countries (Italy, Greece, the former Yugoslavia, the Netherlands, Finland, Japan, and the United States). Study communities were chosen for the relative uniformity of their rural laboring populations and their contrasting dietary patterns. Information on biological risk factors (e.g., serum cholesterol, blood pressure, and antrophotometric measurements) were collected and ECG was taken in addition to a physical examination. Information on diet was collected by use of 7-day food records in small samples of each cohort. The risk factor surveys were repeated after five and ten years. Through central chemical analysis of the foods consumed by randomly selected families as well as diet-recall measures, Keys and his colleagues were able to determine that both the blood cholesterol levels and the heart-attack death rates were highest in societies where fat was a major component of every meal (i.e., the US and Finland). Conversely, blood cholesterol was low and heart attacks were rare in cultures where diets were based on fresh fruit and vegetables, bread, pasta, and plenty of olive oil (i.e., the Mediterranean region). The findings of the seven countries study published in 1970 had a significant impact on CAD prevention, as it described one of the first studies to clearly show that dietary saturated fat leads to CAD, and that the relationship is mediated by serum cholesterol [15].

2.3. Dietary recommendations and clinical trials

2.3.1. Low fat/low saturated fat/increased polyunsaturated diets

Even though the three major preventable risk factors for CAD (elevated serum cholesterol levels, high blood pressure, and smoking) had been identified as early as 1956, the link between cholesterol and CAD required the results of large epidemiology studies before gaining widespread acceptance [16-18].

AHA was one of the first organizations to recommend dietary changes to decrease atherosclerosis [19]. Together with the Society for the Study of Atherosclerosis, the AHA Nutrition committee published their recommendations in 1957 [20]. In brief, it was concluded that diet might play a crucial role in the pathogenesis of atherosclerosis, and the most essential factors in the diet were the fat content and the total calories. It was also thought that the type of the fat, rather than the total or the ratio or balance between the saturated and certain unsaturated fats, might be the determinant. The same year, the AHA Nutrition Committee suggested for the first time that CAD might be prevented by treating obesity with low-fat diet [20]. The recommendations of the committee requested obese individuals to confine caloric consump-

http://dx.doi.org/10.5772/61339

tion by reducing dietary fat consumption. The following year, in 1958, Brown and Page published a paper entitled "Lowering blood lipid levels by changing food patterns" and they offered two dietary ways to treat serum cholesterol, namely, a diet containing minimum animal fat together with an increase in vegetable oil and a strict low fat diet [21]. Afterwards, by 1961, AHA's Ad Hoc Committee on Dietary Fat and Atherosclerosis recommended the reduction or control of fat consumption under medical supervision. Additionally, substitution of polyunsaturated for saturated fats to prevent atherosclerosis and decrease the risks of heart attacks and strokes were also recommended [22]. Thereafter, the importance of substitution of polyunsaturated vegetable oil for saturated fat, instead of a low-fat diet, gained widespread acceptance.

2.3.2. Dietary cholesterol reduction

In 1972, the American Medical Association (AMA) Council on Foods and Nutrition in cooperation with the Food and Nutrition Board of National Academy of Sciences-National Research Council published a joint statement that the blood cholesterol level was linked to the risk of CAD [23]. Similar with AHA guidelines, these two representative councils stressed that reasonable means should be followed to modify the nutritional conditions that contribute to elevated plasma cholesterol and triglyceride levels. The primary goals suggested were reduction in foods rich in cholesterol and partial replacement of saturated with polyunsaturated fats.

2.3.3. Clinical trials for secondary prevention of CHD

The US National Diet-Heart Study was a large, double-blind, two-year study on the effects of diet on blood cholesterol levels in both free-living and closed populations [24]. The results of the study indicated that the average change in blood cholesterol with low saturated fat, low dietary cholesterol diets was 25 and 28 mg/dl or -11 and -12% in a free-living population, while it was 36 mg/dl or -17% in the closed-institutional centers.

2.3.4. Lifestyle intervention studies for reversal of CAD

To date, a number of lifestyle intervention studies have been performed. Obtaining substantial differences in lifestyle and diet between the experimental and control groups is complicated. Moreover, it is almost impossible to avoid an aftereffect of a healthy lifestyle and diet advice from the experimental group to the control group. Therefore, comprehensive controlled trials investigating the combined effects of diet and a healthy lifestyle on disease end points in individuals are difficult to perform and expensive.

In 1948, the Framingham Heart Study—under the direction of the National Heart Institute (now known as the National Heart, Lung, and Blood Institute or NHLBI)—embarked on an ambitious project in health research [25]. The objective of the Framingham Heart Study was to identify the common factors or characteristics that contribute to CAD by following its development over a long period of time in men and women free of these conditions at the outset. The first person was examined in September 1948 and four years later 5,209 persons had received their first examination. The group has now been followed in the study for 24 subsequent biennial examinations. As changes in early detection and treatment of CVD advance, prospective epidemiology is needed to document the value and impact of these changes in an organized fashion. The availability of prospective data on two generations adds to the uniqueness of the Framingham Study among ongoing studies of CAD epidemiology [26].

As a result of corroborative evidence from prospective population studies such as the Framingham study, the scientific community focused on systemic intervention studies to test whether reducing risk factors would reduce disease incidence. Nearly all clinical trials in the 1960s, 1970s, and 1980s compared usual diets with those characterized by low total fat, low saturated fat, low dietary cholesterol, and increased polyunsaturated fats. Unsurprisingly, the reduction in cardiovascular mortality and total mortality was greater in the secondary prevention trials and appeared to be dependent on the baseline cholesterol levels; that is, the higher the baseline risk the greater the obtained benefit.

In 1970, the Oslo Study dealed with 412 men, aged 30 to 64 years, randomized one to two years after a first MI [27]. A diet low in saturated fats and cholesterol,and high in polyunsaturated fats was recommended for the experimental group. After 11 years, a significantly reduced MI mortality in the original diet group was found (32 versus 57, $P = 0.004$). The total number of coronary deaths (fatal MI and sudden death) was 79 in the diet group and 94 in the control group ($P = 0.097$). The CAD mortality was correlated with age, serum cholesterol level, blood pressure, body weight, smoking habits, and a combination of these risk factors.

An early example of a primary prevention trial that used an intervention with regard to more than 1 factor is the first Oslo trial [28]. In this trial, intervention was focused on both diet and smoking. A total of 16,202 men, aged 40 to 49 years, were screened for coronary risk factors. Of these, 1,232 healthy, normotensive men at high risk of CAD were selected for a five-year randomized trial to show whether the lowering of serum lipids and cessation of smoking could reduce the incidence of CAD. These men had high serum cholesterol levels (7.5 to 9.8 mmol/L), were mostly smokers (80%), had systolic blood pressures below 150 mm Hg, and were at very high risk for CAD. They were randomized into two groups; the patients in the intervention group were recommended to lower their blood lipids by change of diet and to stop smoking, and the control group did not receive any advice. The advised diet was low in saturated fat and high in fiber. Saturated fat intake decreased from 18% to 8% of the total energy intake, and saturated fat was partly replaced by n-6 polyunsaturated fatty acids. During the trial, mean serum cholesterol concentrations were approximately 13% lower in the intervention group than in the control group. This difference was in agreement with the difference in fatty acid composition of the diet between the two groups. Besides the difference in diet, 25% of smokers in the experimental group stopped smoking compared with 17% in the control group. At the end of the observation period, the incidence of MI (fatal and non-fatal) and sudden death was 47% lower in the intervention group than in the controls. When the incidence of strokes was added, the difference between the groups was still significant. The reduction in

http://dx.doi.org/10.5772/61339

incidence in the intervention group was correlated with the reduction in total cholesterol, and to a lesser extent, with smoking reduction. It was concluded that, in healthy middle-aged men at high risk of CAD, advice to change eating habits and to stop smoking significantly reduced the incidence of the first event of MI and sudden death.

A large prospective cohort study is the Chicago Heart Association Detection Project in Industry (CHA), which screened blood pressure, cholesterol level, and smoking [28]. Risk factor data were available for 6,766 middle-aged men and women, aged 36 to 64 years. The age-adjusted relative risks of coronary heart disease mortality for low-risk persons compared with those who smoked and had elevated cholesterol and blood pressure levels varied between 0.08 in CHA men aged 18 to 39 years and 0.23 in CHA men aged 40 to 59 years. The life expectancy of persons at low risk was 9.5 years longer in CHA men aged 18 to 39 years and 5.8 years longer in CHA women aged 40 to 59 years compared with persons at elevated risk. These results illustrate the great impact of low risk factor levels on coronary heart disease risk and health in general.

However, the Multiple Risk Factor Intervention Trial (MRFIT), a US multicenter clinical trial, was an unsuccessful large prospective cohort study [29]. The risk factor data were available for more than 360,000 men aged 35 to 57 years. The participants were screened for blood pressure, cholesterol levels, and smoking for 16 years. In the special intervention group, hypertension was treated with standard medications, and smoking cessation was promoted. The dietary goals, reducing saturated fat to less than 8% caloric intake and cholesterol to less than 250 mg/d, with increased polyunsaturated fat (>10%), were nearly accomplished. However, despite the significant reduction in dietary fat, the changes in total cholesterol and low-density lipoprotein cholesterol after seven years of intervention were modest. Total cholesterol decreased by 2.9% in those receiving community care and 5% in those receiving special care. The end points of reduction in total mortality and coronary death were not achieved. This lack of efficacy was striking given that hypertension was better controlled and cigarette cessation was more successful in the special intervention group.

In 1990, Ornish et al. reported a prospective, randomized, controlled trial of 48 patients with angiographically documented CAD [30]. Twenty-eight patients were assigned to an experimental group (low-fat vegetarian diet, stopping smoking, stress management training, and moderate exercise). Follow-up quantitative coronary angiography was performed after intervention and compared with angiograms in 20 usual-care control patients with documented CAD. Overall, 82% of experimental-group patients had an average change towards regression. Additionally, there was angiographic evidence of progression in 53% in the control group. Coronary arteriography was repeated five years later. Additional regression was noted in 20 patients who maintained their lifestyle changes, with further progression in the 15 control patients. These patients followed a very low-fat (10%) vegetarian diet. It was noted that comprehensive lifestyle changes might be able to bring about regression of even severe coronary atherosclerosis after only one year, without use of lipid-lowering drugs.

2.4. Dietary trials for secondary prevention of CAD

2.4.1. Early trials

In 1989, Burr et al. reported the results of the Diet Reinfarction Trial, a randomized controlled trial that investigated the effect of diet on the secondary prevention of MI, involving 2,033 men [31]. The trial had a factorial design, subjects being randomized independently to receive advice or no advice regarding three dietary factors: (1) total fat intake and the ratio of polyunsaturated to saturated fat; (2) fatty fish consumption; and (3) cereal fiber intake. The results suggested that compliance with the advice was reasonably good. There was a slight (3.6%) reduction in cholesterol in those advised to decrease fat. There was no decrease in cholesterol in patients advised to increase fatty fish or cereal fiber intake. None of these three factors influenced the two-year incidence of reinfarction or cardiac death. However, patients counseled to eat fatty fish had a 29% reduction in the two-year all-cause mortality. It was suggested that the difference attributable to advice on fat was somewhat less than anticipated, partly because of failure to comply with the advice and partly because of spontaneous changes in the diets of control subjects.

The Indian Experiment of Infarct Survival Study (1989-1992), a randomized, single-blind, controlled trial, aimed to test whether a fat-reduced diet rich in soluble dietary fiber, antioxidant vitamins, and minerals reduces complications and mortality after acute MI [32]. For this aim, 406 patients with suspected acute MI were randomized to one of two low-fat diets. The experimental group was counseled on a "whole diet approach" that included increased intake of fruits, vegetables, nuts, and fish. Main outcome measures were mortality from cardiac disease and other causes, and serum lipid concentrations and compliance with diet. Total fat was reduced to 24% of daily calories in the experimental group and 28% in control group. Saturated fat was significantly reduced in the experimental group. Dietary cholesterol was 147 mg/d in the experimental group compared with 287 mg/d in the control diet. The experimental group lowered total cholesterol by 13% compared with 5% in the control diet. There was a significant reduction in the combination of nonfatal MI, fatal MI, and sudden death from 82 patients assigned to the control diet to 50 patients on the experimental diet. It was concluded that comprehensive dietary changes in conjunction with weight loss immediately after acute MI might modulate blood lipoproteins and significantly reduced complications and mortality after one year.

In the Lyon Diet Heart Study (1988-1997), a randomized, controlled trial with free-living subjects, 605 survivors of a first MI were randomized to an Mediterranean-type diet (consistent with the new AHA Dietary Guidelines) or a "prudent" low-fat diet on composite measures of the coronary recurrence rate [33]. The Mediterranean-type diet is a whole diet approach that is low in animal products and saturated fat, with an emphasis on the use of olive oil. It is rich in legumes, fruit, vegetables, and fish. Butter and cream were replaced with a canola-based margarine. The saturated fatty acid and oleic acid contents in the margarine were comparable to those in olive oil, with the exception that the margarine was higher in linoleic acid and α-

linolenic acid. Subjects in the experimental group participated in a one-hour counseling session. In contrast, control subjects received no specific dietary advice apart from that generally provided by attending physicians and hospital dietitians. The end points of the Lyon Diet Heart Study were cardiovascular death or nonfatal MI. At the end of the trial, the percentage of daily calories from fat was 30.4% in the Mediterranean diet group and 33.6% in the low-fat/low cholesterol control group. The calories derived from saturated fat were significantly lower in the Mediterranean diet group (8% vs. 11.7%), as was the daily cholesterol intake (203 vs. 312 mg/day). In addition, omega-3 consumption (from vegetables, fish, and margarine) was considerably higher and omega-6 consumption was lower for those on the Mediterranean diet. At the end of the trial, there was no significant difference between the total serum cholesterol or low-density lipoprotein cholesterol levels in those on the two diets. The trial was stopped after 27 months when an intermediate analysis showed that those on the Mediterranean diet had a 73% reduction in CVD deaths and nonfatal MI. After 46 months, despite a similar coronary risk factor profile (plasma lipids and lipoproteins, systolic and diastolic blood pressure, body mass index, and smoking status), subjects following the Mediterranean-style diet had a 50% to 70% lower risk of recurrent heart disease, as measured by three different combinations of outcome measures including (1) cardiac death and nonfatal heart attacks; (2) the preceding plus unstable angina, stroke, heart failure, and pulmonary or peripheral embolism; and (3) all of these measures plus events that required hospitalization.

2.4.2. Contemporary approach for primary prevention of CAD: Mediterranean diet

The Mediterranean diet is considered as one of the most favorable diet for cardiovascular health. It is an evidence-based diet to prevent not only CVD but also some other chronic diseases such as breast cancer, depression, colorectal cancer, diabetes, obesity, asthma, erectile dysfunction, and cognitive decline [34].

The most important feature of the Mediterranean diet seems to be a synergy between the various cardioprotective nutrients and foods [35]. In general, the Mediterranean diet is characterized by a high intake of monounsaturated fats from olive oil, fruits, vegetables, whole grains, legumes, nuts; a moderate intake of fish and poultry; a low intake of dairy products, red meat, processed meats, and sweets [34, 36, 37].

The high concentration of unsaturated fats, such as olive oil, is the most prominent aspect of the Mediterranean diet. Research on the impact of olive oil consumption for CVD prevention has showed that the cardioprotective effects of olive oil are thought to be attributed to the presence of its phenolic compounds, which are potent antioxidants, free radical scavengers, and enzyme modulators [38].

Numerous observational data show a reduction in CVD by increased consumption of fruits and vegetables. The potential benefit of fruits and vegetables could lie in reduced total caloric burden, or in large amount of micronutrients that they provide. The exact evidence establishes the antioxidant properties of fruit and vegetables [39] and the health benefits of increased flavonol intake [40]. The effects of nitric oxide (NO) species, or concomitant weight loss associated with diets high in fruits and vegetables could be alternative mechanisms [34].

An extensive amount of data suggests a beneficial effect of increased whole grains on CVD morbidity and mortality. AHA guidelines indicate that diets high in fiber such as whole grains, oats and barley reduce cardiovascular disease morbidity and mortality through lipid lowering, and recommend a total dietary fiber intake of 25-30 g per day from whole foods [41].

The data about the beneficial effect of moderate nut consumption are positive. Evaluation of observational studies showed that substituting walnuts, peanuts, almonds, or other nuts for a serving of carbohydrates or saturated fats reduced blood lipids, as well as the risk for cardiovascular disease by 30% and 45%, respectively [42].

Estruch et al. designed a randomized trial, the PREvención con DIeta MEDiterránean (PREDIMED) Study, to test the efficacy of two Mediterranean diets (one supplemented with extra-virgin olive oil and another with mixed nuts), as compared with a control diet (advice on a low-fat diet), on primary cardiovascular prevention [37]. A total of 7,447 men and women (age ranged from 55 to 80 years) in Spain who were at high cardiovascular risk at enrollment, but without evidence of cardiovascular disease, were randomized to one of three diets stated above. Participants received quarterly individual and group educational sessions and, depending on group assignment, free provision of extra-virgin olive oil, mixed nuts, or small nonfood gifts. Total fat intake was not restricted in patients on the Mediterranean diet, but the source of fat was predominantly from fatty fish and plants. The low fat diet group was counseled to reduce all types of fat, including olive oil and nuts. The primary end point was the rate of major cardiovascular events (MI, stroke, or death from cardiovascular causes). The trial was stopped after a median follow-up of 4.8 years on the basis of the results of an interim analysis. Total dietary fat was higher in the Mediterranean diet groups. Both groups were similar with regard to saturated fat and dietary cholesterol intake. The primary end point, namely MI, stroke, or death from cardiovascular causes, was reduced by 30% in the Mediterranean diet supplemented with extra virgin olive oil and 28% lower in the Mediterranean diet group supplemented with mixed nuts compared with controls.

Conclusively, Estruch et al. suggested that dietary patterns consistent with the traditional Mediterranean-style diet were particularly cardioprotective [37]. Mediterranean-style diets are widely accepted to be effective in preventing CHD even though they do not decrease total serum cholesterol or low-density lipoprotein cholesterol [43].

3. Dietary fats and cardiovascular/coronary heart disease

3.1. Total fat

Since the beginning of the concern about diet and CVD risk assessment, dietary fat, especially the total fat, is the main point of interest. Till the beginning of the 1990s, the recommendations for the public health was focused on limiting the total fat intake, especially to reduce CVD. As part of the Dietary Approaches to Stop Hypertension (DASH) diet, low-fat dairy intake has been shown to lower blood pressure [44]. However, lowering total cholesterol by replacing dietary total fat with carbohydrate may contrarily increase serum triglyceride concentration

[45]. Moreover, in a meta-analysis of prospective cohort studies, intake of total fat was not found significantly associated with CHD mortality or CHD events [46]. One of the key studies about total fat intake was the Women's Health Initiative Dietary Modification Trial. In this study, dietary intervention that reduced total fat intake did not significantly reduce the risk of CHD or CVD in postmenopausal women and only modest effects on CVD risk factors were achieved [47]. According to the 2006 AHA Diet and Lifestyle recommendations, for decreasing the CVD risk, the recommendations are much about limitations of intake of each type of fat, instead of reducing the total fat intake. Specifically, the AHA recommends to supply 7% of energy from saturated fat and 1% of energy from trans fat [48]. And also, according to the Dietary Guidelines for Americans 2010, lowering the percentage of calories from dietary saturated fatty acids to 7% of calories and replacing them with monounsaturated and/or polyunsaturated fatty acids can further reduce the risk of CVD [49].

3.2. Saturated Fatty Acids (SFA)

The primary SFA sources are animal fat such as meat, milk, and dairy products, some plant oils such as palm and coconut oils, and the industrially-prepared food (cookies, cakes, and pies). Several meta-analyses showed that SFA intake was not significantly associated with risk of CAD or CVD [50-52]. Recent data from meta-analyses of cohort studies and randomized control trials suggest that SFA consumption on CVD risk depends on the replacement nutrient. The latest epidemiologic studies and clinical trials suggest that differing effects depending on the replacement nutrient scenario such as replacing saturated fat with polyunsaturated fat in the diet is more beneficial for CAD risk than with carbohydrates [53]. In a pooled analysis of 11 prospective cohort studies, Jakobsen et al. revealed that consumption of polyunsaturated fatty acid (PUFA) in place of SFA was associated with reduced CAD risk [54]. In another study, Mozaffarian et al. indicated as the result of 8 randomised clinical trials that changing the energy intake from SFA to PUFA by 5% reduced the CAD risk by 10% [55]. Additionally, in the Cochrane Collaboration meta-analysis of 48 RCTs, Hooper et al. revealed that reducing saturated fat by reducing and/or modifying dietary fat reduced the risk of cardiovascular events by 14% [13]. And this study also suggested that the beneficial effects occurred in the case of fat modification rather than reduction of fat intake and in a two-year period. Also, males and population who have moderate or high risk of CVD are more prone to have benefits from dietary fat modification. However, dietary fat modification was not found to be beneficial on CVD mortality [56]. Based on recent evidence, both the AHA and the European Society of Cardiology advise to limit saturated fat intake to <10% and <7% of total daily calories, respectively [6, 57]. According to the 2013 AHA/ACC Guideline on Lifestyle Management to Reduce Cardiovascular Risk, for adults to benefit from LDL cholesterol lowering, only 5%-6% of calories should come from saturated fat (through replacement of PUFA > monounsaturated fat (MUFA) > whole grains > refined carbohydrates). [58]

3.3. Monounsaturated Fatty Acids (MUFA)

The main dietary MUFA is oleic acid, which is abundant in nuts, sunflower oil, olive oil, canola oil, high oleic safflower oil, and avocado. Because olive oil is the essential part of the Mediterranean diet, the role of MUFA in the prevention of CAD has a close interest, especially after Mattson and Grundy showed that high SFA diets increase the LDL cholesterol/HDL cholesterol ratio and changing SFA with MUFA reduces LDL cholesterol levels but not HDL cholesterol [59]. Replacing MUFA with carbohydrates in the diet causes several alterations in the lipid profile, such as TG and VLDL cholesterol decrease and HDL cholesterol and apoA1 increase [60, 61]. However, the epidemiologic data about oleic acid and CAD prevention is controversial. While the Nurses' Health Study (NHS) found remarkable protection, in the Zutphen and Puerto Rico Heart Health Program studies there were no beneficial effects reported between controls and CAD cases [62-64]. In a recent study, Schwingshackl and Hoffmann recapped the most available data about MUFA and CVD risk in which they found no accepted rationale for MUFA recommendation, although there are no significant side effects of diets with rich MUFA up to date [65]. Also, according to the Cochrane meta-analysis by Hooper et al., reduction of SFA intake and replacement with unsaturated fat is advised for the population under risk of CVD [66].

3.4. Trans Fatty Acids (TFA)

Trans fatty acids (TFA) are a type of unsaturated fat that became commonly produced industrially from vegetable fats for use in margarine, snack food, packaged baked goods, and frying fast food. TFA has at least one carbon-carbon double bond in the trans, rather than the typical cis configuration. Early in the 20th century, TFA was invented for increasing the shelf life of oils and consumption of these fats, as margarine increased all over the world. Recently, it has been recognized that it causes elevated cholesterol levels and has a major role in the risk of CAD [67]. Beyond their energy value, TFA does not have any known health benefits and there is an apparent association between TFA consumption and the risk of heart disease. In a meta-analysis of 28 cohort studies, there has been found a highly significant positive association between TFA intake and CAD morbidity and mortality [68]. Energy replacement of TFA with SFA, MUFA, or PUFA 1% resulted in the decrease of the TC: HDL ratio in controlled trials and each 2% replacement would lower CAD risk in prospective cohort studies [69]. Because of this CVD risk increase, the Food and Drug Administration (FDA) and the other Health Regulatory Agencies required food manufacturers to list TFA on the Nutrition Facts and some Supplement Facts sections on the package of food, although TFA levels of less than 0.5 g per serving can be listed as 0 g [70].

3.5. N-3 fatty acids

Because of the low rates of ischemic heart disease in Greenland Eskimos, there was close attention to their diet. This protection was thought to be caused by long-chained PUFA's anti-thrombotic effects, which is an important part of their diet [71]. Prospective cohorts revealed the protective effects of intake of n-3 fatty acids on CAD, and since then evidence suggests that n-3 fatty acid intake may be effective for secondary prevention. The possible effects were thought to be prevention of arrhythmias, as well as lowering of heart rate and blood pressure, decreasing platelet aggregation, and lowering triglyceride concentration [72]. The n-3 fatty acids also decrease hepatic TG secretion and increase clearance from plasma. In diabetic patients, n-3 PUFA are found to reduce TG levels by 25% and VLDL levels by 36%; however, LDL concentrations increased slightly by 5.7% [73]. Since then, several meta-analysis and RCTs have been published about the role of seafood n-3 fatty acids on CVD and CVD mortality. Some of them suggested that n-3 fatty acid intake lowers the CVD risk, but some of them found no significant effect on CVD risk and/or mortality. In the last US guidelines on patients with CAD, fish and/or fish oil supplement is indicated only in the control of a patient's lipid profile (class IIB, level of evidence B) [74]. But in the latest European Society of Cardiology (ESC) guidelines, the protective effects of fish on CVD is associated with n-3 PUFA. Moreover, it is suggested that eating fish at least once a week reduces the CAD risk by 15% [6]. There are controversies between epidemiologic studies and clinical trials, probably due to the different study groups. Epidemiologic observational studies usually evaluate the disease-free population, but clinical trials are often conducted in a population at risk of CVD.

3.6. Plant-based fatty acids

α-linolenic acid (ALA) is a short chain n-3 PUFA found in plant sources such as soybeans, walnuts, rapeseed oil, and flaxseed. It could be an alternative to fish n-3 PUFA because it can be converted to eicosapentaenoic acid (EPA) and docosahexaenoic acid (DHA), which are n-3 PUFAs that are found in fish. But this conversion is limited and the evidence for ALA in CVD protection is limited. In a systematic review of 14 human studies, at least four weeks of supplementation of ALA has no significant effect on the lipid profile [75]. However, since no current specific recommendations for ALA for CAD risk reduction is present, epidemiologic studies suggest a protective role, the diet including ALA (2 to 3 g per day) has been recommended for both primary and secondary prevention of CAD [76]. Further studies need to strengthen the evidence for the effects of ALA on CVD.

3.7. B Vitamins

The main role of B vitamins is principally for energy production, cell metabolism, and nerve function. Beside these, vitamins B12, B6, and folic acid are known to have homocysteine lowering effect. Several studies suggested that high homocysteine levels are associated with increased risk of MI and/or stroke. Because folic acid, B12, and B6 decreased the blood homocysteine level in 20%-40%, from baseline, it has been assumed that these supplements can subsequently reduce CVD risk [77]. The studies about the effects of folic acid and B vitamin supplementation failed to prove that reducing homocysteine level by folic acid and vitamin B supplements decreases CVD incidence. Most of the epidemiologic studies suggested protective effects of B vitamins on CAD but the randomized clinical trials did not show the same beneficial effects. A meta-analysis of 12 randomized trials that has 16,958 participants with pre-existing vascular disease revealed that folic acid supplementation had no effect on CAD risk [78]. After 1996, the US FDA made a regulation for the fortification of grain products (flour, breads, rice, pasta, cornmeal, etc.) with folic acid. Since then, the prevalence of low plasma folate concentrations has decreased [79]. The role of B vitamins and folate are plausible in the prevention of CVD and more studies are needed.

4. Foods and cardiovascular/coronary heart disease

4.1. Fruit and vegetables

Epidemiological studies have suggested that fruits and vegetables reduce CAD risk. A meta-analysis of nine cohort studies (including 129,701 women, 91,379 men, and 5,007 CAD events) showed that each additional fruit serving a day lowered the CHD risk by 7% (RR 0.93, 95% CI: 0.89-0.96; P < 0.001) [80]. Increasing fruit and vegetable consumption to 600 g/day, could reduce the incidence of ischaemic heart disease and ischemic stroke by 31% and 19%, respectively [81]. In the CARDIO2000 study, daily consumption of more fruit was associated with 72% lower risk of CAD (95% CI: 0.11-0.54, P < 0.001) and of more vegetables was associated with 70% lower risk for CAD (95% CI: 0.22-0.40, P < 0.001) [82]. However, the results of the WHI Dietary Modification Trial suggest that an additional portion of vegetables and fruit daily does not influence the risk of CAD [4]. Fruit and vegetable intake are part of the nutritional recommendations in the interventional studies where fruit and vegetable consumption was associated with lower blood pressure only [83] but the association with other CAD risk factors is not apparent. As the intervention studies did not exist, AHA recommends intake of at least eight vegetables and fruits a day [47]. With all these data, vegetables and fruits that are deeply colored (e.g., carrots, peaches, spinach, and berries) are recommended for consumption and preparation techniques that preserve nutrient and fiber content is important. The mechanism of action of their healthy effects is not known, but it can be attributed to their high dietary fiber and antioxidants content.

4.2. Fish

A meta-analysis of 11 cohort studies of 222,364 individuals showed that individuals who consumed fish 2-4 times/week had 23% lower risk of CAD mortality. Moreover, the individuals with higher frequency of fish consumption, i.e., ≥5 times/week, had greater reduction of risk. It is estimated that a daily fish intake of 20 g was associated with 7% lower risk of CAD mortality [84]. The benefit of fish intake for reducing the risk for CAD is due to n-3 PUFA according to the studies showing that fatty fish is associated with protection but lean fish is not. Fatty fish is the primary source of n-3 fatty acids. A prospective cohort study (including 1,373 men) suggested that fatty fish consumption reduces the risk of sudden coronary death risk compared to lean fish consumption [85]. Besides the type and amount of fish consumed, the cooking method of fish is also important. According to the Cardiovascular Health Study, only modest consumption of tuna or other broiled or baked fish was associated with a lower risk of heart failure, but fried fish was not [86]. The most recent Diet and Lifestyle recommendations of AHA for CVD risk reduction include consuming fatty fish at least twice a week [48]. The AHA also recommends eating fish within the recommendations established by the FDA and Environmental Protection Agency to prevent the possible adverse effects due to environmental pollutants such as mercury [87].

4.3. Whole grains

There are many definitions for whole grain present but according to The American Association of Cereal Chemists, a whole-grain ingredient is "...the intact, ground, cracked, or flaked caryopsis, whose principal anatomical components, the starchy endosperm, germ, and bran, are present in substantially the same relative proportions as they exist in the intact caryopsis" [88]. The alternative definition is used by studies that explicitly describe or define whole grain, but do not meet the classical definition of whole grains, by including bran and germ, and studies that do not explicitly use the term "whole grains" but were in fact conducted with individual whole grains such as oats or barley [89]. Whole-grain foods contain fiber, vitamins, minerals, phenolic compounds, phytoestrogens, and other unmeasured constituents. Whole-grain foods may have favorable effects on health by lowering blood pressure and serum lipids, and by also improving glucose and insulin metabolism and endothelial function [90]. They have also beneficial effects by reducing oxidative stress and inflammation.

Recently, many epidemiologic studies have searched the relation between whole grain intake and CVD risk. A meta-analysis of seven large-prospective cohort studies showed that whole grain intake was related with 21% lower risk of CVD for both genders [91]. In the NHS study, among women with type 2 diabetes with 26 years of follow-up, whole grain intake was found to be associated with lower risk of CVD-specific mortality and also bran intake was significantly associated with 35% lower risk of mortality [92]. As recent evidence about the protective role of whole grains in prevention of CVD was strong, FDA declared in Health Claim Notification for Whole Grain Foods that "Diets high in plant foods—i.e., fruits, vegetables, legumes, and whole-grain cereals—are associated with a lower occurrence of coronary heart disease and cancers of the lung, colon, esophagus, and stomach" [93].

Recently, a meta-analysis of 14 studies indicated that the highest whole grain intake amount compared with the lowest amount was significantly associated with reduced risk for CAD. The association was significant in cohort studies but not in case-control studies [94].

4.4. Alcohol

The data on the association between alcohol and CVD come either from short-term interventional studies or from the effects of alcohol on risk factors, as well as long-term observational mortality studies. Many studies suggested that moderate alcohol consumption, compared to no or heavy alcohol consumption, decreased CVD risk in many populations. The evidence suggests a J- or U-shaped relationship between alcohol consumption and risk of CAD [95]. Moderate intake of alcoholic beverages (1 to 2 drinks per day) is associated with a reduced risk of CAD in healthy populations in both men and women [96] and there is no difference between the types of beverages [97]. Different mechanisms have been suggested about the benefit of light-to-moderate alcohol intake on CVD such as an increase in HDL-C, reduction in plasma increase in fibrinolysis, decrease in platelet aggregation, improvement in endothelial function, reduction in inflammation, and promotion of antioxidant effects [98, 99]. However, these are still not enough to prove causality. Despite the evidence from cohort studies about moderate alcohol drinking and CVD, current guidelines do not recommend to begin consuming alcohol for preventing CVD. The recommendations of AHA on alcoholic drinks are that they should limited to no more than two drinks per day for men and one drink per day for women, ideally with meals [48].

5. Conclusions

CHD remains one of the leading causes of morbidity and mortality worldwide, in spite of the advances in pharmacological treatments and better control of risk factors. Diet is a centrally important modifiable risk factor in the prevention and risk reduction of CAD. Progress in understanding the importance of diet on CAD has evolved in the past 100 years. Data on trends in food consumption and ecological studies are the early evidences that showed associations between prevalence and fat intake across and within countries. The last 50 years of clinical trials and nutritional interventions have established a clear link among diet, atherosclerosis, and CAD. Numerous meta-analyses of intervention studies confirm the beneficial effects of replacing saturated with polyunsaturated fatty acid on CAD risk. Moreover, the type of fat, rather than the total or the ratio or balance between the saturated and certain unsaturated fats is determinant. Recent guidelines consider diet as a whole and combine nutrient and energy recommendations into a healthy pattern that is nutrient dense and energy balanced. A "whole diet" approach with equal attention to what is consumed and what is excluded is proven to be more effective in preventing CAD than low-fat, low-cholesterol diets. Dietary patterns consistent with the traditional Mediterranean-style diets with a strong focus on veggies, fruits, fish, wholegrain, olive oil are effective in preventing CAD even though they do not decrease total serum cholesterol.

Author details

Oguzhan Yildiz*, Melik Seyrek and Kemal Gokhan Ulusoy

*Address all correspondence to: oyildiz@gata.edu.tr

Department of Medical Pharmacology, Gulhane Faculty of Medicine, Etlik, Ankara, Turkey

References

[1] Roger VL, Go AS, Lloyd-Jones DM, Benjamin EJ, Berry JD, Borden WB, Bravata DM, Dai S, Ford ES, Fox CS, Fullerton HJ, Gillespie C, Hailpern SM, Heit JA, Howard VJ, Kissela BM, Kittner SJ, Lackland DT, Lichtman JH, Lisabeth LD, Makuc DM, Marcus GM, Marelli A, Matchar DB, Moy CS, Mozaffarian D, Mussolino ME, Nichol G, Paynter NP, Soliman EZ, Sorlie PD, Sotoodehnia N, Turan TN, Virani SS, Wong ND, Woo D, Turner MB. American Heart Association Statistics Committee and Stroke

Statistics Subcommittee. Executive summary: Heart disease and stroke statistics—2012 update: A report from the American Heart Association. Circulation. 2012;125:188-97. DOI: 10.1161/cir.0b013E3182456d46.

[2] Sunar H, Halici U, Canbaz S, Yavuz E, Gur O, Duran E. Effect of obesity on coronary artery bypass surgery. Gulhane Med J. 2003;45:338-342.

[3] Stampfer MJ, Hu FB, Manson JE, Rimm EB, Willett WC. Primary prevention of coronary heart disease in women through diet and lifestyle. N Engl J Med. 2000;343:16-22. DOI: 10.1056/nejm200007063430103.

[4] Yusuf S, Hawken S, Ounpuu S, Dans T, Avezum A, Lanas F, McQueen M, Budaj A, Pais P, Varigos J, Lisheng L. INTERHEART Study Investigators. Effect of potentially modifiable risk factors associated with myocardial infarction in 52 countries (the INTERHEART study): Case-control study. Lancet. 2004;364:937-52. DOI: 10.1016/s0140-6736(04)17018-9.

[5] Akesson A, Larsson SC, Discacciati A, Wolk A. Low-risk diet and lifestyle habits in the primary prevention of myocardial infarction in men: A population-based prospective cohort study. J Am Coll Cardiol. 2014;64:1299-306. DOI: 10.1016/j.jacc.2014.06.1190.

[6] Perk J, De Backer G, Gohlke H, Graham I, Reiner Z, Verschuren M, Albus C, Benlian P, Boysen G, Cifkova R, Deaton C, Ebrahim S, Fisher M, Germano G, Hobbs R, Hoes A, Karadeniz S, Mezzani A, Prescott E, Ryden L, Scherer M, Syvänne M, Scholte op Reimer WJ, Vrints C, Wood D, Zamorano JL, Zannad F. European Association for Cardiovascular Prevention & Rehabilitation (EACPR); ESC Committee for Practice Guidelines (CPG). European guidelines on cardiovascular disease prevention in clinical practice (version 2012). The Fifth Joint Task Force of the European Society of Cardiology and Other Societies on Cardiovascular Disease Prevention in Clinical Practice (constituted by representatives of nine societies and by invited experts). Eur Heart J. 2012;33:1635-701. DOI: 10.1093/eurheartj/ehs092.

[7] Eckel RH, Jakicic JM, Ard JD, de Jesus JM, Houston Miller N, Hubbard VS, Lee IM, Lichtenstein AH, Loria CM, Millen BE, Nonas CA, Sacks FM, Smith SC Jr, Svetkey LP, Wadden TA, Yanovski SZ. American College of Cardiology/American Heart Association Task Force on Practice Guidelines. 2013 AHA/ACC guideline onlifestyle management to reduce cardiovascular risk: A report of the American College of Cardiology/American Heart Association Task Force on Practice Guidelines. J Am Coll Cardiol. 2014;63:2960-84. DOI: 10.1016/j.jacc.2013.11.003.

[8] Connor WE. Diet-heart research in the first part of the 20th century. Acta Cardiol. 1999;54:135-139.

[9] Keys A. Diet and the epidemiology of coronary heart disease. JAMA. 1957;164:1912-1919. DOI: 10.1001/jama.1957.62980170024007e.

[10] Ignatowski AI. Influence of animal food on the organism of rabbits. S Peterb Izv Imp Voyenno-Med Akad. 1908;16:154-176.

[11] Finking G, Hanke H. Nikolajewitsch Anitschkow (1885-1964) Established the cholesterol-fed rabbit as a model for atherosclerosis research. Atherosclerosis. 1997;135:1-7. DOI: 10.1016/s0021-9150(97)00161-5.

[12] Kinsell LW. Dietary modification of serum cholesterol and phospholipid levels. J Clin Endocrinol. 1952;12:909-913. DOI: 10.1210/jcem-12-7-909.

[13] Groen JJ, Tjiong BK, Kamminga CE, Willebrands AF. Influence of nutrition, individuality, and some other factors, including various forms of stress, on serum cholesterol. Voeding. 1952;13:556-587.

[14] de Langen C. Cholesterine-stofwisseling en rassenpathologie. Geneeskundig Tijdschrift voor Nederlansch-Indie (in Dutch). 1916;56:1-34.

[15] Keys A. Seven Countries: A Multivariate Analysis of Death and Coronary Heart Disease.1st ed. Harvard University Press Cambridge, MA London England. 1980.

[16] Rose GA, Thomson WB, Williams RT. Corn oil in treatment of ischemic heart disease. Br Med J. 1965;1:1531-1533. DOI: 10.1136/bmj.1.5449.1531.

[17] Leren P. The Oslo diet-heart study. Eleven-year report. Circulation. 1970;42:935-942. DOI: 10.1161/01.cir.42.5.935.

[18] Woodhill JM, Palmer AJ, Leelarthaepin B, McGilchrist C, Blacket RB. Low fat, low cholesterol diet in secondary prevention of coronary heart disease. Adv Exp Med Biol. 1978;109:317-330. DOI: 10.1007/978-1-4684-0967-3_18.

[19] Dalen JE, Devries S. Diets to prevent coronary heart disease 1957-2013: What have we learned? Am J Med. 2014;127:364-9. DOI: 10.1016/j.amjmed.2013.12.014.

[20] Page IH, Stare FH, Corcoran AC, Pollack H, Wilkinson CF. Atherosclerosis and the fat content of the diet. JAMA. 1957;164:2048-2051. DOI: 10.1001/jama.1957.62980180004013.

[21] Brown HB, Page IH. Lowering blood lipid levels by changing food patterns. JAMA. 1958;168:1989-1995. DOI: 10.1001/jama.1958.03000150031008.

[22] Page IH, Allen EV, Chamberlain FL, Keys A, Stamler J, Stare FJ. Dietary fat and its relation to heart attacks and strokes. Circulation. 1961;23:133-136. DOI: 10.1161/01.cir.23.1.133.

[23] Johnson PE. Diet and coronary heart disease. Prev Med. 1972;1:559-561. DOI: 10.1016/0091-7435(72)90039-4.

[24] Page IH, Brown HB. Some observations on the National Diet-Heart Study. Circulation. 1968;37:313-315. DOI: 10.1161/01.cir.37.3.313.

[25] Mahmood SS, Levy D, Vasan RS, Wang TJ. The Framingham Heart Study and the epidemiology of cardiovascular disease: a historical perspective. Lancet. 2014;383:999-1008. DOI: 10.1016/s0140-6736(13)61752-3.

[26] Millen BE, Quatromoni PA. Nutritional research within the Framingham Heart Study. J Nutr Health Aging. 2001;5:139-43.

[27] Leren P. The Oslo diet-heart study. Eleven-year report. Circulation. 1970;42:935-4. DOI: 10.1161/01.cir.42.5.935.

[28] Hjermann I, Velve Byre K, Holme I, Leren P. Effect of diet and smoking intervention on the incidence of coronary heart disease. Report from the Oslo Study Group of a randomised trial in healthy men. Lancet. 1981;2:1303-10. DOI: 10.1016/s0140-6736(81)91338-6.

[29] Stamler J, Caggiula A, Grandits GA, Kjelsberg M, Cutler JA. Relationship to blood pressure of combinations of dietary macronutrients. Findings of the Multiple Risk Factor Intervention Trial (MRFIT). Circulation. 1996;94:2417-23. DOI: 10.1161/01.cir.94.10.2417.

[30] Ornish D, Brown SE, Scherwitz LW, Billings JH, Armstrong WT, Ports TA, McLanahan SM, Kirkeeide RL, Brand RJ, Gould KL. Can lifestyle changes reverse coronary heart disease? The Lifestyle Heart Trial. Lancet. 1990;336:129-33. DOI: 10.1016/0140-6736(90)91656-u.

[31] Burr ML, Gilbert JF, Holliday RM, et al. Effects of changes in fat, fish and fibre intakes on death and myocardial infarction: Diet and Reinfarction Trial (DART). Lancet. 1989;2:757-761. DOI: 10.1016/s0140-6736(89)90828-3.

[32] Singh RB, Rastogi SS, Verma R, et al. Randomized controlled trial of cardioprotective diet in patients with recent acute myocardial infarction: Results of one year follow-up. BMJ. 1992;304:1015-1019. DOI: 10.1136/bmj.304.6833.1015.

[33] de Lorgeri M, Renaud S, Mamelle N, et al. Mediterranean alphalinolenic-rich diet in secondary prevention of coronary heart disease. Lancet. 1994;343:1454-1459. DOI: 10.1016/s0140-6736(94)92580-1.

[34] Widmer RJ, Flammer AJ, Lerman LO, Lerman A. The Mediterranean diet, its components, and cardiovascular disease. Am J Med. 2015;128:229-38. DOI: 10.1016/j.amjmed.2014.10.014.

[35] Jacobs DJ, Gross MD, Tapsell LC. Food synergy: An operational concept for understanding nutrition. Am J Clin Nutr. 2009;89:1543S-1548S. DOI: 10.3945/ajcn.2009.26736b.

[36] Willett WC, Sacks F, Trichopoulou A, Drescher G, Ferro-Luzzi A, Helsing E,Trichopoulos D. Mediterranean diet pyramid: A cultural model for healthy eating. Am J Clin Nutr. 1995 Jun;61(6 Suppl):1402S-1406S.

[37] Estruch R, Ros E, Salas-Salvadó J, Covas MI, Corella D, Arós F, Gómez-Gracia E, Ruiz-Gutiérrez V, Fiol M, Lapetra J, Lamuela-Raventos RM, Serra-Majem L, Pintó X, Basora J, Muñoz MA, Sorlí JV, Martínez JA, Martínez-González MA. PREDIMED Study Investigators. Primary prevention of cardiovascular disease with a Mediterranean diet. N Engl J Med. 2013;368:1279-90. DOI: 10.1056/nejmoa1200303.

[38] Fuhrman B, Aviram M. Flavonoids protect LDL from oxidation and attenuate atherosclerosis. Curr Opin Lipidol. 2001;12:41-48. DOI: 10.1097/00041433-200102000-00008.

[39] Knekt P, Ritz J, Pereira MA, O'Reilly EJ, Augustsson K, Fraser GE, Goldbourt U, Heitmann BL, Hallmans G, Liu S, Pietinen P, Spiegelman D, Stevens J, Virtamo J, Willett WC, Rimm EB, Ascherio A. Antioxidant vitamins and coronary heart disease risk: a pooled analysis of 9 cohorts. Am J Clin Nutr. 2004;80:1508-20.

[40] Huxley R, Neil HA. The relation between dietary flavonol intake and coronary heart disease mortality: A meta-analysis of prospective cohort studies. Eur J Clin Nutr. 2003;57:904-908. DOI: 10.1038/sj.ejcn.1601624.

[41] Van Horn L. Fiber, lipids, and coronary heart disease. A statement for healthcare professionals from the Nutrition Committee, American Heart Association. Circulation. 1997;95:2701-2704. DOI: 10.1161/01.cir.95.12.2701.

[42] Hu FB, Stampfer MJ. Nut consumption and risk of coronary heart disease: a review of epidemiologic evidence. Curr Atheroscler Rep. 1999;1:204-9. DOI: 10.1007/s11883-999-0033-7.

[43] Collins R, Peto R, Godwin J, MacMahon S. Blood pressure and coronary heart disease. Lancet. 1990;336:370-1. DOI: 10.1016/0140-6736(90)91908-s.

[44] Appel LJ, Moore TJ, Obarzanek E, Vollmer WM, Svetkey LP, Sacks FM, Bray GA, Vogt TM, Cutler JA, Windhauser MM, Lin PH, Karanja N. A clinical trial of the effects of dietary patterns on blood pressure. DASH Collaborative Research Group. N Engl J Med. 1997;336 (16):1117-1124. DOI: 10.1056/nejm199704173361601.

[45] Ma Y, Li Y, Chiriboga DE, Olendzki BC, Hebert JR, Li W, Leung K, Hafner AR, Ockene IS. Association between carbohydrate intake and serum lipids. J Am Coll Nutr. 2006;25:155-63. DOI: 10.1080/07315724.2006.10719527.

[46] Skeaff CM, Miller J. Dietary fat and coronary heart disease: Summary of evidence from prospective cohort and randomised controlled trials. Ann Nutr Metab. 2009;55:173-201. DOI: 10.1159/000229002.

[47] Howard BV, Van Horn L, Hsia J, Manson JE, Stefanick ML, Wassertheil-Smoller S, Kuller LH, LaCroix AZ, Langer RD, Lasser NL, Lewis CE, Limacher MC, Margolis KL, Mysiw WJ, Ockene JK, Parker LM, Perri MG, Phillips L, Prentice RL, Robbins J, Rossouw JE, Sarto GE, Schatz IJ, Snetselaar LG, Stevens VJ, Tinker LF, Trevisan M, Vitolins MZ, Anderson GL, Assaf AR, Bassford T, Beresford SA, Black HR, Brunner RL, Brzyski RG, Caan B, Chlebowski RT, Gass M, Granek I, Greenland P, Hays J, Heber D, Heiss G, Hendrix SL, Hubbell FA, Johnson KC, Kotchen JM. Low-fat diet-

ary pattern and risk of cardiovascular disease: The Women's Health Initiative Randomized Controlled Dietary Modification Trial. JAMA. 2006;295:655-66. DOI: 10.1001/jama.295.6.655.

[48] Lichtenstein AH, Appel LJ, Brands M, Carnethon M, Daniels S, Franch HA, Franklin B, Kris-Etherton P, Harris WS, Howard B, Karanja N, Lefevre M, Rudel L, Sacks F, Van Horn L, Winston M, Wylie-Rosett J. Diet and lifestyle recommendations revision 2006: A scientific statement from the American Heart Association Nutrition Committee. Circulation. 2006;114:82-96. DOI: 10.1161/circulationaha.106.176158.

[49] U.S. Department of Agriculture and U.S. Department of Health and Human Services Dieatray Guidelines for Americans 2010. Available from : http://www.health.gov/dietaryguidelines/dga2010/DietaryGuidelines2010.pdf [Accessed:2015-07-20].

[50] Skeaff CM, Miller J. Dietary fat and coronary heart disease: Summary of evidence from prospective cohort and randomised controlled trials. Ann Nutr Metab. 2009;55:173-201. DOI: 10.1159/000229002.

[51] Mente A, de Koning L, Shannon HS, Anand SS. A systematic review of the evidence supporting a causal link between dietary factors and coronary heart disease. Arch Intern Med. 2009;169:659-69. DOI: 10.1001/archinternmed.2009.38.

[52] Siri-Tarino PW, Sun Q, Hu FB, Krauss RM. Meta-analysis of prospective cohort studies evaluating the association of saturated fat with cardiovascular disease. Am J Clin Nutr. 2010;91:535-46. DOI: 10.3945/ajcn.2009.27725.

[53] Siri-Tarino PW, Sun Q, Hu FB, Krauss RM. Saturated fat, carbohydrate, and cardiovascular disease. Am J Clin Nutr. 2010;91:502-9. DOI: 10.3945/ajcn.2008.26285.

[54] Jakobsen MU, O'Reilly EJ, Heitmann BL, Pereira MA, Bälter K, Fraser GE, Goldbourt U, Hallmans G, Knekt P, Liu S, Pietinen P, Spiegelman D, Stevens J, Virtamo J, Willett WC, Ascherio A. Major types of dietary fat and risk of coronary heart disease: A pooled analysis of 11 cohort studies. Am J Clin Nutr. 2009;89:1425-32. DOI: 10.3945/ajcn.2008.27124.

[55] Mozaffarian D, Micha R, Wallace S. Effects on coronary heart disease of increasing polyunsaturated fat in place of saturated fat: A systematic review and meta-analysis of randomized controlled trials. PLoS Med. 2010;7(3):e1000252. DOI: 10.1371/journal.pmed.1000252.

[56] Hooper L, Summerbell CD, Thompson R, Sills D, Roberts FG, Moore HJ, Davey Smith G. Reduced or modified dietary fat for preventing cardiovascular disease. Cochrane Database Syst Rev. 2012;5:CD002137. DOI: 10.1002/14651858.CD002137.pub3.

[57] Lichtenstein AH, Appel LJ, Brands M, Carnethon M, Daniels S, Franch HA, Franklin B, Kris-Etherton P, Harris WS, Howard B, Karanja N, Lefevre M, Rudel L, Sacks F, Van Horn L, Winston M, Wylie-Rosett J. Diet and lifestyle recommendations revision

2006: A scientific statement from the American Heart Association Nutrition Committee. Circulation. 2006;114:82-96. DOI: 10.1161/circulationaha.106.176158.

[58] Eckel RH, Jakicic JM, Ard JD, de Jesus JM, Houston Miller N, Hubbard VS, Lee IM, Lichtenstein AH, Loria CM, Millen BE, Nonas CA, Sacks FM, Smith SC Jr, Svetkey LP, Wadden TA, Yanovski SZ. 2013 AHA/ACC guideline on lifestyle management to reduce cardiovascular risk. A report of the American College of Cardiology/American Heart Association Task Force on Practice Guidelines. J Am Coll Cardiol. 2013 1;63 (25 Pt B):2960-84. DOI: 10.1016/j.jacc.2013.11.003.

[59] Mattson FH, Grundy SM. Comparison of effects of dietary saturated, monounsaturated,and polyunsaturated fatty acids on plasma lipids and lipoproteins in man. J Lipid Res. 1985;26:194-202.

[60] Mensink RP, Zock PL, Kester AD, Katan MB. Effects of dietary fatty acids and carbohydrates on the ratio of serum total to HDL cholesterol and on serum lipids and apolipoproteins: A meta-analysis of 60 controlled trials. Am J Clin Nutr. 2003;77:1146-55.

[61] Appel LJ, Sacks FM, Carey VJ, Obarzanek E, Swain JF, Miller ER 3rd, Conlin PR, Erlinger TP, Rosner BA, Laranjo NM, Charleston J, McCarron P, Bishop LM. Omni-Heart Collaborative Research Group. Effects of protein, monounsaturated fat, and carbohydrate intake on blood pressure and serum lipids: Results of the OmniHeart randomized trial. J Am Med Assoc. 2005;294:2455-64. DOI: 10.1001/jama.294.19.2455.

[62] Hu FB, Stampfer MJ, Manson JE, Rimm E, Colditz GA, Rosner BA, Hennekens CH, Willett WC. Dietary fat intake and the risk of coronary heart disease in women. N Engl J Med. 1997;337:1491-9. DOI: 10.1056/nejm199711203372102.

[63] Garcia-Palmieri MR, Sorlie P, Tillotson J, Costas Jr R, Cordero E, Rodriguez M. Relationship of dietary intake to subsequent coronary heart disease incidence: The Puerto Rico Heart Health Program. Am J Clin Nutr. 1980;33:1818-27.

[64] Kromhout D, de Lezenne Coulander C. Diet, prevalence and 10-year mortality from coronary heart disease in 871 middle-aged men. The Zutphen Study. Am J Epidemiol. 1984;119:733-41.

[65] Schwingshackl L, Hoffmann G. Monounsaturated fatty acids and risk of cardiovascular disease: Synopsis of the evidence available from systematic reviews and meta-analyses. Nutrients. 2012;4:1989-2007. DOI: 10.3390/nu4121989.

[66] Hooper L, Summerbell CD, Thompson R, Sills D, Roberts FG, Moore HJ, Davey Smith G. Reduced or modified dietary fat for preventing cardiovascular disease. Cochrane Database Syst Rev. 2012;5:CD002137. DOI: 10.1002/14651858.CD002137.pub3.

[67] Willett WC. Trans fatty acids and cardiovascular disease-epidemiological data. Atheroscler Suppl. 2006;7:5-8. DOI: 10.1016/j.atherosclerosissup.2006.04.002.

[68] Skeaff CM, Miller J. Dietary fat and coronary heart disease: Summary of evidence from prospective cohort and randomised controlled trials. Ann Nutr Metab. 2009;55:173-201. DOI: 10.1159/000229002.

[69] Mozaffarian D, Clarke R. Quantitative effects on cardiovascular risk factors and coronary heart disease risk of replacing partially hydrogenated vegetable oils with other fats and oils. Eur J Clin Nutr. 2009;63 (Suppl 2):S22-33. DOI: 10.1038/sj.ejcn.1602976.

[70] FDA, Labeling & Nutrition 2006. Avaliable from: http://www.fda.gov/food/ingredientspackaginglabeling/labelingnutrition/ucm274592.htm [Accessed: 2015-07-20].

[71] Bang HO, Dyerberg J, Hjoorne N. The composition of food consumed by Greenland Eskimos. Acta Med Scand. 1976;200:69-73. DOI: 10.1111/j.0954-6820.1976.tb08198.x.

[72] Harris WS, Miller M, Tighe AP, Davidson MH, Schaefer EJ. Omega-3 fatty acids and coronary heart disease risk: Clinical and mechanistic perspectives. Atherosclerosis. 2008;197:12-24. DOI: 10.1016/j.atherosclerosis.2007.11.008.

[73] Hartweg J, Farmer AJ, Perera R, Holman RR, Neil HA. Meta-analysis of the effects of n-3 polyunsaturated fatty acids on lipoproteins and other emerging lipid cardiovascular risk markers in patients with type 2 diabetes. Diabetologia. 2007;50:1593-602. DOI: 10.1007/s00125-007-0695-z.

[74] Fihn SD, Gardin JM, Abrams J, Berra K, Blankenship JC, Dallas AP, Douglas PS, Foody JM, Gerber TC, Hinderliter AL, King SB 3rd, Kligfield PD, Krumholz HM, Kwong RY, Lim MJ, Linderbaum JA, Mack MJ, Munger MA, Prager RL, Sabik JF, Shaw LJ, Sikkema JD, Smith CR Jr, Smith SC Jr, Spertus JA, Williams SV, Anderson JL. American College of Cardiology Foundation/American Heart Association Task Force. 2012 ACCF/AHA/ACP/AATS/PCNA/SCAI/STS guideline for the diagnosis and management of patients with stable ischemic heart disease: A report of the American College of Cardiology Foundation/American Heart Association Task Force on Practice Guidelines, and the American College of Physicians, American Association for Thoracic Surgery, Preventive Cardiovascular Nurses Association, Society for Cardiovascular Angiography and Interventions, and Society of Thoracic Surgeons. Circulation. 2012;126:e354-471. DOI: 10.1161/cir.0b013e318277d6a0.

[75] Wendland E, Farmer A, Glasziou P, Neil A. Effect of alpha linolenic acid on cardiovascular risk markers: A systematic review. Heart. 2006;92:166-9. DOI: 10.1136/hrt.2004.053538.

[76] Mozaffarian D. Does alpha-linolenic acid intake reduce the risk of coronary heart disease? A review of the evidence. Altern Ther Health Med. 2005;11:24-30 quiz 31, 79.

[77] Eilat-Adar S, Goldbourt U. Nutritional recommendations for preventing coronary heart disease in women: Evidence concerning whole foods and supplements. Nutr. Metab. Cardiovasc. Dis. 2010 Jul;20(6):459-66. DOI: 10.1016/j.numecd.2010.01.011.

[78] Bazzano LA, Reynolds K, Holder KN, He J. Effect of folic acid supplementation on risk of cardiovascular diseases: A meta-analysis of randomized controlled trials. JAMA. 2006;296:2720-6. DOI: 10.1001/jama.296.22.2720.

[79] Jacques PF, Selhub J, Bostom AG, Wilson PW, Rosenberg IH. The effect of folic acid fortification on plasma folate and total homocysteine concentrations. N Engl J Med. 1999;340:1449-54. DOI: 10.1056/nejm199905133401901.

[80] Dauchet L, Amouyel P, Hercberg S, Dallongeville J. Fruit and vegetable consumption and risk of coronary heart disease: A meta-analysis of cohort studies. J. Nutr. 2006;136:2588-2593.

[81] Lock K, Pomerleau J, Causer L, Altmann DR, McKee M. The global burden of disease attributable to low consumption of fruit and vegetables: Implications for the global strategy on diet. Bull World Health Organ. 2005;83:100-8.

[82] Panagiotakos DB, Pitsavos C, Kokkinos P, Chrysohoou C, Vavuranakis M, Stefanadis C, Toutouzas P. Consumption of fruits and vegetables in relation to the risk of developing acute coronary syndromes; the CARDIO2000 case-control study. Nutr J. 2003;2:2. DOI: 10.1186/1475-2891-2-2.

[83] Appel LJ, Champagne CM, Harsha DW, Cooper LS, Obarzanek E, Elmer PJ, Stevens VJ, Vollmer WM, Lin PH, Svetkey LP, Stedman SW, Young DR. Writing Group of the PREMIER Collaborative Research Group. Effects of comprehensive lifestyle modification on blood pressure control: Main results of the premier clinical trial. JAMA. 2003;289:2083-2093. DOI: 0.1001/jama.289.16.2083.

[84] He K, Song Y, Daviglus ML, Liu K, Van Horn L, Dyer AR, Greenland P. Accumulated evidence on fish consumption and coronary heart disease mortality: A meta-analysis of cohort studies. Circulation. 2004;109:2705-11. DOI: 10.1161/01.cir.0000132503.19410.6b.

[85] Streppel MT, Ocke MC, Boshuizen HC, Kok FJ, Kromhout D. Long-term fish consumption and n-3 fatty acid intake in relation to (sudden) coronary heart disease death: the Zutphen study. Eur Heart J. 2008;29:2024-30. DOI: 0.1093/eurheartj/ehn294.

[86] Mozaffarian D, Bryson CL, Lemaitre RN, Burke GL, Siscovick DS. Fish intake and risk of incident heart failure. J Am Coll Cardiol. 2005;45:2015-21. DOI: 10.1016/j.jacc.2005.03.038.

[87] Kris-Etherton PM, Harris WS, Appel LJ. Fish consumption, fish oil, omega-3 fatty acids, and cardiovascular disease. Circulation. 2002;106:2747-57. DOI: 10.1161/01.cir.0000038493.65177.94.

[88] Slavin J. Whole grains and human health. Nutr Res Rev. 2004 Jun;17(1):99-110. DOI: 10.1079/nrr200374.

[89] de Moura F (editor). Whole grain intake and cardiovascular disease and whole grain intake and diabetes. A review. Life Sciences Research Office; 2008.

[90] Anderson JW, Hanna TJ. Whole grains and protection against coronary heart disease: What are the active components and mechanisms? Am J Clin Nutr. 1999;70:307-308.

[91] Mellen PB, Walsh TF, Herrington DM. Whole grain intake and cardiovascular disease: A meta-analysis. Nutr Metab Cardiovasc Dis. 2008;18:283-90. DOI: /10.1016/j.numecd.2006.12.008.

[92] He M, van Dam RM, Rimm E, Hu FB, Qi L. Whole-grain, cereal fiber, bran, and germ intake and the risks of all-cause and cardiovascular disease-specific mortality among women with type 2 diabetes mellitus. Circulation. 2010;121:2162-8. DOI: 10.1161/circulationaha.109.907360.

[93] US Food and Drug Administration, Health Claim Notification for Whole Grain Foods. US Department of Health and Human Services, 1999. Available from: http://www.fda.gov/Food/IngredientsPackagingLabeling/LabelingNutrition/ucm073639.htm [Accessed: 2015-07-20].

[94] Tang G, Wang D, Long J, Yang F, Si L. Meta-analysis of the association between whole grain intake and coronary heart disease risk. Am J Cardiol. 2015 Mar 1;115(5): 625-9. DOI: 10.1016/j.amjcard.2014.12.015.

[95] Marmoy M, Brunner E. Alcohol and cardiovascular disease: The status of the U-shaped curve. BMJ. 1991;303:565-568. DOI: 10.1136/bmj.303.6802.565.

[96] Goldberg IJ, Mosca L, Piano MR, Fisher EA. Nutrition Committee; Council on Epidemiology and Prevention; Council on Cardiovascular Nursing of the American Heart Association. AHA Science Advisory: Wine and your heart: A science advisory for healthcare professionals from the Nutrition Committee, Council on Epidemiology and Prevention, and Council on Cardiovascular Nursing of the American Heart Association. Circulation. 2001;103:472-475. DOI: 10.1161/01.cir.103.3.472.

[97] Marmot MG. Alcohol and coronary heart disease. Int. J. Epidemiol. 2001;30:724-729. DOI: 10.1093/ije/30.4.724.

[98] Brien SE, Ronksley PE, Turner BJ, Mukamal KJ, Ghali WA. Effect of alcohol consumption on biological markers associated with risk of coronary heart disease: Systematic review and meta-analysis of interventional studies. BMJ. 2011;342:d636. DOI: 10.1136/bmj.d636.

[99] Kloner RA, Rezkalla SH. To drink or not to drink? That is the question. Circulation. 2007;116:1306-1317. DOI: 10.1161/circulationaha.106.678375.